A Healthier Tomorrow

Medicare Reform for All Generations

snova
New York

Health Care in Transition Series

Medicare's Prescription Drug Pricing: Inflation, Challenges and Affordability
Lloyd M. Porter (Editor)
ISBN: 979-8-89530-728-1
eBook ISBN: 979-8-89530-803-5

Machine Learning-Based Decision Support Systems for Diabetic Foot Ulcer Care
Mritunjay Rai, PhD, Jay Kumar Pandey, PhD and Abhishek Kumar Saxena
ISBN: 979-8-89530-542-3
eBook ISBN: 979-8-89530-779-3

Tipping the Boundaries: Health and Well-Being of Sustainable Development
Sandeep Poddar, PhD and Waliza Ansar, PhD
ISBN: 979-8-89530-146-3
eBook ISBN: 979-8-89530-378-8

The Future of Universal Health Insurance
Seher Nur Sülkü and Yağmur Tokatlıoğlu
ISBN: 979-8-89530-107-4
eBook ISBN: 979-8-89530-192-0

More information about this series can be found at
https://novapublishers.com/product-category/series/health-care-in-transition/

Robert M. Deaton
Editor

A Healthier Tomorrow

Medicare Reform for All Generations

snova
New York

NOTICE TO THE READER

The Publisher has taken reasonable care in the preparation of this book, but makes no expressed or implied warranty of any kind and assumes no responsibility for any errors or omissions. No liability is assumed for incidental or consequential damages in connection with or arising out of information contained in this book. The Publisher shall not be liable for any special, consequential, or exemplary damages resulting, in whole or in part, from the readers' use of, or reliance upon, this material. Any parts of this book based on government reports are so indicated and copyright is claimed for those parts to the extent applicable to compilations of such works.

Independent verification should be sought for any data, advice or recommendations contained in this book. In addition, no responsibility is assumed by the Publisher for any injury and/or damage to persons or property arising from any methods, products, instructions, ideas or otherwise contained in this publication.

The Publisher assumes no responsibility for any statements of fact or opinion expressed in the published contents.

This publication is designed to provide accurate and authoritative information with regard to the subject matter covered herein. It is sold with the clear understanding that the Publisher is not engaged in rendering legal or any other professional services. If legal or any other expert assistance is required, the services of a competent person should be sought. FROM A DECLARATION OF PARTICIPANTS JOINTLY ADOPTED BY A COMMITTEE OF THE AMERICAN BAR ASSOCIATION AND A COMMITTEE OF PUBLISHERS.

Additional color graphics may be available in the e-book version of this book.

Library of Congress Cataloging-in-Publication Data

ISBN: 979-8-89530-798-4 (Hardcover)
ISBN: 979-8-89530-958-2 (eBook)

Published by Nova Science Publishers, Inc. † New York

Contents

Preface vii

Chapter 1 **Medicare for All: Protecting Health, Saving Lives, Saving Money** 1
Committee on the Budget

Chapter 2 **Medicare Forever: Protecting Seniors by Making the Wealthy Pay Their Fair Share**............217
Committee on the Budget

Index 337

Preface

Since its inception, Medicare has ensured that our nation's seniors do not fall into poverty because of illness. As a result, older Americans live longer, have a higher quality of life, and receive better health care. Nearly all seniors receive the Medicare benefits they earned during their working years, allowing them to retire in health and dignity. The book explores ways to ensure that Medicare remains solvent forever.

Chapter 1

Medicare for All: Protecting Health, Saving Lives, Saving Money*

Committee on the Budget

Thursday, May 12, 2022
U.S. Senate, Committee on the Budget,
Washington, DC.

The Committee met, pursuant to notice, at 11:02 a.m., via Webex and in Room SH–216, Dirksen Senate Office Building, Hon. Bernard Sanders, Chairman of the Committee, presiding.

Present: Senators Sanders, Merkley, Van Hollen, Padilla, Graham, Grassley, Crapo, Johnson, Braun, and Scott.

Staff Present: Warren Gunnels, Majority Staff Director; Nick Myers, Republican Staff Director.

Opening Statement of Chairman Sanders

Chairman SANDERS. Okay, let us get going. Let me thank the Committee members who are here. Let me thank the panelists who are here. I think all are here in person; I think we will have one virtually. Let me thank all of you for attending the very first U.S. Senate Committee hearing on Medicare for All.

* This is an edited, reformatted and augmented version of Hearing before the Committee on the Budget, United States Senate, One Hundred Seventeenth Congress, Second Session, Publication No. S. HRG. 117–260, dated May 12, 2022.

In: A Healthier Tomorrow
Editor: Robert M. Deaton
ISBN: 979-8-89530-798-4

Let me also thank the many dozens of organizations throughout our country who support Medicare for All and the tens of thousands of doctors, nurses, and other health care professionals who support this legislation.

Let me thank the 15 Senate co-sponsors that we have on this bill and the 122 members of the House who support very similar legislation.

And, mostly, let me thank the American people who, by the millions, understand as I do that our current health care system is dysfunctional, it is extraordinarily wasteful and expensive, and it is cruel. The American people understand as I do that health care is a human right and not a privilege and that we must end the international embarrassment of our great country being the only major nation on Earth that does not guarantee health care as a human right to all of its people.

It is not acceptable to me, nor to the American people, that over 70 million Americans today are either uninsured or underinsured. As we speak, right now, this moment, there are millions of people in our country who would like to go to a doctor, who have to go to the doctor, but simply cannot afford to do so. This is unacceptable, this is un-American, and this cannot be allowed to happen in the wealthiest country on Earth.

Bottom line is that your health and your longevity, how long you live, should not be a factor of how much money you have. Health care is a human right that all Americans, regardless of income, are entitled to, and all Americans deserve the best health care that our country can provide.

As Chairman of the Budget Committee, it is not acceptable to me that we end up spending over twice as much per capita on health care as other major countries around the world, something we do not see too much on TV, you do not read in the newspapers, you do not hear it discussed here. My friends are concerned about the budget deficit, concerned about how much money we spend. Well, somebody should talk about why it is that we are spending almost twice as much per capita on health care as do the people of any other major country on Earth while at the same time, despite all of that expenditure, our life expectancy, how long we live, is less than most other major countries and our health care outcomes in a number of areas lag behind other countries.

Unbelievably—and I want the American people to hear this. You know, we talk about budget deficits or anything else here. Unbelievably, according to the Center for Medicare and Medicaid Services, CMS, we are now spending $12,530 per capita on health care. You got that? $12,530 for every man, woman, and child in this country. This is an outrageous and unsustainable sum of money.

And here is the important point. In comparison, let us take a look at what other countries are spending for health care which is as good or maybe better. United Kingdom spends $5,200. Remember, we spend over $12,000. Canada spends $5,300. France spends $5,500 per person. Germany spends $6,700. All of those countries provide universal health care, i.e., for all of their people.

The key question that we should be discussing as a Congress is: How does it happen that we spend so much money for health care but get so little in return?

Frankly, I am tired of talking to doctors—and we will have some here today—who tell me about the patients who have died because they were uninsured or underinsured and walked into their offices too late with untreatable conditions. And let us remember, again, not widely discussed, but we are losing, according to the best studies, over 60,000 Americans every year who die unnecessarily because they are uninsured or underinsured.

I am tired of seeing working-class families and small business pay far more for health care than they can afford, which forces more than 500,000 Americans to declare bankruptcy each year because of medically related expenses. In America, families should not be driven into financial ruin because somebody became seriously ill in that family. Can you imagine that? Some kid comes down with leukemia, and a family goes bankrupt? Does that make any sense to anybody?

I am tired of hearing from Americans who have lost loved ones because they could not afford the unbelievably high cost of prescription drugs, and I think every Senator has talked to patients, has talked to constituents, who tell them what these outrageously high costs of prescription drugs have done. One out of four patients in America cannot afford the prescription drugs their doctors prescribe.

You want to hear about crazy, and you want to hear about an irrational health care system? Crazy is when a patient walks into a doctor's office, gets a diagnosis, doctor writes out a prescription, and the patient cannot afford to fill that prescription, becomes sicker, ends up in the emergency room or the hospital, a greater expense to the system. My friends, that is called crazy.

I am tired of talking with people who are struggling with mental illness but cannot afford the mental health counseling they desperately need. Last year, as you know, a record breaking 100,000 people died of drug overdoses. And I will tell you that in my office, and I suspect the offices of every Senator here, we get desperate calls from constituents who say, "Somebody in my family desperately needs mental health counseling. I am worried," but far too often we cannot help them get the care that they need.

It is not there because in the system, geared toward the profits of the insurance companies rather than the needs of the American people, we do not have enough psychologists and counselors. We do not have enough doctors. We do not have enough nurses. We do not have enough dentists. We do not have enough medical care providers. We spend twice as much as any other major country. We do not have even have the health care providers that we need to take care of our people.

And also, I am tired of seeing people in my own State and around this country who are walking around with teeth rotting in their mouths because they cannot afford the dental care that they need because dental care is health care, and on and on it goes.

But let us be clear about something, and this is maybe the most important point that I want to make. The current debate that we are having on health care and Medicare for All really has nothing to do with health care because in my view this dysfunctional health care system cannot be rationally defended.

What this debate has everything to do with is the unquenchable greed of the health care industry and its desire to maintain a system which fails the average American but which makes the industry huge profits year after year after year. While ordinary Americans struggled to pay for health care during this pandemic—and we will talk about the impacts of the pandemic on health care— the six largest health insurance companies in America last year made over $60 billion in profit, led by United Health Group which made $24 billion in the midst of the pandemic in 2021.

But it is not just the profits of the insurance companies. CEOs make exorbitant compensation packages. CEOs of 178 major health care companies collectively made $3.2 billion in total compensation in 2020, up 31 percent from 2019, all in the midst of the pandemic. According to Axios, in 2020, the CEO of Cigna, David Cordani, took home $79 million in compensation while people died in the middle of the pandemic.

In terms of the drug companies, the pharmaceutical industry, not much different. Last year, Pfizer, Johnson & Johnson, and AbbVie, three giant pharmaceutical companies increased their profits by over 90 percent to $54 billion. The CEOs of those companies also receive huge compensation packages.

So that is what the debate is about. The debate we are having is whether we have a health care system which provides quality care to all in a cost-effective way or do we have a system which makes the drug companies and the insurance companies and their executives very, very wealthy.

Now in order to defeat Medicare for All, these very powerful special interests, the drug companies, the insurance companies, et cetera, have spent millions of dollars against me, against other proponents on 30-second TV ads, full-page magazine ads, and corporate-sponsored studies to frighten the American people about Medicare for All, and I think we are going to hear some of that being discussed this morning.

And this is, by the way, exactly what happened before the passage of Medicare in the 1960s, which was often attacked at that time as being socialism. Meanwhile, Medicare is today the most popular health care program in the country.

Let me give you just a few examples of the kind of power we are up against when we try to create a health care system that guarantees health care for all people. Since 1998, the private health care sector has spent more than $10.6 billion—that is health care money that people paid—$10.6 billion on lobbying, and over the last 30 years it has spent more than $1.7 billion on campaign contributions to get Congress to do its bidding. We pay our health care bills. They take that money and spend it on lobbying and campaign contributions.

The pharmaceutical industry right now, at this moment, has 1,500 paid lobbyists, including the leadership, formal leadership, of the Democratic and Republican party right here on Capitol Hill, doing everything they possibly can to tell us that we should not lower the cost of prescription drugs. That is how business is done in Washington.

Well, I think many of us have a different idea, and that is that maybe, just maybe Congress should represent the American people and not lobbyists and large corporations.

So what does Medicare for All do? What is it that some of my colleagues are so strongly opposed to? Well, this legislation will do, again, what many, virtually every other country on Earth does. It would provide comprehensive health care to all without out-of-pocket expenses and, unlike the current system, would allow freedom of choice regarding health care providers, no more insurance premiums, no more deductibles, no more co-payments. And comprehensive means the coverage of dental care, vision, hearing aids, prescription drugs, and home-and community-based care.

The transition to the Medicare for All program would take place over four years. The first year, the benefits for older people would be expanded to include dental, vision, and hearing, and the eligibility age for Medicare would be lowered to 55. All children under the age of 18 would be covered. And gradually, over a four-year period, those programs would be provided to every American.

Would a Medicare for All health care system be expensive? The answer is yes. But while providing comprehensive health care for all, it would be significantly less expensive than our current dysfunctional system because it would eliminate an enormous amount of the bureaucracy, profiteering, administrative costs, and misplaced priorities inherent in our current for-profit system.

Under Medicare for All, there would no longer be armies of people billing us, telling us what is covered and what is not covered, and insurance agents hounding us to pay our hospital bills. This would not only save substantial sums of money, but it will make life a lot easier for the American people who would never again have to fight their way through the nightmare of insurance company bureaucracy, an experience I think that almost all Americans have gone through.

In fact, the Congressional Budget Office—and we are going to hear from them later this morning—has estimated that Medicare for All would save Americans $650 billion a year. So for my friends who are worried about the deficit, that ain't chump change. $650 billion a year is real money.

Now trust me, I do know these 30-second ads that will be coming from the insurance and drug companies that will tell you that if Medicare for All becomes law your taxes will go up, and they are correct.

But what they will not tell you is that under Medicare for All you will no longer be paying premiums, deductibles, and co-payments to private health insurance companies. And what they certainly will not be telling you is that Medicare for All will save the average American family thousands of dollars a year. Medicare for All will save the average American family thousands of dollars a year.

Guaranteeing health care as a right is important to the American people, not just from a moral and financial perspective. It also happens to be what the majority of the American people want. In 2020, 69 percent of the American people supported providing Medicare to every American.

Let me conclude, and I thank my colleagues for their indulgence, and Senator Graham will have as much time as he wants. This is an issue not just of health care. This is an issue about what kind of nation we are. It is an issue whether we are going to turn our backs on 60,000 people a year who die because they cannot get the health care that they need, turn our backs on the fact that we live shorter lives than people in other countries, turn our backs in that we are spending almost twice as much per capita on health care as the people of other nations.

This is an issue that has to be dealt with. Medicare for All will become the law of the land, if not now, but in the future because this is what the American people want.

And with that, let me thank Senator Graham for being here and give the mic over to him.

Opening Statement of Senator Graham

Senator GRAHAM. Thank you, Mr. Chairman. This is an important debate, important hearing, important topics. It has tremendous budget impact, and I think it is something the nation needs to be talking about.

But how does something become a law? You vote on it. So here is what I would like to see happen. I would like to see a vote on your proposal in this Committee this year. I welcome a vote on Medicare for All in this Committee this year. You have control of the Senate floor. I welcome a vote on Medicare for All on the floor of the United States Senate this year.

You tell your side of the story; we will tell ours. But if you really want this to become law, you need to start voting.

So, Mr. Chairman, I am hoping that after this speech that you will be putting your idea up for a vote. And if not, why not? Because most of your colleagues would jump out the window if they had to vote on this.

After this discussion by Senator Sanders, you are wondering why we need a wall at all. The state of health care described by Senator Sanders, it certainly can be made better and needs to be reformed, absolutely. Can we spend less and get better outcomes? Absolutely. But to believe what was being said, why are so many people coming to America? Why aren't we leaving to go to someplace else where you do not die in the streets?

So the facts you are describing and the activity to the American people really do not matter—match up. If it were as you said, one of the most disgusting examples of health care being provided on the planet, people would be leaving America, not coming to America.

Under your proposal, every doctor and nurse, in case you are watching this, you would become a Federal Government employee because the only game in town would be Medicare. You would be working for the Federal Government because the single provider for health care in this country would be Medicare, which is a government-run program.

The private health care that you have today as an American would go away. Once you get to be 65, Medicare takes over, but below 65, people are insured in the private sector for the most part. That option goes away for you. Everybody in the health care system becomes a Federal Government employee. Everybody in America goes into a single-payer system run by the Federal Government. Let us see where we are at with Medicare as it stands today. Medicare is an important program. I would like to save it. I do not want to sunset it, as some people are talking about. I, sure as hell, do not want to invite hundreds of millions of people onto the Medicare system that have not paid a dime because Medicare for All really becomes Medicare for Nobody over time.

This is what the trustees say. Medicare Part A, which is the hospital part, will become insolvent by 2026. To rectify the $5 trillion shortfall over 75 years, you have to increase taxes by 27 percent or cut spending by 16 percent. Medicare spending is expected to surge from 4 percent of GDP to 6.2 percent by 2045.

We found common ground here. We need to change that narrative. We need to reform Medicare, not invite a bunch of people onto the system that would sink it. So it is in a fiscally unsound situation. I would like to work with Democrats and Republicans to make it sound, which would be a worthy use of our time.

Now just to remind people what life is like in America today, inflation is like beyond through the roof: 22.7 percent for used cars, 43.6 percent increase in gas prices, fruits and vegetables, dairy products. Just go down the list.

We are talking about the most massive increase in spending known to the United States. How would that affect inflation? Not well. So, absolutely would crush an economy that needs some help. So when Americans understand what it means to do away with private health care and replace it with a one-size-fits-all, they are not so happy. Delay in getting medical tests and treatments: 70 percent say they would oppose a system that created greater delay. You know, Americans have become used to certain things. We like to go to the doctor of our choice. We like to have a say about who our doctor is and get timely services.

Our friends in Canada, it takes 19.8 weeks on average to see a doctor. There is 1.2 million Canadians on a waiting list of critical medical care. In the U.K., it takes 62 days for cancer patients to start treatment. 5.8 million British residents were on a waiting list for critical medical treatment. That is their system.

If you think it is hard to get to see a doctor now, Medicare for All would institute delays that I think would be unacceptable to the average American consumer.

Financing for Medicare for All. All right. What would it take? One-size-fits-all for a health care plan could cost as much as $40 trillion over the first 10 years. Taxes would double, or you would have to cut the budget. Health care spending grows to 40 percent. GDP drops by 10 percent because you are crowding out the private sector.

The economic consequences to this plan for the American taxpayer would be unimaginable. And it is hard enough to create a job in America now. You talk about exploding the size and cost of government. This would just absolutely crush the private sector.

There are better ways. Let us save Medicare as it exists. But for people under 65, let us try to get better quality by getting the health care dollars outside of Medicare in the hands of people closer to the patient. Governors are innovative out there right now. Let us get money down to the states, get flexibility and inventing new preventive health care systems, and give consumers a choice they do not have today.

Right now, Medicare is run by people you will never meet, and we need to reform Medicare. We need to save Medicare, but the system outside of Medicare, which is a lot of money, let us get it down to the state level. Let us come up with ideas that would lower costs and increase quality. Let us keep—create competition in the health care sector, where innovation is rewarded, not punished. And I think that is a better way.

I want to put health care in the hands of people that you actually will meet and have responsibility at the ballot box so if you do not like what you are getting you can change the results.

So, Mr. Chairman, this is a debate worth having. I applaud your passion. I do not agree with your idea, but here is what I would suggest to you and others who believe in this idea. Let us vote on it. I am welcoming a debate and a vote.

Now if we do not vote on it, then it makes me wonder about it. If you think it is this great and it is wonderful and it fixes all of our problems, let us vote.

Thank you.

Chairman SANDERS. Thank you very much, Senator Graham.

We have a great panel, five panelists. We have Dr. Adam Gaffney, Dr. Abdul El-Sayed, Ms. Bonnie Castillo, Dr. Charles Blahous, and Ms. Grace-Marie Turner.

Let us begin with Dr. Adam Gaffney. Dr. Gaffney is an assistant professor of medicine at Harvard Medical School, a pulmonary and critical care physician, and a health policy researcher. His research focuses on national health care reform, health care equity, and disparities in lung health.

Dr. Gaffney, thanks very much for being with us.

Statement of Adam Gaffney, MD, MPH, Assistant Professor of Medicine, Harvard Medical School

Dr. GAFFNEY. Thank you, Chairman Sanders, Ranking Senator Graham, and all of the members of the Budget Committee, for the opportunity to discuss this pressing issue with you today.

So for the past two years, I have been treating patients with COVID–19 in the intensive care unit where I work as a critical care physician. Some of them, like one million other Americans, did not survive, but those experiences have reinforced my belief that our nation needs transformative health care reform, a Medicare for All program that would end much of the medical and financial suffering I have witnessed.

One of my patients awakened after a long stretch on a ventilator, and their first words I later learned were an expression of fear about medical bills. Back then, there was at least a Federal program that existed that would cover the cost of COVID–19 treatment for the uninsured. That program is now defunct.

Today, Americans with COVID–19, just like Americans with cancer, with any illness or injury, can face bankruptcy because of medical bills. One in five U.S. households are carrying medical debt, which now exceeds all other forms of debt sent to collection agencies in this, the richest nation in the world. Medical debt should not exist, and in many other countries it basically does not. It is the consequence of the irrational way our country finances medical care.

But the problem is not only families ruined by health care costs. It is worsened health due to inadequate care. Today, 30 million Americans are uninsured. These patients go without needed care day in and day out, and their health suffers because of it.

In the ICU, I have cared for patients critically ill with failing hearts, failing kidneys, fluid in their lungs because they could not afford routine care for common problems, like high blood pressure or diabetes. And my experience is not unique. A multitude of rigorous studies have demonstrated that uninsurance is lethal. Indeed, it causes well more than 30,000 deaths every year.

However, uninsurance is not our only problem. Far from it, in fact. More than 40 million working-age Americans are underinsured. They are covered but still fear unaffordable bills because of high co-pays, deductibles, uncovered services, and out-of-network care. And here, too, conclusive research has found dire consequences, heart attack patients who delay going to the emergency room, risking sudden death, and children who end up hospitalized because their parents could not afford the co-payments for their asthma medications.

Sadly, I have also witnessed the consequences of underinsurance in my work, seniors with lung disease who have rationed their expensive inhalers because of high co-pays, patients who have rationed their insulin and ended up with severe complications of diabetes.

Typically, it is only after becoming severely ill that patients realize that their insurance is riddled with holes. Even if you have coverage, unless you are Elon Musk, you could be one illness or injury away from financial ruin.

Now Medicare for All would solve each of these problems, allowing us to cover everyone and at the same time to improve the quality of coverage, eliminating co-pays, deductibles, and narrow insurance networks. It would finally give patients real choice, not the bogus choice between an Aetna or a UnitedHealth plan, but the real choice of doctor, clinic, or hospital.

Now I have indicated some of the medical benefits of Medicare of All reform, but the economics are, of course, also quite relevant. This reform would uniquely produce the savings needed to cover the costs of such a major expansion of care as I have described without breaking the bank. The simple fact is that there is enormous bureaucratic waste in American health care, waste born by both patients and clinicians.

Of every dollar we spend on health care, 34 cents goes to administration and bureaucracy, twice the proportion in Canada. Much of that waste is inflicted by private health insurers. While 2 percent of traditional Medicare spending goes to overhead, private health insurance companies' profits and overhead consumes 12 percent or more of our premiums, and much of that overhead is spent on contesting claims and denying care for patients.

The bureaucratic burden of American health care explains the CBO's estimate that Medicare for All would achieve more than $400 billion a year in savings by reducing insurance waste alone. And in contrast, some outdated and inaccurate economic analyses have low-balled such savings, leading to spurious claims that single-payer reform would break the bank.

Make no mistake, Senators, the economics matter. And as a health policy researcher, I spend a lot of time thinking about them, but what matters to me most as a physician is creating a health care system that will support me in delivering top quality care to all of my patients during this pandemic and thereafter.

I became an ICU doctor because I wanted to care for the sickest of the sick, but I should not be seeing desperately ill patients who could have avoided the ICU altogether if they had gotten the care they needed. Those patients have been failed by a broken system that puts the prerogatives of health insurance executives over the health and welfare of ordinary Americans.

Medicare for All can solve the problems of our health care system, covering everyone, improving the quality of coverage, expanding choice, controlling costs, and most importantly, improving our health and longevity.

Thank you.

[The prepared statement of Dr. Gaffney appears on page 42.]

Chairman SANDERS. Thank you, Dr. Gaffney.

Our next panelist is Ms. Bonnie Castillo. Ms. Castillo is a registered nurse and the Executive Director of the National Nurses United and of the California Nurses Association National Nurses Organizing Committee. NNU is the largest union and professional association of registered nurses in the United States, representing more than 175,000 nurses.

And I just want to take this opportunity to thank all of the nurses in this country and the doctors as well. We have lost thousands, I think as we all know. I heard this morning at least 5,000 nurses have died in this pandemic alone. These are the real heroes and heroines of our time, and we thank them very much.

Ms. Castillo, thanks very much for being with us.

Statement of Bonnie Castillo, RN, Executive Director, National Nurses United

Ms. CASTILLO. Thank you. Thank you and good morning. And thank you, Chairman Sanders, Ranking Member Graham, and members of the Committee, for holding this critically important hearing today.

As a registered nurse and Executive Director of the nation's largest union of RNs, I can think of nothing more fitting to commemorate International Nurses Day today than by advocating for the urgent transition to a Medicare for All system. For more than two years, nurses across the country have worked on the front lines of the COVID pandemic. We have cared for patients despite atrocious working conditions that put nurses and our families at risk.

If it was ever in doubt before, this pandemic has shown that our current profit-driven and fragmented health care system does not work. It does not provide quality, therapeutic care to millions of Americans. It does not value and protect its own health care workers, and it is unable to provide a comprehensive pandemic response.

Why didn't nurses and health care workers get the protections we needed in the pandemic? It was because our employers value money over our lives.

Why didn't we have the emergency stocks of critical medical supplies that we needed? Because the health care industry plans their supply chains based on maximizing profit, not safeguarding patient care.

We have seen high death rates from COVID across the country. Why? Because there are tens of millions of people in the country who are uninsured or underinsured and who, therefore, do not get the preventive care they need, putting them at much higher risk for severe COVID illness, hospitalization, and death.

But the problems with our health care system far predate this pandemic. For years, nurses have witnessed the tragedies that result from a profit-driven health care system. Nurses watch far too many, so many, patients forego needed care because they cannot afford the cost. They watch as insurance companies deny lifesaving care, overriding the professional judgment of nurses and other medical professionals. Nurses watch as patients come to the emergency room with advanced stages of illness or disease that could have been avoided if they had had access to preventive care.

The system we have now is beholden to the corporate interests that determine who gets treatment and when they get it. The United States spends more money per capita on health care than any other nation in the world, and yet, we have the worst health outcomes when compared to other wealthy countries. This system is unaffordable for our country and for our patients, and the pandemic has shown that our society cannot afford the public health consequences.

The only way to solve the health care crisis is to enact a singlepayer, Medicare for All system. Under Medicare for All, every person living in the United States would get quality, therapeutic health care regardless of the ability to pay. We would transform the profit-driven health insurance system into one that actually prioritizes patient care.

As a registered nurse, I can envision exactly what Medicare for All would mean for patients. Whenever someone needs medical care, they would see the health care provider of their choice without any worry about financial barriers to care. We would no longer see patients suffer because they cannot afford care. Patients would no longer have to actually ration their medications.

For health care workers, we would be able to provide medical and nursing care based on our professional judgment without the interference of insurance companies.

The Medicare for All Act would allow for tangible, practical improvements to the health care delivery, and importantly, it would change the way the hospitals are paid, fundamentally shifting their profit motives so that they prioritize patient care and worker health and safety instead. By paying hospitals through global budgets, the bill would ensure that hospitals have the funding necessary for safe nurse to patient staffing ratios, pandemic preparedness, and occupational safety and health programs.

The programs would ensure that hospitals in rural and underserved areas always get the funding they need to stay open. And, it is designed to address health care inequities at their core by changing the systems that limit health care for low income communities and particularly for communities of color.

As registered nurses, our primary responsibility is to protect the health and well-being of our patients. Our existing health care system does not allow us to do that. Medicare for All is the solution we need to ensure that every patient gets the health care they need.

Thank you.

[The prepared statement of Ms. Castillo appears on page 54.]

Chairman SANDERS. Ms. Castillo, thank you very much.

Our next panelist is Dr. Abdul El-Sayed, who is a physician, epidemiologist, and educator. He is a Towsley Foundation Policymaker in Residence at the University of Michigan Gerald Ford School of Public Policy. Formerly, he was Health Director for the City of Detroit, where he was responsible for the public health needs of over 670,000 people in that city.

Dr. El-Sayed, thank you very much for being with us.

Statement of Abdul El-Sayed, Md, Dphil, Harry A. and Margaret D. Towsley Foundation Policymaker in Residence, Gerald R. Ford School of Public Policy, University of Michigan

Dr. EL-SAYED. Chairman Sanders, Ranking Member Graham, and members of the Committee, thank you for the opportunity to testify before you today.

My name is Dr. Abdul El-Sayed. I trained as a physician and epidemiologist and served the City of Detroit as Health Director, where one of my responsibilities was rebuilding a health department that had been shut down during the Great Recession.

Today, I teach at the University of Michigan's Ford School of Public Policy. There, I find myself explaining the haphazard dysfunction of our current health care system to some of the brightest young minds in the country. What is a deductible? Well, it is like having to pay an extra $19.99 to watch a movie on Netflix that you thought you already paid for only this time it is for your basic health care needs and it is thousands of dollars. They remind me how much nonsense we accept as normal in our health care.

It is partly why I recently wrote a book on the very subject, Medicare for All: A Citizen's Guide, with Dr. Micah Johnson, and I furnished a copy to each one of your offices.

I want to start with the two most obvious problems in American health care, incomplete coverage and spiraling costs. To understand them, I want to correct a basic misunderstanding of how we approach health care in this country. We like to think of ourselves as consumers, as customers, but we are not.

Let me just share how being a customer works, just to review. Let us say you want some tomatoes. You go to your local farmer's market. You find a stall with some you like. You ask the seller for the price, and if that price is too high you walk away. But if it is good, it is fair, you buy. You tender your payment. You get your tomatoes. That is a normal customer experience, but health care is not that.

If I were to have a heart attack right now, in this room, I would be rushed to the nearest hospital with no choice of what hospital I go to. I would have no choice of what doctor I see, what treatment I get. No one shows me a price list, and I have no opportunity to just walk away if I do not like anything. I am having a heart attack after all.

Afterwards, a bill is not sent to me. It is sent to a third party, my insurer. And rather than being the initiator and completer of a financial transaction, I am the reason a financial transaction happens between my insurer and my provider.

So ask yourself, given the usual customer experience, are we as American health care consumers, are we the customers or are we the tomatoes?

Health care is simply just not a market product. The health insurance industry assures that. You might expect insurance companies to want to negotiate health care costs downward. After all, they are the payer. But they do not. It is one of the unintended consequences of the so-called 80/20 rule, requiring health insurance companies to spend at least 80 percent of what they collect on premiums in health care.

After all, ask yourself, what is the best way to grow your 20 percent piece of the pie? Make sure you got a bigger pie. So they make the pie bigger, and they pass those costs back onto us in the form of premiums and deductibles.

Premiums have risen faster than inflation and wages over the past decade, and deductibles have almost doubled, and those are dangerous. One study found that high deductibles was associated with a nine-month delay in getting treatment for breast cancer. The operative part of the word "insurance" is supposed to be "sure," but in our for-profit system you cannot really be sure of anything. And those are the first-class health care citizens. There are, of course, the second-class health care citizens, over 100 million of them, 28 million who are uninsured, 87 million who are on Medicaid, a critical but underfunded lifeline program. Medicaid reimburses far lower than private health insurance so a lot of providers just do not accept it.

Now here is the thing. Reimbursing the same, exact health care services at lower rates reflects an implicit lack of value of the body for which that health care is being provided. You cannot deny it. And those bodies in this country are disproportionately Black and Brown, disproportionately rural. Meanwhile, the prices keep rising. Corporations keep making money when they do.

We spend more than $12,000 per capita per year on health care, more than twice as much as our counterparts in Canada. They live four years longer on average, by the way.

The pandemic demonstrated that coverage and cost are not our only issues. Early on, health care workers struggled without ventilators or beds or basic PPE. Twenty-seven million Americans lost their employer-sponsored health insurance with their jobs. Local and state health departments and the CDC struggled under the weight because they were already anemic from the disinvestment during the Great Recession. So despite the need for more beds, 21 hospitals shut down in 2020 alone. That is including 73 over the past decade, 4 in Senator Graham's South Carolina alone.

But guess what industry had a banner year in 2020. The health insurance industry. They got to keep all of the money that did not get spent on elective procedures, which, by the way, is why those hospitals shut down. American life expectancy dropped 25 years— actually, it dropped by 3 years, wiping out 25 years of growth.

So what did we learn? Even with private insurance coverage, it is not durable. It is liable to be lost to you, precarious, as we saw in the pandemic. American consumers are losing their health care choices through hospital closures and mergers and acquisitions, which, by the way, allow large health care systems to exploit workers, including nurses and doctors, and we are failing to invest in public health.

Now the genius of Medicare for All is not just that it solves coverage and cost. It is that a universal national health insurance program for everyone offers a solution for each of these problems. Medicare for All is the clearest pathway to universal, durable health care insurance, bar none. Cradle to grave coverage would do away with the premiums, co pays, deductibles that leave even privately insured Americans rationing their health care today, just like they do every day in America.

Medicare for All would expand health care choices by limiting hospital mergers, acquisitions, and shutdowns that threaten those choices and empower mammoth health care systems in the process. It would also empower health care workers. And, it finally addresses the misincentives that we have to invest in prevention and public health.

So to conclude, opponents of Medicare for All are going to tell us all the same fear-mongering arguments we have actually already heard today. They are going to say that Medicare for All would eliminate health care choices, but really, it is critical to preserving the choices Americans actually care about, which are the choice of doctor, the choice of clinic, the choice of hospital.

They will say we cannot afford it when American families cannot afford the system that we have today.

What about innovation, they will ask. Well, providers stay private under Medicare for All, never mind the fact that our Federal Government is the most important funder of biomedical research in the world.

What about rationing, they will say. Well, out-of-pocket costs are forcing Americans to ration health care every day in the current system.

They will tell us that Medicare for All is somehow un-American, but what really is un-American is staring at a broken health care system in the face while it is breaking people in the process and choosing to look away.

Today, you are choosing to stare at it in its cruel, indifferent face, and I commend you for doing this. And I hope that I have offered some insights into how and why it is broken and how Medicare for All is the solution to fix it.

Thank you.

[The prepared statement of Dr. El-Sayed appears on page 91.]

Chairman SANDERS. Thank you, Dr. El-Sayed.

Our next panelist is Ms. Grace-Marie Turner, who is President of the Galen Institute, a public policy research organization that she founded in 1995 to promote an informed debate over free market ideas for health reform. Ms. Turner is founder and facilitator of the Health Policy Consensus Group, which serves as a forum for analysts for market-oriented think tanks around the country.

Ms. Turner, thanks very much for being with us.

Statement of Grace-Marie Turner, President, Galen Institute

Ms. TURNER. Thank you, Chairman Sanders, Ranking Member Graham, Senators, for the opportunity to testify today.

Mr. Chairman, I would like to begin by acknowledging my respect for your tireless work on universal coverage. While there are different views about how to reach that goal, I believe there are important values that we share in achieving universal coverage, with care that is affordable, protecting quality and choice, and especially a strong safety net for the vulnerable.

Americans are frustrated with our current health sector, with millions still uninsured. Those with insurance find their coverage costs too much, and deductibles can be so high many people feel they are not even insured.

But the more government gets involved, the more providers must comply with legislative and regulatory demands instead of innovating to respond to the needs of patients, families, and employers. Wharton Professor Mark Pauly finds that the Federal Government exerts a great influence over our health sector today, with government controlled or directed spending totaling 80 percent.

In proposing policy solutions, I believe it is important to begin by clearly defining the problem. The overwhelming majority of Americans today have access to coverage. More than 30 million people are uninsured, but two-thirds of them are eligible for programs that they are not enrolled in, either in the private or the public sector. Among the remaining one third, most of them are undocumented immigrants, which is an immigration problem more than it is a health care problem. Uninsured rates continue to be higher among Latinos and Blacks, people with incomes below the poverty level, and people in states that have not expanded Medicaid. We could work together to make sure these 30 million people that are eligible for coverage have access to care and coverage.

Medicare for All would mean that virtually everyone would lose the plans they have today in exchange for this one government-run health plan, including 173 million Americans who have coverage through their employer that they value and 64 million Americans, on Medicare, seniors, who have paid into the Medicare program throughout their working lives to have medical coverage when they retire.

Several states have tried to implement a single-payer plan, including the Chairman's home State of Vermont. Colorado took a vote on single-payer. And, California most recently shelved their single-payer plans. They learned the proposal would require the largest tax increase in the State's history of more than $12,000 per household annually to meet the $400 billion-plus annual cost.

And according to the Kaiser Family Foundation, as the Chairman said, two-thirds of Americans say they support a plan that would guarantee health coverage for all. But also, as the Ranking Member said, that figure drops to 37 percent when people learn it will raise taxes and eliminate their private health insurance. It drops to 26 percent when people learn they can expect delays in receiving treatment.

As several of our witnesses have said, delayed or denied care can in fact cost lives. Sally Pipes, who runs the Pacific Research Institute and was born and raised in Canada, said her otherwise healthy godson went to Vancouver Emergency Room earlier this year with chest pains. Doctors gave him an electrocardiogram and a chest X-ray, but not a CT scan. CT scans are notoriously difficult to get in Canada because of the scarcity of equipment. They sent him home with some pills. The next morning, he was found dead in his condominium. The autopsy showed a torn aorta which the CT scan would likely have detected and which likely could have been repaired.

Evidence abroad shows that Medicare for All would lead to restricted access to new medicines, diagnostics, and treatments, fewer innovations in personalized care, and lower payment rates. It would force physicians and other providers to curtail services or even close their doors. We saw this happen just up the street at Providence Hospital. It became too reliant on Medicaid funds and, after a century and a half, had to close its doors to acute hospital treatment.

I would like to commend Ranking Member Graham for his hard work on proposals to usher in a new era of health reform by unleashing the innovation and energy pent up in our health sector to solve so many of the problems we are facing. Senator Graham has provided ideas and guidance for the work of policy experts from 82 organizations that have signed on to the Health Care Choices plan. The plan has dozens of recommendations to encourage choice and competition, offering more options for more affordable coverage, more choices, and better care for those who have the greatest health needs.

Thank you for the opportunity to testify. I look forward to your questions.

[The prepared statement of Ms. Turner appears on page 102.]

Chairman SANDERS. Ms. Turner, thank you very much.

We have one more panelist, Dr. Blahous, but before we get to him I would ask unanimous consent that Senator Merkley to be allowed to speak because he has to run to another appointment.

Senator Merkley.

Senator MERKLEY. Thank you very much, Mr. Chairman, and I appreciate this conversation so much because our health care system is so enormously stressful. There are so many cracks, so many different forms of medical care, and people are always falling between them.

Health Care System Performance Compared to Spending

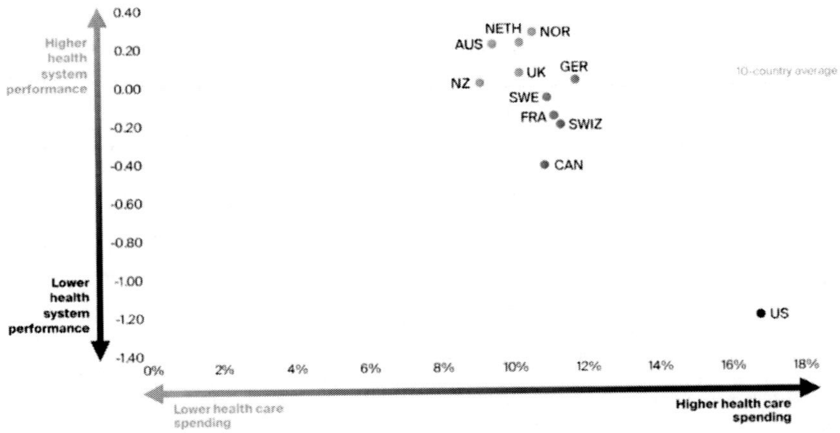

Note: Health care spending as a percent of GDP. Performance scores are based on standard deviation calculated from the 10-country average that excludes the US. See *How We Conducted This Study* for more detail. Data: Spending data are from OECD for the year 2019 (updated in July 2021).

Source: Eric C. Schneider et al., *Mirror, Mirror 2021- Reflecting Poorly: Health Care in the U.S. Compared to Other High-Income Countries* (Commonwealth Fund, Aug. 2021). *https://doi.org/10.26099/01DV-H208*

Just this last weekend, my son was in the emergency room with COVID. He had just turned 26. He is applying for continuation of Health Coverage

(COBRA), but it takes weeks to get that number. And so the first thing he was asked is, where is your insurance card, and he handed over his insurance card. And he was told: Well, we are sorry. This just expired because it is past your birth date.

And, just constantly, people are stressed out by the complexity and the cost of our system.

I thought I would try to quickly address a few of the points that my colleague from South Carolina has made because I see it a little differently. He mentioned the southern border, and we do see a lot of people on the southern border coming from very poor countries where there is a lot of issues and they are seeking a better life, but really, the comparison we are talking about is between other developed countries and the United States.

So I would ask unanimous consent to submit this chart for the record, and I will hold it up for the camera.

Senator MERKLEY. This is the rest of the developed world up here, much better health care, much lower cost. Here is the United States down here in the corner, much higher cost, much lower quality. Well, that is why we are having this conversation. The rest of the developed world has figured out that you can provide much better health care and much lower cost, and that is what Medicare for All is all about.

Second, my colleague made the point that everyone would work for the Federal Government, but this is not a single provider proposal. This is a single-payer proposal. That is completely different: single-payer proposal, like Medicare, the providers are the providers we have today.

And then my colleague mentioned inflation. But, what is worse for America than the inflation we have in the medical system? It is massive because there are not competitive forces to drive it down.

And, my colleague mentioned that competition we should introduce into the system, but as pointed out by our witness, it does not really work in the medical world. And if you want competition, you want everything to be in-network because that way everyone is competing. Well, how do you get in-network? You take Medicare for All. And if you really want competition within the existing system and you did not support Medicare for All, then you support a public option.

We have a public option in my home State of Oregon for insurance in the workplace. It is called the State Accident Insurance Fund. Private business chooses the public option over the private option more than half the time, and that competition actually drove down the cost a lot.

Therefore, if you want competition, you do not want the current existing system.

And then our witnesses talked about the inefficiency. I think about all the providers who say they spend all their time sorting through the many different insurance systems, trying to figure out what they can charge. That is a huge waste in our system.

I think about the businesses that say we spend so much time wrestling with which new insurance plan to try to keep the cost down while still offering insurance through our company. That is a huge waste of time and effort.

And then we heard about medical debt, and we heard about underinsurance, and we heard about medical rationing.

We have enumerable problems in this current system that Medicare for All will address.

And in my one minute remaining, I would like to ask a question to our expert on nursing, Bonnie Castillo. My wife is a nurse, so I take special interest in this. How will the provision of nursing workforce or nursing quality be affected by going to a Medicare for All system?

Ms. CASTILLO. Thank you. You know, obviously, we have been dealing with an industry-created nurse staffing crisis for many years. Right now, we have 1.2 million nurses with active licenses that are not working, and you know, they—so they are not working because many have left because of the poor working conditions, and more and more have left in the last two years in particular, which is because of everything that they are seeing in terms of the denial of care and the fact that they—as I said before, the atrocious conditions in the hospital.

And if the nurses are not able to give good quality care that they are expertly trained to give, that creates great moral distress. And to see so many patients suffering because they are suffering from illnesses that with a little bit of prevention and early care could have prevented a more acute situation for them, that has been very, very difficult.

So providing Medicare for All, getting early care, preventive care, that is going to—that allows us to do what we do as nurses, and that is to provide good, comprehensive care.

Senator MERKLEY. Thank you and just a huge thank you to all the nurses who make the world better one bedside at a time.

Ms. CASTILLO. And if I could add, too, just for the record, that really, Congress needs to pass mandatory minimum safe nurse-to-patient ratios, and they can do that independently now.

Chairman SANDERS. Okay. Senator Merkley, thank you.

Now we are going to get back to regular order, and that is, our last panelist is Dr. Charles Blahous, who is with us virtually. He is the J. Fish and Lillian F. Smith Chair and Senior Research Strategist at the Mercatus Center at George Mason University. Dr. Blahous specializes in domestic economic policy and retirement security, with an emphasis on Social Security as well as Federal fiscal policy.

Dr. Blahous, thanks very much for being with us.

Statement of the Honorable Charles Blahous, Ph.D., J. Fish and Lillian F. Smith Chair and Senior Research Strategist, Mercatus Center, George Mason University

Mr. BLAHOUS. Thank you, Chairman Sanders. Thank you, Ranking Member Graham, members of the Committee. I greatly appreciate this opportunity to discuss the Federal budget costs of Medicare for All.

Now before I summarize my findings, just a brief caveat. My testimony is largely based on analysis that I performed in 2018. Current proposals differ in key respects from the provisions that I studied. So at the end of my statement, I will discuss how recent developments might change these numbers.

Now my study found that Medicare for All would add somewhere between $32.6 trillion and $38.8 trillion in new Federal budget costs over the first 10 years. The $32.6 trillion scenario essentially assumed that every cost containment provision in the bill saved as much as possible. If, instead, things played out more consistently with historical trends, the added cost would be closer to $38.8 trillion.

The study also noted that doubling all currently projected Federal individual and corporate income taxes would be insufficient to finance even the lower bound estimate of $32.6 trillion.

Now the vast majority of these costs arise from the Federal Government's assuming responsibility for health spending that is now done by others, by state and local governments, by private insurance, and by individuals out of pocket. And certain aspects of Medicare for All would add to this health spending while others would seek to bring costs down.

The biggest factor increasing health spending would be Medicare for All's expansion and increased generosity of health insurance coverage. Spending on behalf of the currently uninsured would rise, as one would expect and presumably intend. Additional benefits would be provided that Medicare currently does not, such as dental, vision, and hearing services.

But, most importantly, Medicare for all would provide first-dollar coverage of Americans' health expenses, meaning with only a few exceptions no patient cost sharing. Now this would increase the demand for health services because the more of people's health care that is financed by their insurance, the more they tend to consume. So under Medicare for All, the Federal Government would assume responsibility for financing health care services above and beyond current demand.

Now other provisions of Medicare for All are intended to reduce costs. My study assumed substantial administrative cost savings and bracketed a range of possible outcomes of provisions intended to lower drug prices.

The big variable here is payment rates for health care providers. Current bills envision that payments would be set through processes similar to Medicare's, and Medicare pays providers much less than private insurance does. If Medicare for All paid providers at Medicare rates, payments for services now covered by private insurance would be sharply cut, by more than 40 percent for inpatient hospital care, more than 30 percent for doctors' services and so forth.

Now such payment rates would be substantially below providers' reported costs of providing services. So for this and other reasons, several studies assume Medicare for All must adopt higher payment rates than current Medicare does, and this, of course, leads to higher Federal cost estimates and findings that Medicare for All would further increase national health spending.

Now since my study was published, more recent proposals have generally included additional benefits I did not estimate, such as long-term services and supports, and that pushes costs up.

But other developments would lower the projected costs. Baseline projections for national health expenditures have gone down a little bit. Also, the so-called Cadillac plan tax was repealed, and other health-related taxes have been repealed. And this increases net Federal health subsidies under current law and thus reduces the additional costs posed by Medicare for All.

CBO has also found that many services would continue to be financed outside of a Medicare for All system. When you account for this, that further lowers the Federal cost estimate, but of course, it does not lower national health spending.

Perhaps most importantly, CBO found that much of the new demand for health care under Medicare for All would simply go unmet. Now this also lowers projected costs, but obviously, it is bad news for patients who would be denied care.

It is reasonable to guess that a re-estimate of my realistic payment scenario might drop its 10-year cost from roughly $39 trillion to about $31 trillion. Now this would still be more than we could finance by doubling all projected income taxes, and it would still mean a net increase in national health costs.

One last important point: CBO projects lower administrative costs than mine and most other studies do. For example, they project that 80 percent of nurses' current administrative tasks would be eliminated by Medicare for All and that all the time saved would be reallocated to providing care.

Now the implications of these assumptions are very significant. If we were a little bit less optimistic about the administrative time saved, we would see a much bigger problem with denial of care. For example, if Medicare for All reduced nurses' administrative tasks by 40 percent, which is still quite optimistic, then if we paid providers at Medicare rates, nearly all of the new demand for hospital and physician services under Medicare for All, 97 percent of it, would go unmet.

Now lawmakers would be very unlikely to tolerate that outcome and would probably address it by paying providers more. So that is an additional reason why the actual costs of Medicare for All would probably be much higher than in these various studies' lower-cost projection scenarios.

I hope this information is useful. I thank the Committee again for the opportunity to discuss these important implications of Medicare for All.

[The prepared statement of Mr. Blahous appears on page 131.]

Chairman SANDERS. Dr. Blahous, thanks very much for your testimony.

Okay. I think we begin the questions right now. Let me start off with one very simple question and kind of a "yes" or "no" answer maybe for all of our panelists. Is health care a human right to which all Americans are entitled regardless of their income, Dr. Gaffney.

Dr. GAFFNEY. It absolutely could be.

Chairman SANDERS. Ms. Castillo.

Ms. CASTILLO. Yes.

Chairman SANDERS. Dr. El-Sayed.

Dr. EL-SAYED. Yes, sir.

Chairman SANDERS. Ms. Turner.

Ms. TURNER. Yes, sir, but also the people who are providing that care have an equal right to compensation.

Chairman SANDERS. Dr. Blahous.

Mr. BLAHOUS. I believe everyone is entitled to receive care. It is a necessity.

Chairman SANDERS. Okay. Thank you. Let me start off with a question for Dr. Gaffney. During the pandemic, we saw the absurdity of tying health care to employer-based coverage. Some 27 million people lost their jobs, and when they lost their jobs they lost their health care. In your view, should health care be something that all people are entitled to because they are human beings or should it be, in most cases, attached to their employment?

And when it is attached to their employment, it may well be: I have a good job, and I have great health care coverage. He does not have a good job; his coverage is minimal.

Is that system making sense to you as a physician?

Dr. GAFFNEY. Well, it does not make sense either medically or financially. For one thing, you constantly hear the critique of Medicare for All that it would take away people's private health insurance. As you said, people are losing private health insurance all the time because they got fired, they got laid off, they turned 65 and gained access to Medicare. So it does not make sense.

Furthermore, that sort of churn, as we call it, the constant shifting in and out of medical plans, health care plans, has really adverse consequences for patient care. You can imagine if you have complex medical needs, having to see a number of doctors, having to go to particular hospitals. All of a sudden, your health care plan changes. Now you need to see all new professionals, assuming you still have a new plan. You may be entirely uninsured and unable to see anyone at all.

So it does not make sense, no.

Chairman SANDERS. All right. Let me to go to Ms. Castillo. If we had already adopted Medicare for All before the pandemic, how would things have been different for front-line nurses and their patients? Would our hospitals have been better prepared to protect patients and employees?

Ms. CASTILLO. You know, if—and actually just to relate to the previous questions, imagine, you know, all those folks that lost their jobs in the midst of a deadly pandemic. So if we had Medicare for All before this pandemic started, hospitals would have been better prepared to respond. There would have been a system in place. For years, hospital corporations have used and relied on this just-in-time-staffing and for supplies. And in most of the country, hospitals did not even hire enough nurses for regular patient care, day to day, and that is pre-pandemic. Or, they did not have enough supplies for a public health emergency.

Through the global budgeting payment mechanism that is in your bill, Senator, hospitals would be required to have the minimum—safe minimum nurse staffing levels, and they would be required to have a one-year supply of the critical PPE and all the other medical supplies that were needed. So this—our pandemic response would have been much safer for patients and for health care workers if we had a Medicare for All system.

Chairman SANDERS. Thank you. Dr. El-Sayed, my conservative friends are supposed to worry about how much money we spend, right? That is what being a conservative is about. And I share some of that. You know, I do not like to spend money. I was kind of a cheapskate mayor and try to continue to do that.

So I just do not understand why my Republican friends are not jumping up and down and saying, Bernie, we are with you. It is a little bit crazy that we are spending twice as much per capita on health care as the people of other nations.

And we can argue. You know, I hear, we all hear the scare tactics from Canada or U.K. and so forth, but I would remind my Republican friends that conservative governments have been in power in Canada, in the U.K., here in the U.K. right now, and they would not for a second try to get rid of their national health care system because it is so popular.

But my question, Dr. El-Sayed, is tell us why is it in fact that we are spending over $12,000 a year on health care, twice as much as our Canadian friends, the French, British, countries all over the world, while we live shorter lives and in many cases our health care outcomes are not as good? How does that happen?

Dr. EL-SAYED. Well, we talked a little bit about the tomato scenario and the fact that, you know, in our system nobody has an incentive to save money. If you are a provider, your incentive is to bill more because you make more. And if you are an insurer, your incentive is to grow your piece of the pie, that 20 percent that you get to keep, so you have no incentive to keep it down either. And they keep pushing the bill back onto the rest of us.

But because we have so many payers and so many providers, 700 health insurers in our society——

Chairman SANDERS. How many health insurance companies?

Dr. EL-SAYED. Right around 700.

Chairman SANDERS. Okay.

Dr. EL-SAYED. No one of them has the power to actually rein down the prices even if they wanted to. And on top of that, you have to have a whole bunch of crosstalk, a whole bunch of billers, whether it is on the provider side or the payer side, to be able to make these financial transactions happen. That is overhead in the system that the public pays for.

Chairman SANDERS. All right. Let me ask you this. Does anybody have any idea—we have talked about not having enough doctors and nurses, et cetera. How many people do we have in the system who do nothing else but bill us and drive us crazy that we are late on our bills? Does anyone know that number?

Dr. EL-SAYED. I do not know if Adam has an estimate.

Chairman SANDERS. Do you know, Dr. Gaffney?

Dr. GAFFNEY. I do not have the personnel number, but I do have the overall expenditures of what we spend on administration, and that is one-third of every health care dollar in the United States to administration, double the proportion of Canada.

Chairman SANDERS. So we are spending hundreds of billions of dollars on folks who bill us and drive us crazy but do not provide any health care to us.

Dr. EL-SAYED. That is right.

Chairman SANDERS.

Dr. El-Sayed Dr. EL-SAYED. And so that is one piece of the deep inefficiency in our system.

The other piece is that we just do not invest in the means of prevention almost at all. I told you one of my jobs was to rebuild a health department in America's poorest city. We have fundamentally disinvested in the means of keeping people healthy over the long term, the kinds of things that save money over the long term, in large part because nobody has an incentive to do that. Our system is predicated on a financial transaction after someone gets sick. So if you think about the political economy of it, there is very little incentive to prevent at all.

Chairman SANDERS. In terms of cost savings—and I say this to my conservative friends because I know that they are worried about expenditures—if we lower the cost of prescription drugs in this country to what other countries pay, anyone have any idea how much savings there would be in our system? Dr. Gaffney.

Dr. GAFFNEY. I mean, the CBO estimate was about a 30 percent reduction in drug prices. Other countries pay probably on average about half as much. You are talking about more than a hundred billion dollars, yeah.

Chairman SANDERS. Okay. Senator Graham.

Senator GRAHAM. One, I thoroughly enjoy the Committee. I really do.

Now to my—can I call my liberal friend, socialist friend? What would you like to be called?

Chairman SANDERS. Let us call us friends.

Senator GRAHAM. Okay, a friend. You can call me conservative, and I will not object. So to my friend from Vermont, you are right; we can lower costs and improve quality. The question is: How? Do you agree with that, Ms. Turner.

Ms. TURNER. Absolutely.

Senator GRAHAM. Okay. How do you get innovation in a system, Dr. El-Sayed? Did I say that right? I am sorry.

Dr. EL-SAYED. El-Sayed.

Senator GRAHAM. Yeah, count me in for innovation. Count me in for lowering costs. Count me in for improving quality. Makes all the sense in the world.

But let us talk about tomatoes. Who grows tomatoes in America? Anybody an expert on tomatoes? The government does not grow tomatoes. Tomatoes are grown by the private sector, and there is competition in the marketplace to grow tomatoes, and we do not do collective farming. And the last thing you want in the tomato world is to have the government take over the production of tomatoes and go to the Soviet-style collective farming where everybody eventually starves.

So let us keep tomatoes the way they are, and let us improve health care.

So the bottom line is I am looking for a system that will lower costs, improve quality, and I am begging you to have a vote on your bill. I am begging you. I am encouraging you. I am asking President Biden, in case you are watching, please call Senator Schumer and insist that we have a vote on Medicare for All on the floor of the United States Senate as soon as possible.

And we will not because Democratic colleagues know that it would go over like a lead balloon with the American public. Maybe I am wrong. Maybe you would win the day. But we are not going to fix this problem until we start voting on solutions and alternatives.

Dr. Blahous, is that right?

Mr. BLAHOUS. Yes.

Senator GRAHAM. If every hospital in America went to Medicare reimbursement rates for their primary—their only source of payment, how many hospitals would close?

Mr. BLAHOUS. Well, it is hard to say how many would close. The CMS Medicare actuaries have said that the vast majority of hospitals operate at a negative margin for their Medicare patients, their Medicare treatments.

Senator GRAHAM. So they make it up through the private pay system. Is that correct?

Mr. BLAHOUS. That is correct. And they put out a projection a couple of years ago saying that, you know, roughly 80 percent of facilities would be plunged into negative margins within a few years if all of their reimbursements were at Medicare rates.

Senator GRAHAM. Ms. Turner, what is your view of that? What if in America, all of a sudden, everybody in the hospital arena were reimbursed at Medicare payments, at the current rate, and that was it?

Ms. TURNER. Well, that is a good question to ask the Director of the Congressional Budget Office because the CBO has basically said that a great majority of physician practices and hospitals and clinics would simply not be able to keep their doors open. The private sector, employer-based health insurance in particular——

Senator GRAHAM. If you spent 15 minutes talking to the people in South Carolina in rural areas, their biggest nightmare is to be locked in at Medicare and Medicaid rates because they would have to close because you just cannot pay the costs. And if you start mandating patient-to-nurse ratios, that would increase your costs. So a lot of hospitals would go out of business. There has got to be a better way.

So the idea of having the government as the only source of revenue is, I think, a bad idea because you are no better than the government will allow you to be, and you would have to increase Medicare and Medicaid reimbursement rates or you would shut down a large number of hospitals in this country because they literally cannot operate without a private pay function.

Let me ask this question. Do you all agree that under Medicare for All private health insurance options go away for the American people? Everybody is nodding. Okay. I just want to get that baseline. The question: Is that a good idea or a bad idea?

So what I would like to do, Mr. Chairman, is vote on your proposal. That is—I like the Committee. We talk a lot. We do not vote on much of anything. Let us take your idea and vote on it because if we did that I think you would find out that Medicare for All would be the equivalent of collective farming over time, and I do not want to go down that road.

I would like to do more private sector involvement in health care, not less. I would like to have more competition, not less. I would like to get more innovation, not less.

And I can tell you one thing. The more you consolidate power in the health care arena under the government umbrella, you are going to get less of innovation, you are going to get more on costs, and you are going to get less in quality. You just have to wait longer. You have to ration care because eventually you break the budget to the point it cannot be repaired.

Medicare is in a very tenuous situation. Let us focus on saving Medicare as we have it today, and let us find ways to talk with each other about lowering that cost from $12,000 per patient to something lower and see if you can have an open mind to some of my ideas, and maybe I will have an open mind to some of your ideas. Might be able to fix this thing over time.

But let us start with this idea. We should be voting on this. We should not be talking about it any longer. Let us vote.

Chairman SANDERS. Well, if I could just briefly respond, before I give the mic to Senator Padilla, about voting.

Senator GRAHAM. Can I say one thing I forgot? Unanimous consent to submit letters and an op-ed to the record from FreedomWorks and Council for Citizens Against Government Waste, Americans for Prosperity, Americans for Tax Reform, and the Cato Institute, as well as an article from the Washington Post.

Chairman SANDERS. Without objection.

Senator GRAHAM. Thank you, Mr. Chairman.

[The submitted materials begin on page 167.]

Chairman SANDERS. Senator Graham, you may or may not know that I have been one of the major proponents in the Senate to have more votes. I like votes. I think it brings forth debate. But I think while we are at it, in addition—

Senator GRAHAM. You are the Chairman.

Chairman SANDERS. I am the Chairman of this Committee but not the Majority Leader. I think we should vote on whether we continue massive tax breaks for billionaires so that Jeff Bezos in a given year does not pay a nickel in taxes. I think we should vote on whether we end Citizens United so that billionaires are not able to buy elections as they are doing it right now as we speak. I think we should vote on whether or not Medicare should negotiate prescription drug prices so that we can lower the cost of prescription drugs in this country by half and a lot of other issues. You are talking to the wrong guy here. I like the idea of votes.

Senator GRAHAM. With all due respect, Mr. Chairman, you are the Chairman of the Committee. This is about Medicare for All. If you want to vote on all those things, fine. Let us start with your idea.

Chairman SANDERS. Let us vote on all of them. Good.

Senator GRAHAM. Well, let us start with Medicare for All. Have a vote next week.

Chairman SANDERS. All right. Okay, Senator Padilla.

Senator PADILLA. Thank you, Mr. Chairman, and I want to thank—I want to start by thanking you for your leadership on this issue and for holding this hearing. I am proud to support Medicare for All and look forward to working with you to move this forward.

And I also want to personally thank and recognize our front-line heroes. I see all these scrubs in the audience, and that always puts a smile on my face because I know that you all have been on the front lines in the more than two-year fight against COVID–19.

I also want to say that we have this terminology that came out of the COVID–19 pandemic: essential workers. Let us be clear. Your work was essential long before the pandemic but especially during the pandemic.

We have a few heroes today and some great witnesses, including one that happens to be a California nurse and my personal friend, Bonnie Castillo. Thank you for being here.

Now Ms. Castillo is Executive Director of the National Nurses United and a fierce advocate for equal health care for all, and I am proud that she is here representing California as well as the workforce.

As we have all seen, the COVID–19 pandemic has put a spotlight on what many people of color already knew, and that is the fact that the current health care system does not treat everyone equally. For far too long, communities of color, patients of color have faced discrimination in our health care system. And we can debate whether it is intentional or unintentional, but the facts and the data are clear. And that is one of the reasons why I believe Medicare for All is so important: because it will level the playing field for communities of color.

It is simply a fact that many communities of color living in the United States have less access to health care, have worse health outcomes, and are less insured than other communities, but a significant equalizer has been Medicare. Research has shown that there are substantial reductions in racial disparities and access to care and self-reported health when people reach 65. Now this is striking and should be kept top of mind when we consider this bill. Health care should not be determined by your ZIP Code, and no one should go bankrupt because they cannot afford growing medical expenses.

So I share your conviction, Mr. Chairman. It is frankly unacceptable that as the wealthiest nation in the world we do not guarantee health care for all. Health care is a human right. I am looking forward to taking action here.

Now turning to my questions in the couple minutes I have left, the first is to Ms. Castillo. You know, cost is often cited as a reason to oppose Medicare for All for those who do not believe yet. Yet. But the real question I have is: Cost for whom?

Now I have heard story after story from families across California about how a single illness can be financially crippling for an individual or a family. Families often go into massive debt or even bankruptcy to cover a loved one's health care costs, but it does not have to be this way.

Health care should not be something only the wealthy can afford. No one should go into debt because of rising health care costs or an illness. One example that we are legislating separately, no one should have to ration their insulin or put off critical surgeries because of the price tag.

So with that as the backdrop, Ms. Castillo, as one of the leaders of the largest health care worker unions in the nation, how would Medicare for All help alleviate the racial and income disparities that you see on the ground?

Ms. CASTILLO. Well, thank you and thank you for your leadership, Senator Padilla.

You know, for us as registered nurses, I think, you know, the key words are early, access, prevention, detection, and treatment, and that means removing those barriers. And those barriers are prohibitive, as it has been mentioned for the 30 million uninsured, but for the underinsured that cannot afford to use their insurance, not to mention all those who have lost their jobs and lost their insurance. Insurance does not equal care, and people need to be able to access that care.

And the care—and we on this panel—I mean, we have the expertise and the education to provide that care. That is what we—that is our job, and we do our job every day. You know, during the pandemic we did not run away from the disaster. We ran to it.

But we need the tools, and we need to remove the barriers to care for everyone. You know, COVID does not respect any kind of barrier to care. If it infects one of us, it can infect all of us. And so as providers, we need to—it is important that we address these.

I will also just—I would like to comment on, you know, for instance, hospitals are closing all the time. We, as a union, fight hospital closures because—and they are deciding to close because it is simply not profitable to operate a hospital in the lower-income communities, specifically communities of color, rural communities. And so if we have the global budgeting, where budgeting was based on need, human need, then we would be able to work to decrease those disparities that exist.

Senator PADILLA. Thank you. And, Mr. Chairman, I know my five minutes are up, but if I can, just one quick question. I promise to be brief.

The COVID–19 pandemic has also put enormous stress on the mental health of the American people. Cases of mental illness and substance abuse disorder have sharply risen during the pandemic, and more people are seeking care. Often cost and stigma pose barriers for people seeking mental health treatment. That just should not be the case.

Medicare for All, I believe, can also help level the playing field for those suffering from mental illness, not just physical illness. Dr. El-Sayed, how can Medicare for All help those suffering from mental illness and substance abuse disorder?

Dr. EL-SAYED. Yeah, Senator Padilla, I really appreciate the question. We are suffering a second pandemic of mental illness in this country, and unfortunately, our health care system has done this thing where we basically decapitate the head from the body. We say if it is in the head, whether it is mental health or it is dental health or it is vision or hearing, then we are going to pay for it separately. And one of the best pieces of Medicare for All and the Chairman's bill is that it reminds us that making Medicare whole is really the first step to extending Medicare for everybody. Covering these critical needs is critically important.

The second point here is that because we have such a different system of reimbursement for mental health we systematically lag in terms of capacity. My own spouse is a mental health provider. She is a psychiatrist, and every day she talks about caring for students who would not have care except for that they happen to be students at the university and get it through their university.

And so putting the head back on the body of health care and making health care whole through Medicare for All, ending the differentiation between the head and the body, I think, is critical, and Medicare for All would do just that.

Senator PADILLA. Thank you.

Thank you, Mr. Chairman.

Chairman SANDERS. Senator Johnson and Senator Padilla, would you mind chairing while I run down and vote?

Senator Johnson.

Senator JOHNSON. Thank you, Mr. Chairman. You are going to miss some good stuff here.

The first step in solving any problem is admitting you have one, and we all admit we have one, right? Then you have to promptly diagnose this, and I think that is where things break down pretty quick.

Seems like the Chairman says it is all about profitability of the industry, and he rattled off a bunch of numbers that totaled up $117 billion. Dr. Gaffney, you talked about lowering drug costs, $100 billion. We spend over $4,000 billion a year in health care.

Even if you get after-tax profitability of 10 percent, which I think is probably high if you take a look at the entire industry, that would be about $400 billion, and you would still end up with over $11,000 per person. So the profits, yeah, if you squeeze out all profitability, you could lower health care costs but not that substantially.

What astounds me is the people that promote Medicare for All, the faith in government you have. I mean, let us face it. The pandemic has exposed an awful lot. Our response to the pandemic was largely driven by government agencies. Agencies, I would say, have been corrupted and captured by big pharma.

You know, there is not one therapy, there is not one vaccine that is generic that has been recommended. Everything is either the novel, patentable drugs, starting at about 500 bucks for PAXLOVID, $700 for molnupiravir, $3,500 for remdesivir. Okay? But this cornucopia of widely available generic drugs was ignored.

And how many times have we talked about early treatment? Get in there early. And yet, National Institutes of Health (NIH) guidelines today: Get tested and do nothing. Go home, afraid.

We not only ignored our agencies, the government not only ignored early treatment, they sabotaged it.

And I do not see how anybody can take a look at our response to—the government response to this pandemic—a million people dead, the human toll and the economic devastation of these ill-advised, widespread shutdowns, shutdowns that did not work, what we have done to our children, how anybody could say that was a success. It has been a miserable failure.

So why in the world would anybody want to put government more in charge of health care?

Let us properly diagnose the problem by just looking at history. Okay? 1940: 80 cents of every dollar was paid for by the consumer. We had consumerism in health care.

What has happened since then is now you got government paying for 55 percent, insurance paying for 35 percent, and the consumer only pays for a dime out of every dollar spent in health care.

Now I come from the private sector. I would have loved to have been a monopolist, but because I was not my prices were a lot lower, my quality was a lot higher, as was my customer service. That is what the free market provides: the lowest possible cost, the best possible level of quality and customer service.

We need to introduce consumerism. We have got to reintroduce the discipline of a free marketplace. Having government take it over will not do that.

Ms. Turner, I want to ask a question. One of the reasons people do like Medicare is because it is heavily subsidized, not just by government payments but by the private sector, correct? The cost sharing makes our hospital systems actually work because oftentimes, certainly with Medicaid and Medicare, they are not reimbursed even for their costs. So talk about that cost sharing and how that would all go away and all of a sudden government care for all would not look that pretty.

Ms. TURNER. Private health coverage, primarily through employers but also through private plans, pay higher rates in order to get hospital and, physician care for their members, and those higher payment rates are what allow hospitals and physician practices to actually keep their doors open.

I had a physician friend in Florida who said that he wanted to take Medicaid patients, and he did, and he had a patient needing treatment for complicated lung problems. He said, ordinarily, private health insurance would pay him $750 for this course of care. When he got his check from Medicaid, the check was for 6 cents. He said, "How many Medicaid patients can I afford to see when I get those kinds of reimbursement levels?"

Senator JOHNSON. I think another issue is, as I have talked to hospitals and people coming in during the pandemic, and now that those rules that were suspended—you know, things like telemedicine, which makes sense, that is a market-driven innovation, right? All of a sudden, you will not be able to practice telemedicine.

So all the innovations that we were able to implement during the pandemic to relieve the health care system of the bureaucratic rules—I mean, again, those of you pushing Medicare for All, what makes you think there will be lower bureaucracy with governmentrun health care? There will be greater bureaucracy, greater rules, more regulations, less innovation, and higher costs. Would you agree with that, Ms. Turner?

Ms. TURNER. And less, even less, transparency. I agree with Dr. El-Sayed that we need to have much more transparency. Four trillion—400,000 billion dollars—are sloshing through our health care system, and so few people feel they have any control over that spending and that they can make their own decisions about how to get the best care at the lowest prices from quality providers. That is what we all need.

Senator JOHNSON. I have 37 oversight letters into the agencies, covering a wide range of subjects in terms of this mismanagement of the pandemic. I have gotten almost zero responses because the health agencies have not been honest; they have not been transparent.

And so, again, to think government is going to be more transparent and is going to be more efficient, that health care is going to—you know, all of a sudden, everything is going to be coming up roses I think is complete misdiagnosis of what a possible solution might be.

Thank you, Mr. Chairman.

Senator PADILLA [presiding]. Thank you.

Senator Scott.

Senator SCOTT. I want to thank everybody for being here today. You know, I grew up in a country where a kid like me growing up in public housing, born to a single mom, could go out and try anything because it was a capitalist system that created opportunities for us. We had to get a good education. You had to work hard. I mean, I started working at seven. My family, we all worked hard, and we were able to achieve the dream.

Right now, if you are—look at what is going on in this country right now. Let us look at where the economy is right now. Today, PPI numbers came out, 11 percent. The inflation number is up, over 8 percent. I look at our GDP; it is negative. Think about it. In the United States of America, you cannot get baby formula if you are a young mom. I have talked to young moms that had to drive around all weekend last week trying to get baby formula for their kids. So we have a supply chain crisis. We got interest rates going up. We got the stock market going down.

So the socialist agenda that the Democrats are pushing, it is not working. You cannot spend money you do not have. We have $30 trillion in debt. Medicare is going bankrupt. Social Security is going bankrupt. We are not prefunding any programs in this country. There was a bill that got passed that put Medicare actually in a worse position. We removed retiree benefits from the Postal Service to Medicare when we know Medicare is not funded.

So now we are talking about Medicare for All, which I think it ought to be called Medicare for None. The bill that we are talking about today will abolish the current Medicare—well, here is what we are talking about. Abolish the current Medicare program and make private insurance illegal. Think about that. The goal is to make private insurance illegal.

They do not want to wildly expand government. They want to make it illegal to have your private health insurance. We ought to just all read the bill and understand exactly what is happening.

So the horrible proposal will ruin the Medicare program because right now, as we know, it is not funded, right, and we are running trillion-plus-dollar deficits. The Biden agenda takes our debt to $45 trillion. Tell me how we are going to pay the interest expense on what we already have.

It is going to throw 150 million—150 million—people off the private insurance program. Over 24 million people have Medicare Advantage programs, which they like because they get additional benefits. That is gone.

According to independent estimates, it will cost upwards of $30 trillion over the next 10 years. I do not know where the money is coming from.

So, one, it makes private insurance illegal. It lets government decide what procedures you get, when, and when you get to have them, which ones are covered, which ones you get to have. You want the government to make these choices for you.

It pays doctors less, health care workers significantly less. We already have a worker shortage. You pay people less. Guess what? You are going to get fewer of them.

If you care about health care for this country, it does not make any sense at all.

So, Ms. Turner, advocates of Medicare for All keep using U.K. and Canada as examples of great socialized health care. Can you talk about the problems of wait times in the U.K. or Canada and how it impacts, you know, how it impacts somebody's individual health?

Ms. TURNER. Well, and as you say, because of a resource shortage, they do; people wind up with long waiting times. The Fraser Institute in Canada has been studying wait times for 30 years. When they started, the average wait time from seeing a practitioner to getting referred to a specialist and getting your treatment was about nine weeks. It is now 26 weeks, half a year, and in some areas it is a year.

In the U.K., the U.K. has so many people on waiting lists for care that the U.K. Health Secretary says if you spend more than 18 months on the waiting list then you can go to a private payer in order to get care.

But it is not just there. Any place where you see resource constraints—and that is absolutely what will have to happen with this, with a government-run health care system. In California, health officials just announced that fines for $55 million—Mr. Padilla's home State. The Los Angeles County Government. For low-income residents' treatment plan, they found that people were having to wait an average of 90 days, which is 6 times longer than the 15-day limit.

So it happens anywhere that you have global budgets and resource constraints and are not able to pay enough people and not have enough facilities to provide the care. Universal coverage does not mean universal care.

Senator SCOTT. Oh, you get it. So take the U.K. If you are rich, do you have to go through the U.K. system? No. There is a separate system for the rich. They can go to private hospitals.

So if you are poor, you have to wait, if you get the care in time to stay alive. But if you are rich, you can either go to the U.K. or you can actually come to the United States, which like a lot of Canadians come to the United States.

So I mean, what this will do is if you want care for everybody, this will mean you will get care, way less care, for people and you will wait longer for your care.

Thank you.

Senator PADILLA. Thank you, Senator Scott. Welcome back, Chairman Sanders.

Chairman SANDERS [presiding]. My apologies for having to run. It is kind of a party line vote and it is a 50/50 Senate so every vote matters.

Let me just take the opportunity to ask a couple more questions.

Under an employer-based health care system, does anybody have a guess as to how many people are staying at their jobs today not because they enjoy their jobs or feel productive in their jobs, but because they see work right now as the only way they can get decent health care coverage? Any thoughts on that? I see some hands in the audience. Dr. El-Sayed, is that something you have thought about?

Dr. EL-SAYED. Absolutely something I have thought about. It is hard to get an estimate of that, simply because job markets are in such flux and people's preferences are complex.

Although, I think about the impact—and, frankly, the CBO has thought about these things, too—the impact on the economy. Our Republican colleagues love to talk about what is good for the economy. You think about the impact on the economy, all the businesses that go unbuilt, all of the new careers that go unestablished because people are worried about what might happen if they leave their job and lose their health insurance.

On top of that, small businesses, almost every single small business owner you talk to, and you ask them what are their biggest challenges? They will rate, according to survey after survey, health insurance for their employees as one of the worst.

And so it is hard to pitch a counterfactual in terms of numbers, but it is important for us to ask what would be the effect if you did not have to worry about that, doing that entrepreneurial thing, that thing that America is supposed to be known for, that that would mean you and your family losing the health insurance in the process.

Chairman SANDERS. Anybody else want to respond to that? Ms. Turner?

Ms. TURNER. Senator, employers try so hard and they get so beat up on because they really are trying hard to find good health insurance that is as affordable as possible for their employees. And actually, a study by the Heritage Foundation found that 5.7 million more people had coverage in December of 2020, a year into the pandemic, than did in 2019. So employers tried very hard to keep their employees on the payroll as much as they could.

Many people also enrolled in coverage through the Affordable Care Act (ACA). So there are safety nets.

Chairman SANDERS. No, I do not think that it is a question of beating—nobody here, I do not think, is beating up on small business. I think the point that Dr. El-Sayed was making—and I remember this, as being a mayor. We had the same problem as any small business. We had to search for the best, most cost-effective health insurance. We spent an enormous amount of time and money trying to figure it out.

And what I think is not well known is what Medicare For All will do is take that burden off of small business because all of their employees will have quality health care and they can maybe go about their business of doing what they do, rather than spending so much time and energy on worrying about having to get affordable health care.

Dr. EL-SAYED. If I may, Mr. Chairman, far from beating up on small business owners, the question I keep asking is what would make it easier to be a small business owner? And I think taking off the mental space that goes into asking how do I make sure that my employees are covered today, would make it far easier to focus on whatever the business is.

But it is not just small business. It is also big business. I am from Metro Detroit where, during the Great Recession, the automotive bailout was the single most important question on everybody's mind. And one of the big questions was how do we pay for private health insurance not just for employees but for retirees at GM? And what ended up happening is a number of the jobs that would have stayed in the United States actually got off-shored to Canada because folks could get their health insurance paid for. It was not a line item off the top of every employee that you had to employ.

So these questions are dogging businesses, whether large or small, in this country. And if we are serious about investing in our economy, taking the overhead of having to think about health care for every single employee you have off the top of business decisions, I think would be pro-growth and pro-economic empowerment in this country.

Chairman SANDERS. Let me ask another question.

We do not talk about, you know, generally speaking, the more important the issue is, the less we talk about it. In our Nation, our life expectancy is shorter than most other industrialized countries. But even within our Nation, there is a huge disparity in life expectancy.

I read an article somewhere that in Southern West Virginia, which is five hours away by car from Fairfax, Virginia. Southern West Virginia very poor, Fairfax rather wealthy. Life expectancy for males I think was something like 15 years different. And right here in Washington, D.C., depending on which part of the city you live in, the life expectancy will be significant.

Why is that? Some thoughts? Dr. Gaffney?

Dr. GAFFNEY. Well, obviously health is more than a reflection of medical care alone. And I think that speaks to the gross inequality in our society that affects people in terms of their housing, in terms of their exposure to COVID–19, for that matter, in terms of occupational safety, in terms of exposure to pollution.

But I do think medical care matters. It matters a great deal in these inequalities. And we know that because researchers—you can look at life expectancy but you can also look at something called treatable mortality, which is deaths that we think are preventable through medical care.

And if you compare, for instance, a country like Canada to the United States in its treatable mortality, we have about 50% higher treatable mortality than Canada.

So the fact of the matter is that we need to fix a lot in our society to rectify the kinds of gross inequalities you are describing. But a big part of that is fixing our medical care system to make it accessible, to make it universal, and to make sure that people can have access to the best care regardless of their race, ethnicity, or income.

Dr. EL-SAYED. If I can build on what Dr. Gaffney shared, if you think about the way we calculate life expectancy, you think about the contribution of every life, on average. The lives that contribute the most to reducing our life expectancy are the lives that are lost the earliest. Those are the babies that pass. And you think about keeping a baby alive, that is a real complex question because you are talking about two lives. You are talking about the life of the person that bore that baby and you are talking about the life of that baby theirselves.

I was health director in the City of Detroit. We had one of the highest infant mortality rates in the entire country. We were also the poorest city in America. Those two things are not unrelated.

Chairman SANDERS. If I recall, those infant mortality rates are not dissimilar from some really poor Third World countries; is that correct?

Dr. EL-SAYED. Across our country, our infant mortality is not dissimilar from very poor lower-income countries. But in Detroit, in particular, yes. My family comes from Egypt. I had a grandmother who lost two infants before the age of one, from among eight to whom she gave birth. She had a personal infant mortality rate of 25 percent.

And the crazy thing is that I would go to Egypt when I was a kid, I would go 15 hours. I could go 15 minutes from where I grew up in Detroit and go to a place where the infant mortality rate was quite similar to where it was in Egypt.

And so, if we are serious about investing, and I know my colleagues, my conservative colleagues here care a lot about the lives of children they say. And if we are serious about that, then what we would make sure is that every single mother had health insurance regardless of her circumstances so that she could access prenatal care services. That every single baby would have the basic services it needed should it fall ill.

But too often, in cities like Detroit, because we had hospitals go from being public hospitals to being nonprofits to being, finally, forprofits where they are constantly asking how can I skimp a dollar out of Medicaid because it is such a low-income community, too many people in effect get locked out because of the churn of trying to stay on Medicaid at that moment where they are trying to safely bear a child and bring it to life.

So if we are serious about the well-being of infants, if we are serious about our life expectancy, then we ought to be serious about making sure that that transition into life is done with the full investment in health care for that mother and that baby.

Chairman SANDERS. I see Senator Braun is here. Senator Braun.

Senator BRAUN. Thank you, Chairman Sanders, for letting me be able to speak. I had a lot of stuff going on.

I am glad we convened this because I come from Indiana, viewed health care as the most important benefit for my own employees, ran a company for 37 years. And probably the proudest thing I did was covered pre-existing conditions and no caps on coverage, and turned my employees into health care consumers along the way.

What Senator Sanders is talking about in Medicare For All is because we have got a broken health care industry. I have fought with it in trying to get good coverage for my own employees. There is two things in life, generally, when you are spending money. You have to aspire to what you know is a need and then do it in a way that is affordable.

Ironically, all other countries have not found a way to get the markets to work. And that is why you have them doing something that is either a two-tiered system or what Senator Sanders is talking about.

I personally think that we could cascade into that. And I have talked to a lot of CEOs, most of whom never took it as seriously as I did, brought it into the C-suite. And I will tell you what we accomplished. We cut costs by close to 50 percent. You would normally think well, that means people were not getting covered. No, they were getting covered. And along with doing it, I removed the coinsurance part of insurance, to where outside of my employees' deductible, they are never going to go broke because they get sick or have a bad accident. That should be the attitude of every company.

When you are not taking care of things in the private sector, you are going to look to government to do it. Whether that is the eventual thing that happens here remains to be seen.

I would love to see the health care industry actually reform itself, embrace transparency, embrace competition, embrace educating a health care consumer and see if you can take costs out of the system before government ends up paying for it or to where you have got a broken health insurance system increasingly dominated by huge corporations that even when you are a decent sized company like mine you cannot even wrestle with them.

So it is either going to be a solution that the problem generators fix by embracing competition, embracing transparency, knowing that health care, along with education, are the two most important things for families. Ironically, they are the two most expensive things in our system. And when that happens, government gets more involved.

I think that we need to converge from two different directions. I think Medicare For All will win the day and it is a solution that most other countries had to go to some version of. But I think we have got the possibility of keeping the unique best things about our health care system. But it is going to be totally up to the big hospital corporations, big health insurance, even practitioners to embrace transparency, give health care consumers choice.

And pharma, which gets a lot of the blame, they deserve it. They do an excellent job on the R&D and then they come up with some monstrosity middle man that sucks out billions and billions of dollars, that keep insulin high. So it is broken in almost every facet.

There is entrepreneurialism happening. In Indiana, a clinic was started by some anesthesiologists. It cuts the red tape of government and big corporations. Give this example, a gall bladder operation. In our State, the negotiated rate is $18,000. The surgeon, whoever is doing the work, gets paid a very, very small amount of it. If you are uninsured but you can afford it, it is going to cost you $32,000. They are going to do it for $8,000.

That is the kind of restructuring we need and it needs to be the providers of health care. Insurance should almost be out of the question. The pool for insurance would be all Americans. And it ought to be easy like that because it is the number one most important thing, especially as you age. And sadly, too, we have got work to do here within our own government. The programs that depend, the elderly and especially those that cannot afford insurance, Medicare and Medicaid, are going the wrong direction, not sustainably.

I really do not have a question because I have been working on this so long. I just want to let you know that you can have two different points of view but we ought to at least agree on the problem, that health care as we know it is not accessible to enough people, it sends too many people to bankruptcy court. And if the people that run these big entities now do not do something about it, they should not have anyone to complain to because government will be the solution.

I think if we did do some legislation that forced transparency, competition, they say they are free market. Let us do it. It would make government-provided health care less expensive. And maybe we could take it from 20 percent of our GDP down to 12 and have our cake and eat it, too.

The way it looks, they are so intransigent, I have been speaking about it, I do not know if they will accept changing themselves. That would be a better solution and we ought to probably try to work on a few ways to do that, as well.

Thanks for listening.

Chairman SANDERS. Senator Braun, thanks very much.

Let me just thank the panel. We have kept you here for a very long time. But I appreciate all of the work that all of our panelists are doing. As Senator Braun indicated, there is probably no issue more important to the American people than health care.

So thank you all very much.

Our next panelist is going to be the Director of the Congressional Budget Office, Director Phil Swagel. Thank you.

Dr. Swagel is going to be with us virtually. He is the Director of the Congressional Budget Office, a position he has held since 2019. Previously, he was a Professor at the University of Maryland School of Public Policy and a Visiting Scholar at the American Enterprise Institute and the Milken Institute.

Dr. Swagel has served as Assistant Secretary for Economic Policy at the Treasury Department and as Chief of Staff and Senior Economist at the White House Council of Economic Advisors.

Dr. Swagel, thanks very much for being with us.

Statement of the Honorable Phillip Swagel, Ph.D., Director, Congressional Budget Office; Accompanied by Chapin White, Ph.D., Director of Health Analysis, Congressional Budget Office; and Jeffrey R. Kling, Ph.D., Research Director, Congressional Budget Office

Mr. SWAGEL. Thank you, Chairman Sanders.

Chairman Sanders, Ranking Member Graham, and members of the Committee, thank you for inviting CBO to testify about single payer health care systems based on the Medicare Fee-For-Service program.

Now I am testifying by video because I have a little time yet in isolation. I am fine and I look forward to emerging.

I am joined today by my colleagues Chapin White and Jeff Kling and I am grateful to Chairman Sanders and to your Committee staff for arranging this remote testimony.

CBO has analyzed five options illustrating the effects of differences in providers' payment rates, patients' cost sharing, and the system's coverage of long-term services and supports.

The system proposed by Chairman Sanders in S. 1129, the Medicare For All Act of 2019, is like these five options in some ways and different in some others. We have not analyzed S. 1129 in particular.

CBO found the following effects relative to what would occur under current law:

Federal subsidies for health care in 2030 would be significantly larger, with the increases in subsidies ranging from $1.5 trillion to $3.0 trillion, depending on the option.

National health expenditures would change by amounts ranging from a decrease of $0.7 trillion to an increase of $0.3 trillion, again depending on the system's design features. The most important factors tending to reduce national health expenditures are lower payment rates for providers and reductions in payers' administrative spending.

Conversely, the most important factor tending to increase expenditures is increased use of care. And that is especially if longterm services and supports are a covered benefit, as is the case in one of our five options. So health insurance coverage would increase, with virtually all U.S. residents covered by health insurance.

Total out-of-pocket costs would also be lower.

The supply of health care would increase because of fewer restrictions on utilization, less money and time spent by providers on administration, and providers' responses to increased demand for care. The amount of care used would rise, and in that sense, overall access to care would be greater in the single-payer systems we analyzed.

The increase in demand for health care would exceed the increase in supply, in our analysis, resulting in greater unmet demand than under current law. Though higher overall access to care and increased unmet demand would occur simultaneously because people would use more care and would have used even more had it been supplied. The increase in unmet demand for care would correspond to increased congestion in the health care system. That would mean more delays and forgone care.

Turning to the economic effects, I will describe the outcomes under the five options that CBO analyzed if the system was financed by either a payroll tax or an income tax. And the estimates on those economic effects depend on the type of tax used for financing.

So our projections for the effects relative to what would occur under current law are as follows:

Gross domestic product (GDP) would be approximately 1 percent to 10 percent lower by 2030, and aggregate nonhealth consumption per capita would change by amounts ranging from an increase of 3 percent to a decline of 7 percent.

Lifetime nonhealth consumption would rise among lower-income households and decline among higher income households, and the number of lifetime hours people choose to work would be lower for most households across the income distribution.

The net reductions in GDP occur primarily because of the effects of the increased taxes on labor and capital income. If the system was financed by other types of taxes, by government borrowing or reductions in other types of government spending, the net effect on the economy and, of course, the distributional implications would be different.

In addition to the effects of the system's financing, other effects would occur, and these are other economic effects:

For example, workers would see increased taxable wages as employers would no longer provide health care benefits and would pass along the savings to employees, again through higher cash wages.

Higher longevity and labor productivity would result with the improvements in health care.

CBO has published a series of reports and working papers underlying the summary I have provided today in the written testimony.

My colleagues and I would be happy to talk about the details of that analysis and to answer any questions.

Thank you, very much.

[The prepared statement of Mr. Swagel appears on page 143.]

Chairman SANDERS. Dr. Swagel, thanks very much for being here and thanks very much for all of your work. We hope you get well quickly.

In December of 2020, CBO released a 209-page working paper on single-payer health care. CBO considered five options of moving to a single-payer system and found that in four out of the five scenarios, a single-payer program would save the American people between $42 billion and $743 billion a year, beginning in 2030.

The option that most resembles the Medicare for All bill that I introduced, which is option three, would save the health care system $650 billion a year beginning in 2030 while covering every man, woman, and child in our country with no premiums, no deductibles, and no copayments.

So Dr. Swagel, am I correct in stating that option three, which is the option most closest to what I have introduced, would save $650 billion a year beginning in 2030?

Mr. SWAGEL. Yes, sir, Mr. Chairman.

National health expenditure would go down by $650 billion in 2030 in option three. That has the lower payments to providers, lower cost-sharing, has long-term services and supports, what is in Medicaid but not beyond what is currently in Medicaid.

Chairman SANDERS. Speak a bit about the nature of administrative savings. How does a Medicare For All move closer to what other countries spend on administration? How much are we spending now compared to what we would spend under Medicare For All?

Mr. SWAGEL. I might ask my colleagues to jump in with additional details, as well.

So option three, which is the one that you had mentioned before, would result in a $414 billion reduction in administrative costs. There would be an additional $508 billion savings from changes in the payments to providers.

The administrative costs would be on two sides, both on the provider side that with a single payer system and essentially universal coverage, providers such as doctors and hospitals would spend much less time in a sense figuring out the sorts of things they figure out now with insurance companies. So that is on the provider side.

Chairman SANDERS. Let me ask you this, if I could. I am sorry to interrupt you, but I do not know if you have it on the top of your head right now. What does Medicare spend on administration compared to the private health insurance industry right now?

Mr. SWAGEL. Chapin, do you have that off the top of your head?

Mr. WHITE. Sure. In our analysis, the Medicare Fee-For-Service program had administrative expenses of about 2.3 percent, compared to private insurers, which were more in the range of around 12 percent.

Chairman SANDERS. And there are some, obviously, private insurance companies that spend a lot more than 12 percent. I hope everybody understands what we are talking about. The goal of health care is to put doctors and nurses and health care professionals into contact with patients. Administration is the buffer in between. That is shuffling papers.

And what we are talking about now, according to the CBO, on average the private sector spends about 12 percent and Medicare spends 2.3 percent. When you add that to the entire health care system, we are talking about hundreds of billions of dollars in savings.

Not to mention, Dr. Swagel, I do not know how you quantify this, but I think people throughout this country go crazy in trying to argue with insurance companies about what they are entitled to and why they were covered or why they were not covered.

Do we have any—are there economic analyses as to what that costs in terms of the amount of time the American people have to spend in arguing with insurance companies?

Mr. SWAGEL. We looked carefully at the experience and the literature in the U.S. and we looked at the experience of other countries, such as Canada, at those savings. And that is our lower administrative costs.

As you say, there would be immense savings, both from the provider side and for families. And that would result in more care, essentially the time freed up by those administrative savings would mean more time providing care to beneficiaries.

Chairman SANDERS. Let us talk a little bit about prescription drugs and the savings that would occur under Medicare for All. I believe, and the American people overwhelmingly believe that Medicare should negotiate prescription drug prices. The fact that we do not do that is the reason that we pay by far the highest prices in the world for our medicine right now.

Do you have estimates about how much Medicare For All would save through prescription drug negotiations with the industry?

Mr. SWAGEL. We do have lower savings from negotiated prescription drug costs. Again, I am sorry, I do not have that off the top of my head. Chapin, do you remember the——

Mr. WHITE. It depends on the specification. We had a higher payment scenario and a set of lower payment scenarios. In the lower payment scenarios, prices for prescription drugs would be about 27 percent lower than under current law. But the volume of prescription drugs used would be higher because of lower cost-sharing. And so the total spending on prescription drugs would go down under either of those scenarios.

Chairman SANDERS. Okay.

Now one of the reasons that Medicare For All is expensive is because it does what should be done, and that is make sure that every American has health care, provides quality care to all of our people.

How many more people—what, in your judgment, would be the impact in terms of accessibility to health care for a Medicare For All system? How many more people would be getting health care who today simply cannot afford to get that?

Mr. SWAGEL. Under the single-payer system, virtually all people residing in the U.S. would be covered. This would mean improved access to care and, importantly, be for both those who are uninsured under current law in 2030 and those who are insured. Even those who would be insured would have access to greater networks and lower out-of-pocket costs and therefore would use more health care.

And of course, for people who would be uninsured that would be even a bigger difference in terms of their access and lower costs.

Chairman SANDERS. Has the CBO done any work in taking a look at what the impact on the economy would be if all Americans were guaranteed health care and would no longer have to stay at a job that they did not want to stay in just because they get good health care at that job? Is that something you guys have looked at?

Mr. SWAGEL. It is and we put out a report going through the macroeconomic effects of the advent of the single-payer system, as well as the financing that I mentioned in the opening remarks. There would be many economic effects.

One I mentioned is increased cash wages as employers shifted the——

Chairman SANDERS. Let me stop you.

Mr. SWAGEL. Yes, please.

Chairman SANDERS. What that means right now that employers spend a whole lot of money providing health care to their employees. And without having to do that, there would be the opportunity to pay their workers higher wages; correct?

Mr. SWAGEL. That is exactly right. And there would be other effects, greater job mobility I think was mentioned.

Chairman SANDERS. Yes, talk about that job mobility. Do you have any guess—I know this is a hard question and nobody will have an exact answer. But I go all over the country and talk to people who say I am on my job not because I really want to be there. I want to do something different. My wife is ill and I have got good health care coverage right now. I cannot afford to leave that job.

Do you have any sense of how many people we are talking about who are at their job for health care? And what it would mean for the economy if they were able to do what they wanted to do and retain health care for the family?

Mr. SWAGEL. I will give an initial answer and then my colleagues can jump in. There is solid economic evidence for this, the phenomenon of job lock, and that reducing that would increase mobility, increase choices for families, but also increase entrepreneurship. That would increase productivity and economic growth.

I do not know the quantification offhand but maybe my colleagues do. But the evidence is pretty solid there.

Mr. WHITE. I think that CBO's assessment is that people do tend to stay in jobs longer and it is a phenomena called job lock. Our assessment is that that phenomenon is real but we have not quantified the number of people or the effects of increased job mobility on GDP or earnings.

Chairman SANDERS. But we are in agreement that if everybody in this country were guaranteed comprehensive health care, people would be freer to leave their jobs and do what they really wanted to do? Are we in agreement on that?

Mr. SWAGEL. That is right, and that would boost productivity and entrepreneurship.

Chairman SANDERS. Okay, that is about it for me and I do not see any of my colleagues here. So Dr. Swagel and your team, let me thank you all for the very important work you have done on this issue. Thanks very much.

Mr. SWAGEL. Thank you, Mr. Chairman.

Chairman SANDERS. Before we close, I would like to ask unanimous consent that a statement for the record by Eagan Kemp, a health care policy advocate at Public Citizen, be entered into the hearing record.

Without objection, that will happen.

[The submitted statement appears on page 157.]

Chairman SANDERS. Let me just again thank all of the witnesses here, as well as Dr. Swagel and his team, for being with us.

This debate is, in my view, maybe the most important debate facing our country. I just want to thank all of you for the work you are doing and have done and I know will do.

As information for all Senators, questions for the record are due by 12:00 noon tomorrow, with signed hard copies delivered to the Committee Clerk in Dirksen 624. Email copies will also be accepted. Under our rules, the witnesses will have seven days from receipt of our questions to respond to answers.

With no further business before the Committee, this hearing is adjourned.

[Whereupon, at 1:13 p.m., the Committee was adjourned.]

Additional Material Submitted for the Record

[Prepared statements, responses to written questions, and additional material submitted for the record follow:]

Hearing before the Senate Budget Committee, "Medicare for All: Protecting Health, Saving Lives, Saving Money," Thursday, May 12, 2022, Written Testimony of Adam Gaffney, MD MPH, Assistant Professor, Harvard Medical School

Thank you Chairman Sanders and all of the members of the Budget Committee for the opportunity to discuss the pressing issue of Medicare for All. In the testimony that follows, I outline the benefits of Medicare for All from a medical perspective, and then explore the salient economic issues raised by national health insurance reform.

Covering Everyone: A Medical and Moral Imperative

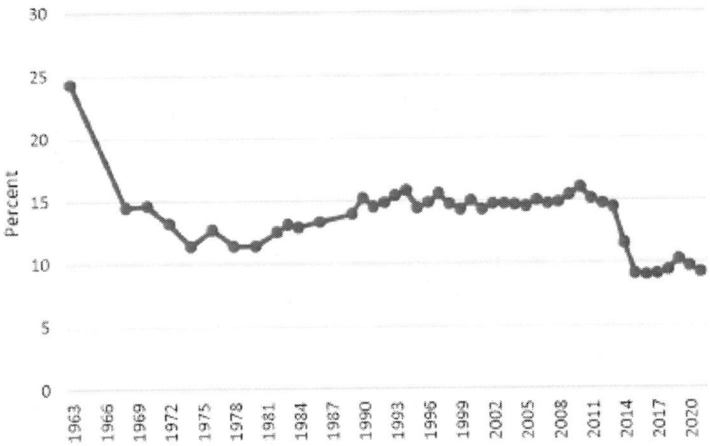

Source for data before 2010: Council of Economic Advisers, "Methodological Appendix: Methods Used to Construct a Consistent Historical Time Series of Health Insurance Coverage," 2014, Available from: https://obamawhitehouse.archives.gov/sites/default/files/docs/longtermhealthinsuranceseriesmethodologyfinal.p df.

Source for data from 2010 – 2021: Early Release Estimates from the National Health Interview Survey, multiple years. Available at: https://www.cdc.gov/nchs/data/nhis/earlyrelease.pdf. Note that there was a change in survey methodology in 2019.

Figure 1. Uninsured, 1963 – 2021.

Universal coverage is a medical and moral imperative, yet it remains an unfulfilled dream in the United States. As a result of passage of Medicare and Medicaid in 1965, and the Affordable Care Act in 2010, the uninsurance rate has fallen over the past six decades (Figure 1). Yet despite progress, 30 million Americans remained uninsured in 2021, or 9.2% of the US population.[1]

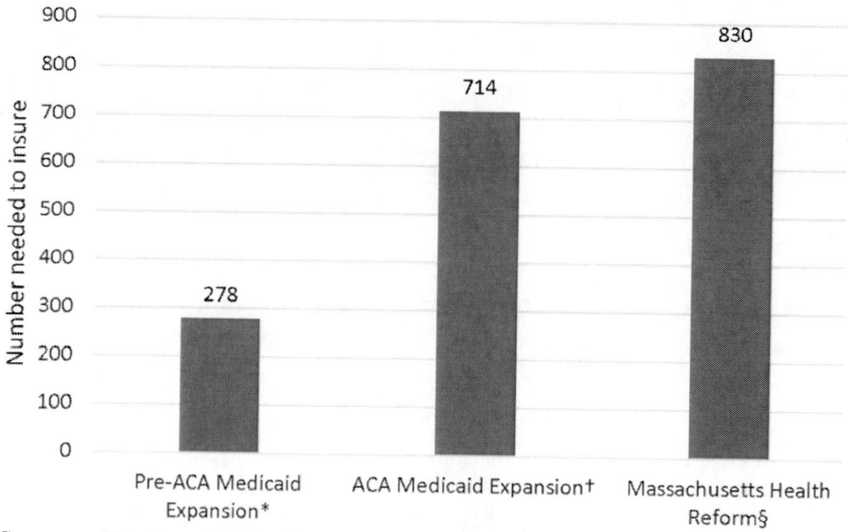

* Sommers BD. State Medicaid Expansions and Mortality, Revisited: A Cost-Benefit Analysis. American Journal of Health Economics 2017; 3: 392–421. Figure is midpoint of estimates provided by Sommers.

† Calculated from age 19-64 subgroup from: Miller S, Altekruse S, Johnson N, Wherry LR. Medicaid and Mortality: New Evidence from Linked Survey and Administrative Data. National Bureau of Economic Research, 2019 DOI:10.3386/w26081. Figure is calculated from Miller et al.'s finding for the age 19-64 subgroup.

§ Sommers BD, Long SK, Baicker K. Changes in mortality after Massachusetts health care reform: A quasiexperimental study. Annals of internal medicine 2014; 160: 585–93. Figure of 1/830 is estimate provided by Sommers et al.

Figure 2. Number needed to insure (NNI) to prevent one death annually in 4 Quasi-Experimental/Experimental Studies.

Uninsurance does not affect all groups equally: Black, Hispanic, and lower income individuals are uninsured at substantially higher rates than others.[1] The consequences for patients' health and wellbeing can be severe. Lack of health coverage leads to medical debt, financial strain, foregone

---

[1] Cohen RA. Health insurance coverage: Early release of estimates from the National Health Interview Survey, 2021. Published online 2021:24.

medical care, worse health, and premature death.[2,3,4,5,6,7] Quasi-experimental studies have demonstrated that for every 278 830 patients we leave uninsured, one dies annually (Figure 2). This translates into more than 30,000 deaths every year due to lack of health insurance, an entirely unnecessary toll of suffering and death.

By covering all US residents, Medicare for All would leave no one uninsured in the nation. It would, however, accomplish much more.

The Need to Improve Coverage for All

Alongside persistent uninsurance runs an even more common problem: inadequate quality of coverage, i.e., coverage with such high copays and deductibles, narrow networks of providers, and inadequate benefits that it leaves enrollees medically and financially vulnerable. In 2020, 26% of adults in the US went without a doctor visit in the past year due to costs, five-fold higher than the proportion of Canadians.[8] And about 1 in 5 Americans went without a needed prescription drug, four-fold higher than persons in United Kingdom and more than double the rate in Canada.[8]

The proportion of working age adults with medical insurance who are classified as underinsured due to high exposure to medical costs rose from 9%

---

[2] McWilliams JM, Meara E, Zaslavsky AM, Ayanian JZ. Use of health services by previously uninsured Medicare beneficiaries. *New England Journal of Medicine*. 2007;357(2):143-153. doi:10.1056/NEJMsa067712.

[3] Finkelstein A, Taubman S, Wright B, et al. The Oregon health insurance experiment: evidence from the first year. *Q J Econ*. 2012;127(3):1057-1106.

[4] Woolhandler S, Himmelstein DU. The relationship of health insurance and mortality: Is lack of insurance deadly? *Annals of internal medicine*. Published online 2017. doi:10.7326/M17-1403.

[5] Miller S, Altekruse S, Johnson N, Wherry LR. *Medicaid and Mortality: New Evidence from Linked Survey and Administrative Data*. National Bureau of Economic Research; 2019. doi:10.3386/w26081.

[6] Goldin J, Lurie IZ, McCubbin J. *Health Insurance and Mortality: Experimental Evidence from Taxpayer Outreach*. National Bureau of Economic Research; 2019. doi:10.3386/w26533.

[7] Sommers BD, Gawande AA, Baicker K. Health Insurance Coverage and Health — What the Recent Evidence Tells Us. *New England Journal of Medicine*. 2017;377(6):586-593. doi:10.1056/NEJMsb1706645.

[8] Doty MM, Tikkanen RS, FitzGerald M, Fields K, Williams RD. Income-Related Inequality In Affordability And Access To Primary Care In Eleven High-Income Countries. *Health Affairs*. 2020;40(1):113-120. doi:10.1377/hlthaff.2020.01566.

in 2003[9] to 21% in 2020, or 41.1 million Americans.[10] As with uninsurance, underinsurance has major adverse consequences for patients. The underinsured are more likely to be contacted by collection agencies for medical debt, and to go without needed prescription drugs and doctor visits.[10]

Numerous well-designed studies have conclusively tied cost-sharing to worse health. Copays and deductibles worsen blood pressure control, as demonstrated in one randomized trial.[11] They lead to more recurrent vascular events after heart attacks, as seen in another.[12] They cause serious delays in care for patients with cardiovascular[13] or ocular[14] complications of diabetes. Low socioeconomic status individuals with high-deductible health plans even avoid the ER when suffering from high-severity conditions.[15] Highdeductibles cause women with breast cancer to delay imaging, biopsies, and even chemotherapy.[16] When copays are high, seniors with multiple sclerosis and rheumatoid arthritis go without critically important drugs that keep their diseases at bay.[17] Cost-sharing causes asthmatics and those with chronic

---

9 Collins SR, Bhupal HK, Doty MM. *Health Insurance Coverage Eight Years After the ACA: Fewer Uninsured Americans and Shorter Coverage Gaps, But More Underinsured.* Commonwealth Fund; 2019. Accessed November 25, 2019. https://www.commonwealthfund.org/sites/default/files/2019-08/Collins_hlt_ins_coverage_8_years_after_ACA_2018_biennial_survey_sb_v2.pdf.

10 Collins S, Gunja MZ, Aboulafia G. U.S. Health Insurance Coverage in 2020: A Looming Crisis in Affordability — Findings from the Commonwealth Fund Biennial Health Insurance Survey, 2020. Published online 2020. Accessed November 22, 2020. https://www.commonwealthfund.org/sites/default/files/2020-08/Collins_looming_crisis_affordability_biennial_2020_sb.pdf.

11 Persaud N, Bedard M, Boozary AS, et al. Effect on Treatment Adherence of Distributing Essential Medicines at No Charge: The CLEAN Meds Randomized Clinical Trial. *JAMA Intern Med.* Published online October 7, 2019. doi:10.1001/jamainternmed.2019.4472.

12 Choudhry NK, Avorn J, Glynn RJ, et al. Full Coverage for Preventive Medications after Myocardial Infarction. *New England Journal of Medicine.* 2011;365(22):2088-2097. doi:10.1056/NEJMsa1107913.

13 Wharam JF, Lu CY, Zhang F, et al. High-Deductible Insurance and Delay in Care for the Macrovascular Complications of Diabetes. *Annals of Internal Medicine.* Published online November 20, 2018. doi:10.7326/M17-3365.

14 Wharam JF, Wallace J, Argetsinger S, et al. Diabetes Microvascular Disease Diagnosis and Treatment After High-Deductible Health Plan Enrollment. *Diabetes Care.* Published online September 29, 2021. doi:10.2337/dc21-0407.

15 Wharam JF, Zhang F, Landon BE, Soumerai SB, Ross-Degnan D. Low-socioeconomic-status enrollees in high-deductible plans reduced high-severity emergency care. *Health Affairs.* 2013;32(8):1398-1406. doi:10.1377/hlthaff.2012.1426.

16 Wharam JF, Zhang F, Wallace J, et al. Vulnerable And Less Vulnerable Women In High-Deductible Health Plans Experienced Delayed Breast Cancer Care. *Health Affairs.* 2019;38(3):408-415. doi:10.1377/hlthaff.2018.05026.

17 Li P, Hu T, Yu X, et al. Impact of Cost-Sharing Increases on Continuity of Specialty Drug Use: A Quasi-Experimental Study. *Health Services Research.* 2017;53(S1):2735-2757. doi:10.1111/14756773.12744.

obstructive pulmonary disease (COPD) to avoid taking their inhalers[18] — likely driving worse disease control and an increase in hospitalizations.[19,20] A recent quasi-experimental study found that even relatively low copays and deductibles led seniors to forgo needed medications, causing a 32.7% increase in mortality.[21]

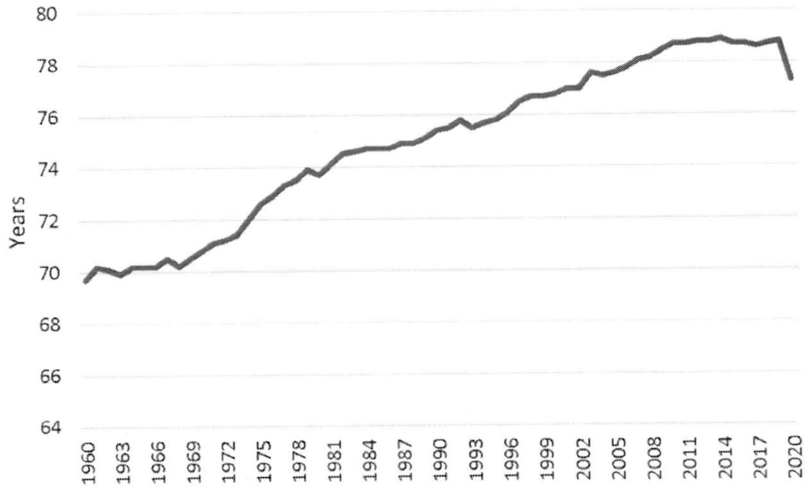

Source of data:

1960-2018: NCHS Data Visualization Gallery Mortality Trends in the United States. 2020. https://www.cdc.gov/nchs/data-visualization/mortality-trends/index.htm.

2019-2020: Arias E, Betzaida T-V, Ahmad F, Kochanek K. Provisional Life Expectancy Estimates for 2020. National Center for Health Statistics (U.S.); 2021. Available from: https://stacks.cdc.gov/view/cdc/107201. Note 2020 data is provisional.

Figure 3. Life Expectancy at Birth in the United States, 1960-2020.*

---

[18] Castaldi PJ, Rogers WH, Safran DG, Wilson IB. Inhaler Costs and Medication Nonadherence Among Seniors with Chronic Pulmonary Disease. *Chest*. 2010;138(3):614-620. doi:10.1378/chest.09-3031.

[19] Dormuth CR, Maclure M, Glynn RJ, Neumann P, Brookhart AM, Schneeweiss S. Emergency hospital admissions after income-based deductibles and prescription copayments in older users of inhaled medications. *Clinical Therapeutics*. 2008;30, Part 1(0):1038-1050. doi:http://dx.doi.org/10.1016/j.clinthera.2008.06.003.

[20] Gaffney A, White A, Hawks L, et al. High Deductible Health Plans and Healthcare Access, Use, and Financial Strain in Those with COPD. *Annals ATS*. Published online October 10, 2019. doi:10.1513/AnnalsATS.201905-400OC.

[21] Chandra A, Flack E, Obermeyer Z. The Health Costs of Cost-Sharing. *National Bureau of Economic Research Working Paper*. https://www.nber.org/papers/w28439.

Such cost barriers no doubt contribute to inferior health in America. And indeed, recent health trends in the US are alarming. Even prior to the COVID-19 pandemic, life expectancy plateaued in the US in the past decade, ending decodes of progress (Figure 3).

Of course, multiple factors in addition to inadequate medical care contribute to poor health. Yet relative to other wealthy nations, "treatable mortality" — that is to say, deaths potentially preventable with medical care — is also higher in the US (Figure 4), a gap that has widened in the past two decades. Moreover, medical control of high blood pressure[22] and diabetes[23] has also worsened in recent years.

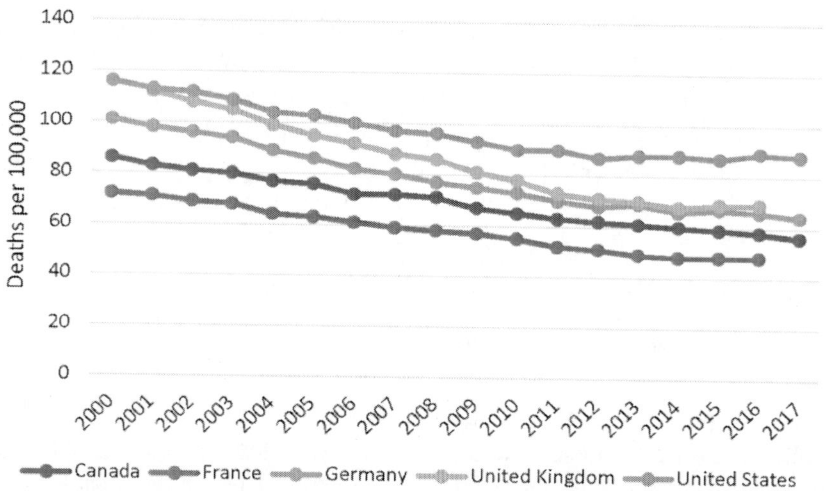

Rates are standardized. Source: OECD.Stat, Accessed March 11, 2022. Data points after 2017 were available only for Germany and so were omitted. Available at: https://stats.oecd.org/#.

Figure 4. "Treatable Mortality" in 5 Nations, 2000-2017.

---

[22] Muntner P, Hardy ST, Fine LJ, et al. Trends in Blood Pressure Control Among US Adults With Hypertension, 1999-2000 to 2017-2018. *JAMA*. 2020;324(12):1190-1200. doi:10.1001/jama.2020.14545.

[23] Fang M, Wang D, Coresh J, Selvin E. Trends in Diabetes Treatment and Control in U.S. Adults, 1999– 2018. *New England Journal of Medicine*. 2021;384(23):2219-2228. doi:10.1056/NEJMsa2032271.

Cost-sharing is not necessary. In Canada, doctor visits, tests, and hospital care are free-at-point of use. This is also the case in the United Kingdom. In Scotland and Wales, all medicines are additionally free-at-point-of use; even hospital parking is free for patients. As the experience of these nations illustrates, the imposition of high out-of-pocket can be avoided at the same time costs are contained. Medicare-for-All would eliminate nearly all out-of-pocket expenses, ensuring that all patients can get the care they need when they need it, improving both their health and financial welfare.

It could also realize a historic expansion in benefits by covering long-term care for everyone — a benefit that relatively few Americans have today. According to the Congressional Budget Office (CBO), a Medicare for All inclusive of long-term care benefits would approximately double the number of eligible Americans receiving covered home-and community-based services.[24] Medicare for All would also expand coverage of other benefits traditionally neglected by current insurance plans, such as dental coverage.

In sum, by covering the uninsured, and improving coverage for everyone else, Medicare for All could greatly improve the health and longevity of Americans.

Realizing Universal Care Affordably

An expansion of health protection to all Americans is clearly urgent. However, healthcare reform must also be affordable. Despite leaving so many uncovered, or with paltry and inadequate coverage, the US healthcare system is far more costly than that of other high-income nations, a difference that has widened since the 1970s (Figure 5).

Uniquely among healthcare reform proposals, Medicare for All would achieve the savings needed to cover the cost of a generous coverage expansion that provides first-dollar coverage to all US residents. I review some of the major factors affecting the price tag of Medicare for All below.

---

[24] Congressional Budget Office. *How CBO Analyzes the Costs of Proposals for Single-Payer Health Care Systems That Are Based on Medicare's Fee-for-Service Program.*; 2021. https://www.cbo.gov/publication/56811.

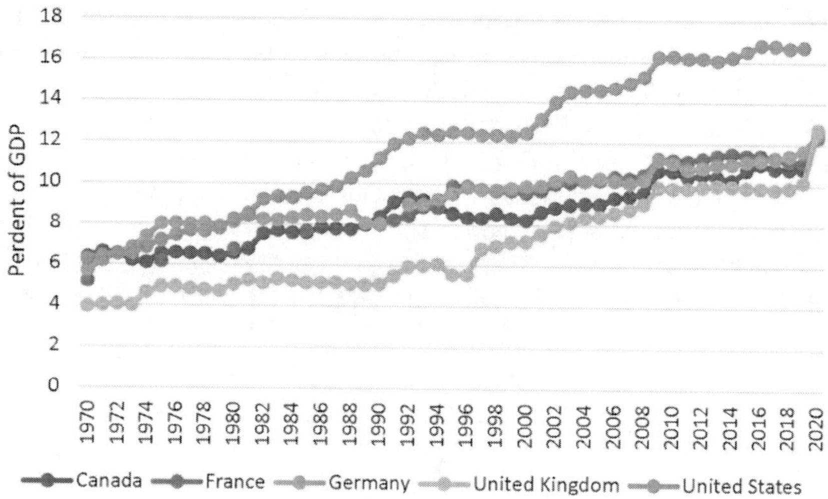

Source: OECD.Stat, Accessed March 11, 2022. There is a series break in 1975 for Canada; in 1995, 2003, and 2006 for France; in 1992 for Germany; and in 1997 for the United Kingdom. The 2019 Canadian estimate and the 2020 United Kingdom and Germany estimates are reported as "provisional." The 2020 US value is reported as an "estimated value." Available from: https://stats.oecd.org/#.

Figure 5. Healthcare spending in five wealthy nations, 1970-2020.

Savings on Payer-Side Administration

One key driver of high US healthcare costs is our system's inordinately high administrative costs, an issue appropriately recognized by the CBO and some other analysts, but inaccurately modelled by some previous economic analyses.

In 2017, 34% of healthcare spending was devoted to administration in the US — approximately twice the proportion spent on administration in Canada's single-payer national health insurance system.[25] Much of this administrative expense stems from the wasteful bureaucracy inherent to private health insurance. Compared to a public insurer like traditional Medicare, private insurers inflict numerous added costs, including profits for shareholders, bloated executive salaries, product and benefit design, marketing, and burdensome processes for disputing claims (needed to maximize profit). The CBO estimates that private insurance plans take 16.0% of their premium

[25] Himmelstein DU, Campbell T, Woolhandler S. Health Care Administrative Costs in the United States and Canada, 2017. *Ann Intern Med.* Published online January 7, 2020. doi:10.7326/M19-2818.

revenues for their overhead and profit.[24] The National Health Expenditure Accounts (NHEA) historical year data provides a slightly lower estimate of 12% (author's calculation; 2018-2020 three-year moving average). Publicly-funded plans operated by private health insurance companies, e.g., Medicare Advantage, have overhead similar to those of other commercial health insurance plans. An estimate from the Government Accountability Office (GAO) put overhead for Medicare Advantage plans (inclusive of profit) at 13.6% in 2011.[26] Today, the share may even be higher. Using the 2020 NHEA estimate of Medicare net private health insurance costs (i.e., overhead) of $63.4 billion divided by 2020 estimates from the 2021 report of Medicare Trustees of $422[27] in Medicare Part C + D spending gives a similar overhead of 15%. In comparison, traditional Medicare has an overhead of approximately 2% (author's calculation from the 2021 Medicare Trustees report[27]); a similar proportion is estimated by the CBO for overhead under Medicare for All.[24] Nations with national health insurance systems, including Canada, have a similarly low insurance overhead.[28] In other words, reducing insurance overhead of the overall US healthcare system to that of traditional Medicare could unlock enormous savings — funds that can then be used to cover the costs of a generous coverage expansion for all.

And indeed, the CBO has estimated savings from such a reduction in insurance costs at over $400 billion annually.[24] Some analyses have come to lower savings because they incorrectly projected that overhead of a single-payer system would be more than three times higher than that projected by the CBO.[24]

Savings on Provider-Side Administration

Payer-side administrative savings are only part of the equation, however. To contend with a multitude of different insurance plans, each with unique payment systems and standards, providers must also spend large amounts of resources on administration. One study, for instance, found that at a large

---

[26] Office USGA. Medicare Advantage: 2011 Profits Similar to Projections for Most Plans, but Higher for Plans with Specific Eligibility Requirements. 2014;(GAO-14-148). Accessed March 27, 2019. https://www.gao.gov/products/GAO-14-148.

[27] The Boards of Trustees, Federal Hospital Insuance and Federal Supplementary Medical Insurance Trust Funds. 2021 Annual Report of the Boards of Trustees of the Federal Hospital Insurance and Federal Supplementary Medical Insurance Trust Funds. Accessed September 16, 2021. https://www.cms.gov/files/document/2021-medicare-trustees-report.pdf.

[28] Jiwani A, Himmelstein D, Woolhandler S, Kahn JG. Billing and insurance-related administrative costs in United States' health care: synthesis of micro-costing evidence. *BMC health services research*. 2014;14:556. doi:10.1186/s12913-014-0556-7.

academic medical center, billing costs consumed 14.5% of the professional revenue it received for a primary care visit, and 25.2% of the revenue for an ER visit.[29] US hospitals hire armies of billers and coders to process claims and maximize payments, and consequently spend 25% of their revenue on administration; these costs are effectively bundled into the "price" of each healthcare service.[30] In comparison, nations with single-payer systems including Canada and Scotland that use hospital global budgets — or lump sums to cover all operating expenditures — spend only about 12% of their revenue on administration.[30]

Other providers also accrue excessive administrative costs because of the needlessly complex US insurance system. For instance, US physician practices spend more than $80,000 annually, per physician, to cover the costs of interactions with insurers — almost four-fold higher than Canada.[31] Yet even these figures may not fully account for time spent by physicians in onerous documentation efforts required (or incentivized) by our complex payment systems. A study by colleagues and I, for instance, estimated that US physicians spent 125 million hours on documentation outside office hours in 2019 — much of it driven by insurers' demands regarding billing — an enormous expenditure of time and resources.[32] A time-motion study examining time spent by 57 physicians found that about half of the work day was expended on the electronic health record (EHR) and desk work.[33] An analysis of EHR's found that internal medicine doctors spent more than 3 hours daily on "desktop medicine."[34] In addition to consuming healthcare resources, such busywork likely contributes to the epidemic of physician

[29] Tseng P, Kaplan RS, Richman BD, Shah MA, Schulman KA. Administrative Costs Associated With Physician Billing and Insurance-Related Activities at an Academic Health Care System. *JAMA*. 2018;319(7):691-697. doi:10.1001/jama.2017.19148.

[30] Himmelstein DU, Jun M, Busse R, et al. A Comparison Of Hospital Administrative Costs In Eight Nations: US Costs Exceed All Others By Far. *Health affairs*. 2014;33(9):1586-1594. doi:10.1377/hlthaff.2013.1327.

[31] Morra D, Nicholson S, Levinson W, Gans DN, Hammons T, Casalino LP. US physician practices versus Canadians: spending nearly four times as much money interacting with payers. *Health Aff (Millwood)*. 2011;30(8):1443-1450. doi:10.1377/hlthaff.2010.0893.

[32] Gaffney A, Woolhandler S, Cai C, et al. Medical Documentation Burden Among US Office-Based Physicians in 2019: A National Study. *JAMA Internal Medicine*. Published online March 28, 2022. doi:10.1001/jamainternmed.2022.0372.

[33] Sinsky C, Colligan L, Li L, et al. Allocation of Physician Time in Ambulatory Practice: A Time and Motion Study in 4 Specialties. *Ann Intern Med.* 2016;165(11):753. doi:10.7326/M16-0961.

[34] Tai-Seale M, Olson CW, Li J, et al. Electronic Health Record Logs Indicate That Physicians Split Time Evenly between Seeing Patients and Desktop Medicine. *Health Affairs*. 2017;36(4):655-662. doi:10.1377/hlthaff.2016.0811.

burnout, which itself imposes costs on the healthcare system. Moreover, such analyses entirely neglect the burden, in time and resources, imposed on *patients* from bureaucratic burdens. US workers may collectively spend as much as half a billion hours a year on the phone with health insurers annually.* Moreover, there may be health impacts on patients: about 1 in 4 nonelderly adult patient reports foregoing or delaying healthcare because of administrative burdens.[35]

Overall, the CBO estimates that under single-payer, provider-side administrative expenses (as a share of total revenue) would fall from 19% to 12% for hospitals, from 15% to 9% for physician/clinical services, and from 9% to 6% for other services.[24] The CBO models these savings by assuming that healthcare providers could deliver more care within existing budgets, but these reductions are indeed clear cut savings.

Moreover, because the CBO does not model global budgeting of hospitals, but instead payment through a fee-for-service system similar to traditional Medicare, achieved savings might even be higher.

Savings on Pharmaceuticals

Compared to other high-income nations, the US pays far more for the same prescription drugs. A single-payer program, particularly if it included aggressive price control tools such as compulsory licensing or public drug development programs, could hence achieve large savings on pharmaceuticals.[36] Under a "high price" single-payer scenario, the CBO estimated only a 7% reduction in drug prices by 2030. However, their "lower price" scenario, which envisions a 30% reduction in drug prices, is entirely realistic – as my colleagues and I have shown[36,37] and would also bring US drug prices closer to those of other nations.

---

* I extrapolated this figure from: Pfeffer J, Witters D, Agrawal S, Harter JK. Magnitude and Effects of "Sludge" in Benefits Administration: How Health Insurance Hassles Burden Workers and Cost Employers. Academy of Management Discoveries 2020;6(3):325–40. My calculation follows authors' assumptions: mean time per worker per week * 130.6 million full-time workers * 50 weeks per year, downwardly adjusted for 7.2% uninsured workers. This figure excludes part time workers.

35 Kyle MA, Frakt AB. Patient administrative burden in the US health care system. *Health Services Research*. n/a(n/a). doi:10.1111/1475-6773.13861.

36 Gaffney A, Lexchin J, The US/Canadian Pharmaceutical Policy Reform Working Group. Healing an ailing pharmaceutical system: prescription for reform for United States and Canada. *BMJ*. 2018;361:k1039. doi:10.1136/bmj.k1039.

37 US / Canadian Pharmaceutical Working Group. *Table 7: Estimated Effects of Proposed Reforms on US National Pharmaceutical Expenditures, 2017*. Accessed September 4, 2018. http://www.pnhp.org/sites/default/files/Pharma_Table7.pdf.

Costs for Increased Use of Care

Covering the uninsured and providing better coverage for the insured is expected — and indeed, intended to increase the use of healthcare, which all else equal will increase healthcare spending, partially offsetting some of the aforementioned savings. Some previous analyses, however, have projected enormous increases in healthcare utilization under single-payer that would actually exceed administrative savings.[38] Such surges in hospitalizations, surgical procedures, and office visits, however, are improbable and likely impossible. An analysis by colleagues and I of 13 historical universal coverage expansions in the US and other nations found that increases in healthcare use due to those expansions have been modest and sometimes non-existent.[39] A major error in some previous analyses has been a neglect of the supply-side of the equation: because the number of hospitals and physicians is finite, coverage expansions tend to deliver more care to the newly insured, with small, nearly imperceptible reductions in low-value care among the well-insured.[40] The CBO does model supply-side factors, although it errs in contextualizing constrained increases in use as unmet demand rather than salubrious reductions in the large amounts of unnecessary and even harmful care that are currently delivered.

How Would Providers Fare?

Some previous analyses have suggested that healthcare providers would fare poorly under Medicare for All indeed, that they might even face financial failure. Some of these same analyses have simultaneously suggested that costs would rise under Medicare for All. These two outcomes cannot simultaneously be true: if healthcare spending rises, so too does provider revenue. In truth, however, neither outcome is likely.

Table 1 provides a previously published estimate by colleagues and I[41] of changes in revenue per practicing physician under Medicare for All that builds

---

[38] Blumberg LJ, Holahan J, Buettgens M, et al. From Incremental to Comprehensive Health Insurance Reform: How Various Reform Options Compare on Coverage and Costs. Published online 2019. https://www.urban.org/research/publication/incremental-comprehensive-health-reform-how-various-reform-options-compare-coverage-and-costs.

[39] Gaffney A, Woolhandler S, Himmelstein D. The Effect of Large-scale Health Coverage Expansions in Wealthy Nations on Society-Wide Healthcare Utilization. *J GEN INTERN MED*. Published online November 19, 2019.

[40] Gaffney A, Himmelstein DU, Woolhandler S, Kahn JG. Pricing Universal Health Care: How Much Would The Use Of Medical Care Rise? *Health Affairs*. 2021;40(1):105-112. doi:10.1377/hlthaff.2020.01715.

[41] Gaffney A, Himmelstein D, Woolhandler S. Congressional Budget Office Scores Medicare-For-All: Universal Coverage For Less Spending. *Health Affairs Blog*. Published online

on CBO estimates. Under both the "low" and "high" payment rate scenarios envisioned by the CBO, revenues per practicing physician actually increase.

Table 1. Modeling CBO's low-cost sharing scenario: Ramifications for physicians

	Low Payment Rates	High Payment Rates
Increased Total Physician and other Clinical Service revenues	$43 billion	$170 billion
Increased Revenues Per Practicing Physician*	$39,816	$157,412

* Based on AAMC estimate of 840,000 practicing physicians in 2030, and the assumption that physician payments account for 77.78% of payments in the "Physician and other Clinical Service" category, as they did in 2018 according to the National Health Expenditure Accounts. This table is reproduced in full from reference[41]

Table 2 provides projections for hospitals' clinical (i.e., non-administrative) revenue. Again, funds available for patient care would increase, not decrease, under both the CBO's "low" and "high" payment rate scenarios.

Table 2. Modeling CBO's low-cost sharing scenario: Ramifications for hospitals' revenues and clinical operating budgets

	Low Payment Rates	High Payment Rates
Change in Hospitals' Gross Revenues	-$187 billion	$144 billion
Hospital administrative spending relative to current law (excluding savings on nursing time)**	-$178 billion	-$139 billion
Net change in hospital clinical (non-administrative) funding excluding savings on nursing time	*-$9 billion*	*$283 billion*
Hospital's Savings on RN and LPN Administrative Time***	$59 billion	$59 billion
Net change in hospital clinical (non-administrative) funding accounting for savings on nursing time	*$50 billion*	*$342 billion*

** Based on the CBO estimate that hospitals' spending on administration (excluding RN and LPN time spent on administration) would be reduced from 19% to 12% of hospital revenues.

*** Based on (1) BLS estimate of number of RNs and LPNs employed in hospitals and average RN and LPN wages in 2019; (2) the assumption that benefit costs = 20% of wages; (3) the assumption that nursing costs would rise at the same rate as overall hospital costs; and (4) CBO's estimate that RNs and LPNs devote 23% of time to administration and that single payer would reduce that time by 80%. This table is reproduced in full from reference:[41]

February 16, 2021. Accessed October 23, 2021. https://www.healthaffairs.org/do/10.1377/hblog20210210.190243/full/.

Clearly, providers would not suffer under Medicare for All. And while increased funding for safety net providers or primary care physicians may be appropriate, huge windfalls to already highly profitable providers seems inappropriate, suggesting that, if anything, costs would likely be even lower than projected by the CBO.

Conclusion

Medicare for All is the one healthcare reform that can accomplish the goal of expanding and improving coverage for everyone in the nation while simultaneously containing costs. Less comprehensive healthcare reforms, in comparison, will either provide less generous coverage, impose higher costs, or both. Systems similar to Medicare for All have been implemented around the world and have led to improved population health, better protection against the costs of illness, and lower national healthcare expenditures. Such a reform is urgently needed and achievable in the US today.

Testimony of Bonnie Castillo, RN, on Behalf of National Nurses United, before the Senate Committee on the Budget, May 12, 2022, Hearing on "Medicare for All: Protecting Health, Saving Lives, Saving Money"

Good morning and thank you, Chairman Sanders, Ranking Member Graham, and members of the committee for holding this critically important hearing today on Medicare for All. My name is Bonnie Castillo. I am a Registered Nurse and Executive Director of National Nurses United (NNU), the largest union and professional association of RNs in the United States. NNU proudly represents over 175,000 members who work as bedside health care professionals.

I'm particularly pleased to be joining you all today on International Nurses Day. I can think of nothing more fitting to commemorate International Nurses Day than by advocating for the quick and urgent transition to a Medicare for All system that would guarantee health care to every person in the United States.

For more than two years, nurses across this country have worked on the frontlines of the Covid-19 pandemic. We have been caring for patients despite atrocious working conditions in which the health and safety of nurses and their families have constantly been put at risk.

Nurses continue to bear witness every day to the ravages of this pandemic. We have seen unfathomable levels of death, physical illness, as well as the despair and grief that comes with severe illness and death, particularly when patients are isolated from their loved ones. And we have worked through this pandemic far too often without the protections we need to do our jobs safely.

In my testimony today, I will use the experiences of registered nurses from across the country to illustrate how the current healthcare system is fundamentally unable to provide the therapeutic quality care that our patients need and deserve. By erecting financial barriers to care, it provides starkly disparate care to different people and communities and, for many, provides no care at all. It is also financially inefficient and wasteful for the country as a whole. The only way we can guarantee every person living in this country receives the healthcare they need with a single standard of excellent care is by adopting a single-payer, Medicare for All system.

If it was ever in doubt before, this pandemic has shown that our current profit-driven and fragmented health insurance system does not work. It does not provide quality therapeutic care to millions of Americans, and it does not value and protect its own health care workers. Critically, the current fragmented system of health insurance is unable to provide the comprehensive pandemic response that we have needed for more than two years.

Why didn't nurses and health care workers get the protections we needed in the pandemic? Because our employers value money over our lives. More than 5,104 nurses and other health care workers have died as a result.

Why didn't we have the emergency stocks of critical medical supplies that we would need in a pandemic? Because the hospital and healthcare industry has long-employed a "just-in-time" supply and personnel model, where they plan their supply chains and staffing based on maximizing profit, not improving and safeguarding patient care.

We have seen high death rates from Covid-19 across the country. The United States population makes up less than five percent of the world's total population, but U.S. Covid-19 fatalities comprise 16 percent of total global Covid-19 fatalities. Our hospitals have been consistently overrun with critically ill patients. There are 30 million people in this country who are uninsured and tens of millions more who are underinsured, who therefore do not get the medical care they need. Without consistent access to high-quality care, including preventive and primary care, our patients are at higher risk of underlying medical conditions, which in turn, puts them at higher risk for severe Covid-19 illness, hospitalization, and death.

We do not have the health care infrastructure we need to effectively respond to this pandemic or prepare for future surges. This is because profit-driven hospital systems have decided where to open and close hospitals based on how much money they can make from the patients in those communities. As a result, rural, low-income, and Black, Indigenous, and people of color (BIPOC) communities lack access to medical care. If our health care infrastructure had been built to provide equitable health care to all communities, our response to the Covid-19 pandemic would have looked very different.

The problems with our health care system far predate this pandemic. For years, nurses have witnessed the preventable tragedies that result from this profit-driven system. Nurses watch as too many patients forgo needed medications, procedures, or care because they cannot afford the costs. They watch as insurance corporations refuse to cover critical care that is required for the health and well-being of patients. Insurers override the professional judgment of licensed health care professionals, and nurses can do little about it when our patients do not get the care that they need. Nurses watch as patients finally come to the hospital emergency room with advanced stages of illness or disease that could have been prevented if they had access to treatment earlier.

The system we have now is beholden to the corporate interests that determine who gets treatment, and what treatment they get. It is deeply inefficient and unsustainable because it prioritizes short-term financial returns rather than long-term investments in our health. This leads to a system that is unaffordable for our country and for our patients. Many patients cannot afford the costs of their care individually, and the country cannot afford the financial burdens of a system with built-in inefficiencies, administrative waste, and needless profiteering. The Covid-19 pandemic, with nearly one million recorded fatalities in the U.S., has shown clearly that our society cannot afford the consequences this has on public health. Any delay in fundamentally transforming our health care system costs money, but more importantly, we pay with our health and with our lives.

The United States leads the world in health care spending. We spend more money per person on health care than any other nation in the world even though millions of people do not get the health care they need. Instead of providing health care for all people in the U.S., we waste hundreds of billions of dollars each year on unnecessary administrative costs, huge profit margins for corporations, and inefficiencies. Despite paying top dollar for our health care, we get poor results. Our country ranks near the bottom among industrialized nations on many international health indicators, including on critical barometers such as average life expectancy, infant mortality, maternal mortality, and death from preventable diseases. High costs and poor health outcomes persist because access to an insurance plan is not the same as guaranteed health care for all.

The only way to solve the health care crisis in this country, is to enact a single-payer, Medicare for All system.

By moving to a single-payer system, we would transform the profit-driven health insurance system into a health care system that prioritizes patient care. Under the Medicare for All Act of 2022, the existing Medicare program would be improved and then expanded to cover every person living in the United States. Medicare for All would immediately reduce inefficiencies in the current fragmented insurance system by cutting unnecessary administrative expenses associated with billing countless insurance providers, negotiating in-network and out-of-network payments, and fighting against high copays, prior authorization barriers, and unexpected expenses. Medicare for All would also remove the huge amounts of money that are funneled into insurance industry executive pay and corporate profits instead of being spent on our health.

Study after study has shown that a single-payer system is the only way that our country can provide guaranteed health care to all, with comprehensive benefits, while also reducing the amount of money we spend on health care overall. In other words, with Medicare for All, we would get more, cover everyone, pay less, and experience better health care outcomes. Economic analyses have shown that our country would save between two and five trillion dollars over ten years if we implemented a single-payer Medicare for All program.

Medicare for All would save us hundreds of billions of dollars each year by eliminating the administrative complexity and profiteering in our current system and by leveraging our collective buying power under a single-payer to negotiate fairer prices for everyone. Through bulk negotiations, Medicare for All would end high prescription drugs prices. Instead of payments going towards inflated prices, administrative complexity, and health industry profiteering, our health care dollars would be redirected to providing quality patient care.

As a registered nurse, I can envision exactly what Medicare for All would mean for patients in this country. Whenever someone needs medical care, they would see the health care provider of their choice without any worry about financial and insurance barriers to care — about insurance networks, copayments, deductibles, coinsurance, preauthorization requirements, limits on health care spending, or surprise billing. Every patient would receive the care they need free at the point of service.

We would no longer see patients who could not get lifesaving care because their insurance provider denied them coverage, or because they did not have insurance to begin with. We would no longer see huge numbers of patients who present with severe illness or disease because they could not afford the care they needed months or years earlier. Patients would no longer have to ration their medication.

And for those of us who are health care workers, we would be able to provide medical and nursing care based on our professional judgment, without the interference of insurance companies who are not licensed health care providers and whose interests are in reducing claims to increase returns.

The Medicare for All Act would allow for tangible and practical improvements to health care delivery for registered nurses and other health care workers at hospitals across the country. Importantly, the bill would change the way that hospitals are paid for their services. This payment model would fundamentally shift the profit-motives of hospital corporations and ensure that they focus on patient care while simultaneously investing in their caregiver workforce and protecting worker health and safety.

The Medicare for All Act would pay all institutional providers through a global budget that would allow them to provide quality patient care for their communities. Aligning hospital payments with costs, these global budgets would be tailored to meet and reflect the care and access needs of the patients served by each hospital. Through the global budgeting model, payments would more closely reflect the actual costs of providing health care to patients, and those payments would ensure equity across health care institutions.

Through global budgeting, the Medicare for All program would also use targeted funding to ensure that hospitals are providing for the health and safety of their patients and their health care workforce. For example, the bill explicitly requires that hospitals have the funding necessary for safe nurse-to-patient staffing ratios, for pandemic preparedness costs, for safe patient handling, and for other occupational health and safety programs.

Providers would be accountable for their spending and would no longer be able to overcharge the Medicare program. Importantly, the global budgeting model requires transparency and allows the public to track where our health care dollars are going. We can ensure that rural hospitals and hospitals in underserved areas always get the funding they need to stay open.

Providers must also report all relevant data associated with operational costs and justify their spending. With periodic audits and review, providers would be held accountable for their projected spending and the program could monitor whether the provider is meeting program goals and standards.

Importantly, the Medicare for All budget and payment system would greatly improve health equity and would decrease the health disparities we see for rural and low-income communities and for communities of color.

If Medicare for All was in place before the pandemic, we would have been better prepared to respond to Covid-19 with sufficient nurses, doctors, respiratory therapists, and other staff as well as beds, equipment, and medical supplies. The Medicare for All national health budget would also include "a reserve fund to respond to the costs of treating an epidemic, pandemic, natural disaster, or other such health emergency."

If we had a Medicare for All system, health care workers would not needlessly become infected, hospitalized, or die because of the health care industry's reliance on the "just-in-time" supply model. This model, which prioritizes profits over worker health and safety, failed to get health care workers the necessary PPE and other critical medical supplies that would have kept them and their patients safe. Instead, the global budget payments for hospitals and skilled nursing facilities would include funding for infectious disease response preparedness. These facilities would be required to maintain a one-year stockpile of personal protective equipment, and to provide occupational testing and surveillance, medical services for on-the-job infectious disease exposure, and contact tracing.

Medicare for All would not only save money and improve the health of patients, but it would also improve the lives and practice of our healthcare professionals — our doctors, nurses, and other clinicians.

As registered nurses, our primary responsibility is to protect the health and wellbeing of our patients. Our existing health care system does not allow us to do that. We cannot expect a system that is designed to profit off illness, pain, and suffering, to work in the interests of our patients. Medicare for All is the solution we need to ensure that every patient gets the health care they need.

Thank you.

Attachments

1) Issue Brief, Medicare for All Act of 2022: The Nurse Staffing Crisis & the Urgent Need for Health Care Redesign
2) Issue Brief, Medicare for All Act of 2022: Covid-19, Future Pandemics & Medicare for All
3) Issue Brief, Medicare for All Act of 2022: Program Design
4) Issue Brief, Medicare for All Act of 2022: Ensuring Access to Care
5) Issue Brief, Medicare for All Act of 2022: Eliminating Health & Health Care Disparities
6) Issue Brief, Medicare for All Act of 2022: Global Budgets & Other Reimbursements
7) Issue Brief: Medicare for All Act of 2022: Cost & Savings Analyses
8) Issue Brief: Medicare for All Act of 2022: Canada, Taiwan & U.S. Comparison

Medicare for All Act of 2022: The Nurse Staffing Crisis & the Urgent Need for Health Care Redesign

For decades, the hospital and health insurance industries have operated on a model with one goal: maximize net revenue. These profits come at the expense of both patient care as well as worker health and safety — a hospital is not a factory, and health care workers are not machines. Covid-19 has exacerbated the industry-created staffing crisis, which has been decades in the making as health care corporations have deliberately understaffed hospitals to cut costs and prioritize profits over safe working conditions and patient care. Talk of a "nursing shortage" has become ubiquitous during the Covid-19 pandemic. In reality, there is no shortage of nurses in the U.S., only a shortage of nurses willing to risk their licenses or their patients' lives by working in the unsafe conditions that have become prevalent in today's hospital industry.

This brief discusses the link between the intentional profit-maximizing practices of the hospital industry and high rates of nurses leaving the bedside — or leaving the nursing profession altogether — to protect themselves, their nursing licenses, their families, and their patients. Because hospital employers fail to protect nurses on the job and fail to provide nurses with the staff and resources needed for them to give safe, therapeutic care, nurses face profound levels of moral distress, preventable workplace dangers, and job dissatisfaction. Medicare for All is a key solution to this problem; targeted hospital payments for nurse-to-patient staffing ratios and occupational health and safety protections would allow nurses to provide quality patient care in a safe and sustainable environment.

A Shortage of Good Nursing Jobs, Not a Shortage of Nurses

There is no shortage of registered nurses. As of November 6, 2021, the National Council of State Boards of Nursing reported that there are over 4.4 million RNs with active licenses,[42] yet according to the U.S. Bureau of Labor Statistics, there are only 3.2 million people who are employed as RNs, with 1.8 million employed in hospitals.[43] In addition, except for a handful of states, there are sufficient numbers of registered nurses to meet the needs of the country's patients, according to a 2017 U.S. Department of Health and Human Services (HHS) report on the supply and demand of the nursing workforce from 2014 to 2030.[44] Moreover, HHS projected that most states (43) would have surpluses in 2030.[45] Rather, there is a shortage of good permanent nursing jobs where RNs are fully valued for their work at the bedside through safe patient staffing levels, strong union protections, and safe and healthy workplaces.

Importantly, registered nursing can be a pathway to good union jobs for people from Black, Brown, Indigenous, and other communities of color (BIPOC) and other underserved communities, but hiring and educational policies by the hospital industry have restricted the pipeline of nurses from socioeconomically diverse and underserved communities. Although there is no general nursing shortage, the lack of racial, ethnic, cultural, linguistic, and

---

[42] National Council of State Boards of Nursing. "Active RN Licenses, A Profile of Nursing Licensure in the U.S." National Council of State Boards of Nursing (2022) (Last updated May 20, 2022). Accessed May 10, 2022. https://www.ncsbn.org/6161.htm. As the National Council of State Boards of Nursing data excludes Michigan RNs, their number of active RN licenses reflects the number of RNs employed in Michigan which is less than the number of RNs licensed in Michigan. National Council of State Boards of Nursing uses Michigan data from U.S. Bureau of Labor Statistics. "May 2020 Occupational Employment and Wages." U.S. Department of Labor (2021). Available at https://www.bls.gov/oes/home.htm.

[43] U.S. Bureau of Labor Statistics. "May 2020 Occupational Employment and Wages." U.S. Department of Labor (2021). Available at https://www.bls.gov/oes/home.htm.

[44] Health Resources and Services Administration. "National and Regional Supply and Demand Projections of the Nursing Workforce: 2014-2030." U.S. Department of Health and Human Services (2017). Accessed on May 10, 2022. https://bhw.hrsa.gov/sites/default/ files/bureau-health-workforce/data-research/nchwa-hrsa-nursing-report.pdf.

[45] *Ibid.*

socioeconomic diversity within the current nursing workforce reflects the need for increasing the numbers of and support for socioeconomically diverse registered nurses from BIPOC communities and other underserved communities. Racial and socioeconomic diversity within the nursing workforce is crucial for both improving our nation's health and achieving health equity.[46]

How Hospital Industry Practices Drive Nurses Away from the Bedside

To reduce labor costs and to increase profits, the hospital industry deliberately refuses to staff our nation's hospitals with enough nurses to care for patients safely and optimally, harming both nurses and patients in the process. Even before Covid-19, the hospital industry had driven nurses away from direct nursing care at the bedside by adopting policies that result in high patient caseloads and unsafe working conditions, such as the intentional understaffing of units. Understaffing, a deliberate practice in which hospital management does not schedule an adequate number of nurses to safely care for patients in a hospital unit, is driven by a desire to increase hospital profits. Employers do not maintain a robust pool of nurses from which they can increase staffing when patient loads increase, hospitals repeatedly cancel or "call-off" nurses who are scheduled to work and are slow to fill permanent RN positions.

Unsafe staffing levels and poor working conditions make it impossible for nurses to meet their ethical and professional obligations as RNs to provide safe, effective, and therapeutic nursing care.

Studies have shown that adequate staffing levels through RN-to-patient ratios result in better patient outcomes, and health and safety programs not only protect workers, but improve the health and safety of patients as well. Further, hospital employers consistently fail to protect nurses from health and safety dangers in the hospital including infectious diseases, workplace violence, and musculoskeletal injury.

Additionally, the hospital industry devalues RNs' professional practice and restricts their autonomy in myriad ways. Most notably, the industry focus on patient satisfaction scores and the routinization that breaks holistic nursing

---

[46] National Advisory Council for Nurse Education and Practice. "Achieving Health Equity through Nursing Workforce Diversity." U.S. Department of Health and Human Services (2013). Accessed May 11, 2022. https://www.hrsa.gov/sites/default/files/hrsa/advisory-committees/nursing/reports/2013-eleventhreport.pdf.

care into discrete tasks have been particularly troublesome for nurses. Both trends are driven by the industry goal of maximizing net revenue and restricts the autonomy nurses have to use their knowledge and experience to care for their patients.

Employers' disregard for and mistreatment of nurses has increased during the pandemic. However, throughout the pandemic, there has been a jarring contradiction between the saccharine and excessive celebration of nurses as heroes for risking their and their families' lives and the utter disregard of nurse safety by the hospital industry. The disposability of nurses during the pandemic can be plainly observed as hospital employers refuse to provide necessary optimal personal protective equipment, mandate endless shifts, refuse sick or quarantine leave and pay, refuse employees Covid-19 tests, demand nurses work even if they have been exposed to Covid-19, and discipline nurses who speak out about unsafe conditions for workers and their patients.[47]

For hospital employers, the Covid-19 pandemic has become the ready excuse to waive their legal duties as employers to protect nurses and other workers who provide essential, life-sustaining labor, and their duty to provide optimal, therapeutic care to their patients. Registered nurses are a critical public health resource. The pandemic should be a reason to provide them more, not an excuse to provide them less.

In sum, hospital employers' utter disregard for the lives of nurses, their patients, their families, and their professional autonomy during the pandemic has resulted in both a physical and psychological toll on nurses. The failure by hospital employers to staff appropriately and provide the resources needed to provide safe, therapeutic patient care has caused nurses to experience severe moral distress and injury (often incorrectly labeled "burnout"); mental health issues such as stress, anxiety, depression, and post-traumatic stress disorder; and physical exhaustion. As a result, many nurses are leaving the bedside. If hospitals protected nurses with safe working conditions and safe staffing rather than pushing nurses to do more with less, we could keep better retain practicing nurses and bring nurses back to the bedside.

[47] National Nurses United. "Deadly Shame: Redressing the Devaluation of Registered Nurse Labor Through Pandemic Equity." National Nurses United (Dec. 2020). Accessed May 10, 2022. https://www.nationalnursesunited.org/sites/default/files/nnu/graphics/documents/1220_Covid19_DeadlyShame_PandemicEquity_WhitePaper_FINAL.pdf.

Medicare for All Removes Profit-Driven Insurers from Health Care

The increased corporatization of health care and the continued devaluation of nursing labor can only be addressed by removing the profit motive from health care. Under Medicare for All, we will transform our profit-driven health insurance system into a health care system that prioritizes patient care and, by extension, the nursing profession. Medicare for All would end the fundamental inequality that all systems of private health insurance, as structures organized to maximize corporate profits, are built on.

In a Medicare for All system, no patient will go without necessary and lifesaving preventive care because they can't afford it. Patients will never have to ration their medication. Doctors and nurses will be able to provide care based on their best professional judgment without insurance company interference. We must realign our health care system to meet the needs of patients rather than the aims of the health care industry's bottom line; doing so will improve the working conditions of nurses. Valuing the labor and lives of nurses will increase the number of RNs who choose to remain at the bedside and the number of people who choose to enter the profession.

The Medicare for All Act of 2022 importantly includes explicit provisions to ensure that hospitals and other health care facilities have the funding necessary for safe nurse-to-patient staffing ratios, for optimal staffing levels for physicians and other health care workers, for pandemic preparedness costs, for safe patient handling, and for other occupational health and safety programs.[48] In other words, Medicare for All would curtail health care employers' ability to divert revenue from investments in their caregiving workforce and protecting worker health and safety. Through targeted funding, health care employers would be held accountable for both safe patient care and occupational health and safety. Under the Act, the Office of Health Equity would also be established, which would be responsible for both tracking barriers to health care access resulting from the lack of health care professional staffing and recruitment and would be responsible for implementing policies to address such staffing inequities in our health care system.[49]

Additionally, to end the nurse staffing crisis and to bring nurses back to the bedside, Congress must adopt federal policies that value the vital work of direct patient care RNs and that ensure employers meet their legal obligations to provide safe and healthy workplaces, such as safe staffing standards,

---

[48] Medicare for All Act of 2022 §§ 611(b)(2)(D), 611(d)(1)(A), 611(d)(1)(G).
[49] Medicare for All Act of 2022 § 615.

optimal workplace safety protections, fair wages, and robust union rights — including conditioning future pandemic relief funding for the hospital industry on implementing nurse retention measures. This unprecedented crisis of the Covid-19 pandemic provides us the opportunity to fight for the protections, pay, and dignity that nurses deserve as well as guaranteed health care for all.

Medicare for All Act of 2022: Covid-19, Future Pandemics and Medicare for All

As of May 11, 2022, the United States is verging on 1 million confirmed deaths from Covid-19. The Covid-19 pandemic demonstrated just how harmful our profit-driven health care system can be for both patients and our health care workforce. The unfathomably high death, hospitalization, and infection rates during this pandemic were enabled and worsened by a health care system that is fragmented by profit-seeking insurers and that denies care to millions of patients. Although many have become numb to the impact of the Covid-19 pandemic, people continue to be infected, hospitalized, and, in some cases, to die.

The pandemic is a tragedy of avoidable exposures and deaths caused by a lack of preparedness, inadequate hospital capacity and supplies, and uncoordinated, uneven availability of tests, contact tracing, vaccines, treatments, and personal protective equipment (PPE). It also deepened racial and socioeconomic health inequities that have existed for decades, inequities that Black, Indigenous, Latinx, and other communities of color, working class communities, and other underserved communities have experienced for generations and continue to experience daily.

The pandemic is also a tale of utter indifference by employers, particularly health industry employers, and our public health agencies to the health and safety of nurses, doctors, other health care workers, and essential workers who have been risking their lives to keep everyone else safe. Nurses did not have the protections they needed in the pandemic because our profit-driven health care system values profit more than the lives of its workers.

But not everyone is suffering; many hospital systems and private insurers profited during the pandemic. The hospital industry, despite raking in billions of dollars in federal relief, has continued to knowingly place nurses, doctors, and other health care workers at risk of exposure to Covid-19 without adequate protection. The first year of the Covid-19 pandemic, 2020, was the second most profitable year for the hospital industry ever, with a total net income of almost $92 billion in the U.S. alone.[50] The health insurance industry also continued its trend of skyrocketing profits in 2020, taking in $31 billion in net earnings and increasing profit margins by 3.8%, which represented the highest returns in at least decade.[51]

The comprehensive solution to the failures of our profit-driven health care system during the Covid-19 pandemic is to expeditiously implement Medicare for All. The Covid-19 pandemic gave clear reason for lawmakers to act decisively and with all due urgency to transform our fragmented system of health insurance into a single, government-run insurance system that priorities equitable provision of patient care under a single standard of high-quality care.

The Pandemic Exposes the Fractures in Our Multi-Payer System of Insurance

Millions of families in the United States who were uninsured or underinsured during the past two years of the pandemic delayed or skipped care, both Covid-19 and non-Covid-19 care, because of costs. But foregoing treatment for Covid-19 harms everyone as the virus continues to spread, prolonging the pandemic and increasing morbidity and mortality. Moreover, because families in the United States have long struggled to afford and access high-quality health care, far too many people in the country have chronic and underlying health conditions which have made them more susceptible to severe Covid-19 illness, hospitalization, and death.

In 2020, during the beginning of the Covid-19 pandemic, one poll found that 68% of adults said that out-of-pocket costs related to treatment would be a factor in their decision on whether to seek treatment for Covid-19.[52] Almost two years later in December 2021, another survey by the Kaiser Family

---

50 *See* American Hospital Association. "AHA Hospital Statistics Database." *AHA Data & Insights* (Updated 2022). Accessed May 9, 2022. https://www.ahadata.com/aha-hospital-statistics.

51 American Hospital Association. "NAIC 2020 Health Insurance Industry Analysis Report." National Association of Insurance Commissioners (2021). Accessed May 9, 2022. https://content.naic.org/sites/default/files/inline-files/2020-Annual-Health-Insurance-Industry-Analysis-Report.pdf.

52 Collins, S. et al. "What are Americans' views on the Coronavirus pandemic? NBC News/Commonwealth Fund Health Care Poll." Commonwealth Fund (March 20, 2020). Accessed May 9, 2022. https://www.commonwealthfund.org/publications/surveys/2020/mar/what- are-americans-views-coronavirus-pandemic.

Foundation reported that half of adults in the United States said they delayed or skipped health care or dental care in the past year because of costs, with larger percentages reported by Black, Latinx, or low-income adults.[53] Three in ten (29%) adults reported not taking their medicines as prescribed at some point in the past year because of the cost, nearly half (46%) of insured adults reported difficulty affording their out-of-pocket costs, and one in four (27%) insured adults reported difficulty affording their deductible.

The economic squeeze of the pandemic also fell squarely on working people, particularly working people of color, and resulted in disproportionate losses of job-based health insurance coverage. The Commonwealth Fund estimated that about 14.6 million people lost some or all of their health insurance coverage between February and June 2020 alone.[54] They found that 7.7 million workers lost jobs that provided employer-sponsored insurance, with an additional 6.9 million dependents covered by these employer-sponsored plans. Moreover, the loss of employer-based coverage disproportionately impacted families of color. For example, even accounting for pre-pandemic disparities, Black adults were more likely to experience losses of income or job loss in the first year of the pandemic[55] and, thus, were more likely to be pushed through the enormous gaps of our employer-sponsored health insurance system.

The Pandemic's Disproportionate Impact on Black, Indigenous, People of Color (BIPOC) and Working Families

Covid-19 has forced the United States to finally acknowledge the enduring, destructive, and deadly economic and racial gaps in our health care system and in our society. As SARS-CoV-2 spread across the globe, health care disparities in the United States were exacerbated by our fractured health care system in

---

[53] Kearney, A. et al. "Americans' Challenges with Health Care Costs." Kaiser Family Foundation (Dec. 2021). Accessed May 9, 2022. https://www.kff.org/health-costs/issue-brief/americans-challenges-with-health-care-costs/.

[54] Fronstin, P., Woodbury, S. "How many Americans have lost jobs with employer health coverage during the pandemic?" Commonwealth Fund, Issue Briefs (Oct. 2020). Accessed May 9, 2022. https://www.commonwealthfund.org/publications/issue-briefs/2020/oct/how-many- lost-jobs-employer-coverage-pandemic.

[55] Monte, L., Perez-Lopez, D. "Covid-19 Pandemic Hit Black Households Harder Than White Household Event When Pre-Pandemic Socio-Economic Disparities are Taken into Account." U.S. Census Bureau (Jul. 2021). Accessed May 9, 2022. https://www.census.gov/library/stories/2021/07/how-pandemic-affected-black-and-white-households.html.

which different health care providers, health care corporations, and public health care programs do not coordinate with each other. Without universal publicly run health care coverage, there was a failure of strategic planning and preparedness to respond to the pandemic in communities, particularly BIPOC communities and other communities that faced health care disparities before the pandemic.

Although these health and health care disparities have been evident for decades, the racial and ethnic disparities in exposure, severe illness, and death from Covid-19 pandemic brought renewed and widespread attention to the issue. The Centers for Disease Control and Prevention (CDC) found large disparities in age-adjusted risk of infection, hospitalization, and death for American Indian and Alaska Native (AI/AN), Black, and Latinx people compared to white people.[56] As shown in the chart below, AI/IN people had the largest disparity in cases, hospitalizations, and deaths with Black and Latinx people also having large disparities compared to white people.

Table 1. Selected statistics adapted from CDC Covid-19 age-adjusted data (April 2022)[57]

Rate ratios compared to white, non-Hispanic persons	American Indian or Alaska Native, Non-Hispanic persons	Black or African American, Non-Hispanic persons	Hispanic or Latinx persons
Cases	1.6x	1.1x	1.5x
Hospitalization	3.1x	2.4x	2.3x
Death	2.1x	1.7x	1.8x

Existing disparities in health for BIPOC communities, reduced access to health care during the pandemic, and greater occupational exposure to the virus all played key roles in the racial and ethnic disparities in Covid-19 infections, hospitalizations, and deaths.[58] BIPOC communities are on average less likely to have health insurance, less likely to see a doctor regularly, and

[56] "Hospitalization and Death by Race/Ethnicity." Centers for Disease Control and Prevention (Updated Apr. 29, 2022). Accessed May 9, 2022. https://www.cdc.gov/coronavirus/2019-ncov/covid-data/investigations-discovery/hospitalization-death-by-race-ethnicity.html.

[57] *See ibid.*

[58] *Ibid.* Note that studies have shown that racism directly worsens physical and mental health, rather than only affecting health status indirectly. *See* Singh M. "'Long overdue': lawmakers declare racism a public health emergency." *Guardian* (Jun. 12, 2020). Accessed May 9, 2022. https://www.theguardian.com/society/2020/jun/12/racism-public-health-black-brown-coronavirus.

less likely to receive preventive care.[59] Many BIPOC adults were likely to be essential workers exposing themselves day in and day out during the past year. During the pandemic, Latinx, Black, Native American, and Pacific Islander men were the most likely male workers to have frontline occupations, and Vietnamese, Latinx, and Filipinx women were the most likely female workers to hold frontline occupations.[60]

As a result of the long-standing structural racism of our health care system, BIPOC communities were more vulnerable to the devastation of both the virus itself and the economic impact of the pandemic.

Covid-19's Impact on Nurses and Other Health Care Workers

The science of aerosol transmissible disease and occupational safety and health have long taught us how to prevent exposure to airborne diseases, like Covid-19, at work but health care workers have experienced high rates of exposure, infection, and death from Covid-19. Workplace risks of exposure, infection, and death from Covid-19 were unnecessary and preventable. While no national government agency tracks health care worker infections and deaths from Covid-19, as of April 19, 2022, National Nurses United (NNU) has recorded nearly one and a half million health care worker cases and the deaths of at least 5,104 health care workers from Covid-19, with at least 492 deaths of registered nurses from Covid-19 in the United States.[61] This is undoubtedly an undercount of health care worker infections and deaths.

Like the impact of Covid-19 overall in the U.S., there have been racial and ethnic disparities in the impacts of Covid-19 for health care workers of color. A recent *Kaiser Health News* and *Guardian* report found that two-thirds of the 3,600 health care worker deaths they were able to identify were health

---

[59] Ariga, S., Hill, L., Orgera K. "Health Coverage by Race and Ethnicity, 2010-2019." Kaiser Family Foundation (Jul 2021). Accessed May 9, 2022. https://www.kff.org/racial-equity-and-health-policy/issue-brief/health-coverage-by-race-and-ethnicity/.

[60] Goldman, N. et al. "Racial and ethnic differentials in COVID-19-related job exposures by occupational standing in the US." *PLoS One*, 16(9): E0256085 (Sept. 2021). Accessed May 9, 2022. https://www.ncbi.nlm.nih.gov/pmc/articles/PMC8409606/.

[61] As tracked by National Nurses United using the methodology outlined in "Sins of Omission: How Government Failures to Track Covid-19 Data Have Led to More Than 3,200 Health Care Worker Deaths and Jeopardize Public Health." National Nurses United (Updated Mar 2021). Accessed May 9, 2022. https://www.nationalnursesunited.org/sites/default/files/nnu/documents/0321_Covid19_SinsOfOmission_Data_Report.pdf.

care workers of color.[62] When NNU looked at registered nurse (RN) deaths, we found a disproportionate impact in the deaths of RNs of color. Nearly half of the nurses who have died of Covid-19 were nurses of color, who represent about 24% of the RN workforce. More than 17% of registered nurses who have died from Covid-19 were Black although Black nurses only make up 12% of nurses. And nearly one-quarter of all registered nurses who have died from covid were of Philippine descent, despite making up only 4% of RNs in the U.S.[63]

Health Care Industry "Just-in-Time" Resourcing Results in Lack of Workplace Protections

The hospital industry's "just-in-time" supply and personnel model, which tightly manages inventory and staffing based on short-term financial returns rather than long-term investments and preparedness, has been disastrous during the Covid-19 pandemic.[64] Although infectious disease surges are unpredictable, they are inevitable. Hospitals should have been better prepared, given the initial outbreak in China in late 2019. Yet because employers prioritized profits over preparedness, RNs were forced to choose between staying on the job and caring for their patients, who are also at risk of infection from nurses' lack of PPE,[65] or staying home to protect themselves and their families.

The horror stories from health care workers about the failures of their employers to protect them and their patients were numerous throughout the

---

[62] "Lost on the Frontline: Thousands of US healthcare workers have died fighting Covid-19. We count them and investigate why." *Kaiser Health News / The Guardian* (Apr. 2021). Accessed May 9, 2022. https://www.theguardian.com/us-news/ng-interactive/2020/dec/22/lost-on-the-frontline-our-findings-to-date.

[63] National Nurses United. "Sins of Omission: How Government Failures to Track Covid-19 Data Have Led to More Than 3,200 Health Care Worker Deaths and Jeopardize Public Health." National Nurses United (Updated Mar 2021). Accessed May 9, 2022. https://www.nationalnursesunited.org/sites/default/files/nnu/documents/0321_Covid19_SinsOfOmission_Data_Report.pdf.

[64] *See* National Nurses United. "Protecting Our Front Line: Ending the Shortage of Good Nursing Jobs and the Industry-Created Staffing Crisis." National Nurses United (Dec. 2021). Accessed May 9, 2022. https://www.nationalnursesunited.org/sites/default/files/nnu/documents/1121_StaffingCrisis_ProtectingOurFrontLine_Report_FINAL.pdf.

O'Leary, L. "The Modern Supply Chain is Snapping." *The Atlantic* (Mar. 19, 2020). Accessed May 9, 2022. https://www.theatlantic.com/ideas/archive/2020/03/supply-chainsand-coronavirus/608329/.

[65] Jewett, C. "Patients Went into the Hospital for Care. After Testing Positive There for Covid, Some Never Came Out." *Kaiser Health News* (Nov. 4, 2021). Accessed May 9, 2022. https://khn.org/news/article/hospital-acquired-covid-nosocomial-cases-data-analysis/.

pandemic. Nurses were forced to go without or to wear PPE manufactured for a single use for days on end. Some nurses were forced to use garbage bags when their employer ran out of surgical gowns.[66] Those who did have access to PPE in the pandemic's early stages generally had to fight for it. Although PPE was a key issue for nurses, it was far from the only issue. Employers also failed to screen and test patients for Covid-19,[67] to notify nurses of a Covid-19 exposure,[68] and to provide testing and sick leave while awaiting test results. This is not an exhaustive list of their failings.

As of April 2022, National Nurses United has conducted seven surveys of RNs over the course of the pandemic. We have continuously found that hospital employers fail to prepare for Covid-19 surges and fail to invest the resources necessary to protect nurses and other health care workers from the significant risk of Covid-19.[69] Even two years into the pandemic, National Nurses United's latest survey of RNs, published in April 2022, found that health care employers are still not protecting RNs on the job from Covid-19. Our survey found:

- Only 71.8 percent of hospital RNs reported wearing a respirator for every Covid-positive patient encounter.
- 62 percent of hospital RNs reported having to reuse single-use PPE.

---

[66] *See*, e.g., Sanchez, T. "Coronavirus: Nurses are Wearing Trash Bags at One Bay Area Hospital Facing a Protective Equipment Shortage." *San Francisco Chronicle* (Apr. 2, 2020). Accessed May 9, 2022. https://www.sfchronicle.com/bayarea/article/Coronavirus-Nurses-are- wearing-trash-bagsat-one-15172777.php.

[67] Jewett, C. "Patients Went into the Hospital for Care. After Testing Positive There for Covid, Some Never Came Out." *Kaiser Health News* (Nov. 4, 2021). Accessed May 9, 2022. https://khn.org/news/article/hospital-acquired-covid-nosocomial-cases-data-analysis/.

[68] Gold, J., Hawryluk, M. "Hospital Workers Complain of Minimal Disclosure After COVID Exposures." *Kaiser Health News / The Guardian* (May 13, 2020). Accessed May 9, 2022. https://khn.org/news/hospital-workers-complain-of-minimal-disclosure-after-covid-exposures/.

[69] *See, e.g.*, National Nurses United. "New survey of nurses provides frontline proof of widespread employer, government disregard for nurse and patient safety, mainly through lack of optimal PPE." National Nurses United (May 2020). Accessed May 9, 2022. https://www.nationalnursesunited.org/press/new-survey-results.

National Nurses United. "National nurse survey exposes hospitals' knowing failure to prepare for a Covid-19 surge during flu season." National Nurses United (Nov. 2020). Accessed May 9, 2022. https://www.nationalnursesunited.org/press/national-nurse-survey-4-exposes- hospitals-knowing-failure-prepare-covid-19-surge.

National Nurses United. "National nurse survey reveals that health care employers need to do more to comply with OSHA emergency temporary standard." National Nurses United (Sept. 2021). Accessed May 9, 2022. https://www.nationalnursesunited.org/press/national- nurse-survey-reveals-health-care-employers-need-to-do-more-to-protect-workers.

- Only 32 percent of hospital RNs reported that their employer has sufficient PPE stock to protect staff from a rapid Covid surge.
- Less than a quarter (24 percent) of hospital RNs reported that their employer notifies them of Covid-19 exposures in a timely manner.
- 17.8 percent of RNs report that access to testing has declined since the beginning of the pandemic.
- Only 24 percent of hospital RNs reported that their employer has an overflow plan to place additional, trained staff to safely care for Covid patients in isolation.[70]

Intentional Understaffing and Lack of Resources Leads to Moral Injury, Moral Distress, and Emotional Exhaustion for RNs and Other Health Care Workers

With the onset of the pandemic, the hospital industry compounded the issues discussed above by its flagrant refusal to protect nurses from exposure and infection from Covid-19, treating RNs as disposable. Nurses caring for Covid patients experience both high rates of infections and deaths and high rates of acute stress, anxiety, depression, and post-traumatic stress as well as moral distress and moral injury, causing them to leave the bedside at high rates. NNU describes in more detail nurse experiences on the pandemic's front lines, the failures of health care employers to protect nurses and our patients, and the impact on nurses in our report, "Deadly Shame: Redressing the Devaluation of Registered Nurse Labor Through Pandemic Equity."[71]

During the pandemic, nurses have experienced high levels of distress due to fears of contracting Covid-19 or infecting their family members. Nurses have also experienced moral distress because crisis standards of care implemented by their employers prevent them from providing optimal patient care. For example, throughout the pandemic, employer policies of PPE rationing have led to care rationing, forcing nurses to provide care in unsafe practice conditions in conflict with their professional obligations to provide safe, therapeutic care to their patients.

---

[70] National Nurses United. "National nurse survey reveals significant increases in unsafe staffing, workplace violence, and moral distress." National Nurses United (Apr. 2022). Accessed May 9, 2022. https://www.nationalnursesunited.org/press/survey-reveals-increases-in-unsafe-staffing-workplace-violence-moral-distress.

[71] National Nurses United. "Deadly Shame: Redressing the Devaluation of Registered Nurse Labor Through Pandemic Equity." National Nurses United (Dec. 2020). Accessed May 9, 2022. https://www.nationalnursesunited.org/sites/default/files/nnu/graphics/documents/1220_Covid19_DeadlyShame_PandemicEquity_WhitePaper_FINAL.pdf.

Key findings from NNU's most recent survey of RNs demonstrate how the impact of the pandemic and employers' failures to protect nurses are long-lasting beyond the physical toll of Covid-19 infection, hospitalization, and death. From NNU's February and March 2022 survey results, RNs reported the following:

- 66.8 percent of hospital RNs fear they will contract Covid-19.
- Nearly three-quarters (74.6 percent) are afraid they will infect a family member.
- Nearly 60 percent (58.4 percent) are having more difficulty sleeping.
- 83.5 percent feel stressed more often than before the pandemic.
- 77.2 percent feel anxious more often than they did before the pandemic.
- 68.7 percent feel sad or depressed more often than they did before the pandemic.
- More than half (56 percent) feel traumatized by their experiences caring for patients.
- 23 percent sought treatment for a mental health condition related to caring for patients during the pandemic.[72]

Medicare for All is the Solution to Pandemic Readiness and the Future of Public Health

The Covid-19 pandemic provided a clear reason for Congress to act decisively and expediently to end our fragmented system of profit-driven health insurance and implement Medicare for All. With Medicare for All, hospitals and our health care system would have been better prepared to respond to Covid-19 with adequate beds, equipment, and staffing levels needed to respond to the pandemic, and our health care system would have been better coordinated to respond to outbreaks more effectively and to stop them from happening in the first place. As a coordinator of pandemic response, the Medicare for All program also could have been the centralized purchaser of

[72] National Nurses United. "National nurse survey reveals significant increases in unsafe staffing, workplace violence, and moral distress." National Nurses United (Apr. 2022). Accessed May 9, 2022. https://www.nationalnursesunited.org/press/survey-reveals-increases-in-unsafe-staffing-workplace-violence-moral-distress.

PPE and other supplies rather than having hospitals, counties, and states bid against each other for supplies, driving up costs.

Importantly, Medicare for All would address underlying disparities in health and health access, which greatly contributed to the disparate racial, ethnic, and other impacts of the pandemic. By ensuring health care funding and resources are equitably distributed across the country, historically underfunded safety-net providers would be fully resourced in every community, ultimately reducing and managing chronic conditions that left people more susceptible to Covid-19.

The Medicare for All Act of 2022 also includes several provisions that are relevant to pandemic readiness and infectious disease response.

Pandemic Preparedness Funding in National Health Budget

The bill requires the Secretary of Health and Human Services to "establish and maintain a reserve fund to respond to the costs of treating an epidemic, pandemic, natural disaster, or other such health emergency" within the national health budget.[73] With Medicare for All, the country would also have more equitably addressed the pandemic and avoided the disproportionate deaths and infections in Native American, Black, and Latinx communities because health care would be accessible to all without financial barriers to care.

PPE Stockpile and Pandemic Preparedness Funding in Hospital Global Budgets

With Medicare for All, our hospitals and health care facilities would have been better prepared to respond to Covid-19 with sufficient nurses, doctors, respiratory therapists, and other staff as well as beds, equipment, and medical supplies. Global budget payments to hospitals and other institutional providers include several provisions related to pandemic preparedness, including funding for "[c]osts for infectious disease response preparedness, including maintenance of a 1-year […] stockpile of personal protective equipment, occupational testing and surveillance, medical services for occupational infectious disease exposure, and contact tracing."[74]

Under Medicare for All, hospitals and other health care facilities would have had reliable funding for supplies and equipment needed to respond to the pandemic. Nurses and other health care workers would not have unnecessarily

---

[73] Medicare for All of 2022 § 601(a)(5).
[74] Medicare for All of 2022 § 611(d)(1)(D).

become infected, been hospitalized, and died from Covid-19 because health care employers failed to provide necessary PPE and other precautions that would have kept them and their patients safe.

Funding for Emergent or Unexpected Infectious Disease Outbreaks
Finally, under Medicare for All, we could have more effectively targeted funding for emergent Covid-19 outbreaks and inequities in pandemic response. The bill includes funding for hospitals in the global budgets provision for costs related to infectious disease outbreaks.[75] The bill also allows hospitals and other health care facilities to request interim funding and additional funding in upcoming budgets, ensuring the Medicare for All program can effectively and quickly direct emergency funds to hospitals based on need due to in community outbreaks.

Medicare for All Act of 2022: Program Design

How Would the Government Administer a Single-Payer Health Plan?

- *Federal Governance.* The Secretary of the U.S. Department of Health and Human Services (Secretary) would oversee the Medicare for All Program (Program) at the federal level and would be responsible for developing policies, procedures, and regulations to carry it out. In so doing, the Secretary would consult with a broad range of entities including federal agencies, professional organizations, and labor unions. Program accountability measures include requiring the Secretary to provide annual reports to Congress and audits by the U.S. Comptroller General every 5 years.[76]
- *Regional Administration.* The Secretary would establish regional offices and appoint regional directors as well as deputy directors to represent Native American and Alaska Native tribes in each region. The Secretary would incorporate the existing offices of the Centers for Medicare & Medicaid Services (CMS) where possible. The regional directors would be responsible for performing health care needs assessments, recommending changes in provider payments,

[75] Medicare for All of 2022 § 611(a)(4)(A)(ii) and Sec. 611(b)(2)(G).
[76] Medicare for All Act of 2022 §§ 401-404.

and establishing quality assurance mechanisms in their respective regions. Finally, the Secretary would appoint a beneficiary ombudsman to receive complaints and grievances and provide assistance to individuals entitled to Program benefits.[77]

Who Would Be Eligible for the Plan, and How Would People Enroll?

- *Four-year eligibility phase-in.* The Program has a four-year transition period. In the first year, persons under the age of 19 and over the age of 55 would be eligible for Medicare. In the second year, persons over the age of 45 would be eligible for Medicare, and in the third year, persons over the age of 35. In the fourth year, all people living in the United States would be eligible for full benefits under the Medicare for All Program.[78]
- *Enrollment.* The Program would include a mechanism for automatic enrollment at birth and upon immigration into the U.S. or attainment of qualified resident status. Eligible individuals would be able to enroll for benefits and obtain a Medicare card in order to receive services under the Program. The Program could build on the current Medicare enrollment system.[79]

What Health Care Services Would the Plan Cover?

- *Universal benefits.* Current Medicare benefits would be expanded and improved in order to provide comprehensive health care coverage to all Program enrollees.[80]
- *Comprehensive benefits.* The benefits would include all primary and preventive care; hospital and outpatient services; prescription drugs; dental; vision; audiology; women's reproductive health services; maternity and newborn care; long-term services and supports, including home and community based services and supports; pediatrics, including early and periodic screening, diagnostic, and

[77] Medicare for All Act of 2022 §§ 401-404.
[78] Medicare for All Act of 2022 §§ 106, 1002.
[79] Medicare for All Act of 2022 § 105.
[80] Medicare for All Act of 2022 §§ 201, 204.

treatment services; prescription drugs; mental health and substance abuse treatment; laboratory and diagnostic services; emergency services; and more.[81]

What Cost Sharing, if Any, Would the Plan Require?

The plan prohibits cost sharing for all covered benefits. No premiums, deductibles, coinsurance, copayments, or balance billing are allowed except for high-and middle-income families some cost-sharing for prescription drugs may be permitted but capped at $200 per year.[82]

What Role Would Private Health Insurance Have?

The bill allows private health insurance coverage only for benefits that are not covered under the Program but prohibits private health insurance coverage for covered benefits. Because the Program provides comprehensive benefits and coverage, private health insurance is expected to have only a small role (e.g., non-medically necessary care or for international tourists).[83]

What Role Would Other Public Programs Have?

After the four-year transition period, all those receiving health care coverage through Medicare, Medicaid, the State Children's Health Insurance Program, or health marketplaces established under the Patient Protection and Affordable Care Act would be covered by the Medicare for All Program.

These programs would sunset. School-related health programs and existing medical benefits or services under the Department of Veteran Affairs and the Indian Health Service would be maintained, though veterans and Native Americans would also be entitled to full Program benefits.[84]

---

[81] Medicare for All Act of 2022 §§ 201, 204.
[82] Medicare for All Act of 2022 § 202.
[83] Medicare for All Act of 2022 § 107.
[84] Medicare for All Act of 2022 §§ 901, 902.

What Rules Would Participating Providers Be Required to Follow?

To become a participating provider under the Program, the provider must be eligible to participate and must enter into a participation agreement with the Secretary which includes, as described below, disclosure requirements and other checks on provider participation.[85]

- *Provider qualifications.* Providers are qualified to participate in the Program if they have the requisite license from the state in which they practice and meet minimum provider standards adopted by the Program, including adequate facilities, safe staffing, and patient access. Providers are only eligible to be participating providers for care that they provide directly to individuals.[86]
- *Private contracting limitations.* Participating providers are prohibited from entering into private contracts for covered services with individuals eligible for Program benefits. Any provider that furnishes covered services through a private contract will be ineligible to participate in the Program for one year. Participating providers may enter into private contracts with individuals who are ineligible to enroll in the Program and may enter into contracts with any individual for noncovered services. Disclosure requirements are established for private contracts.[87]
- *Prohibitions on discrimination.* Providers are prohibited from denying benefits, reducing benefits, or otherwise discriminating against patients based on race, color, national origin, age, disability, marital status, citizenship status, primary language use, genetic conditions, previous or existing medical conditions, religion, or sex, including sex stereotyping, gender identity, sexual orientation, and pregnancy and related medical conditions including termination of pregnancy.[88]
- *Prohibition on balance billing.* Participating providers are prohibited from balance billing or otherwise charging a Program enrollee for any covered benefit.[89]
- *Data reporting requirements.* Participating providers are required to furnish information necessary for establishing reimbursements,

[85] Medicare for All Act of 2022 § 301.
[86] Medicare for All Act of 2022 § 302.
[87] Medicare for All Act of 2022 § 303.
[88] Medicare for All Act of 2022 §§ 104, 301(b).
[89] Medicare for All Act of 2022 § 202(b), 301(b).

quality review, and other data reporting, including current data reported under Medicare or state programs, data on costs, quality, outcomes, health equity, and financial data.[90]

- *Application of existing anti-fraud and abuse statutes.* The bill applies existing Medicare and Medicaid measures against provider fraud and abuse to the Program, including prohibitions on self-referrals.[91]
- *Prohibited uses of reimbursements.* To ensure that provider reimbursements are used for the provision of benefits under the Program, the bill prohibits program funds from being used for compensation for any institutional provider employee, contractor, or subcontractor above existing compensation caps established for federal contractors under the Bipartisan Budget Act of 2013.[92]

Who Would Own the Hospitals and Employ the Providers?

Hospital ownership and provider employment would be unchanged. Thus, most of the health care delivery system would remain in the private sector.

How Would a Single-Payer System Pay Providers and Set Payment Rates?

- *National Health Budget.* The Secretary would establish a national health budget that would be allocated regionally. Regional allocations would include payments for the region's providers, capital expenditures, special projects, health professional education, administrative expenses, and prevention and public health activities.
- *Institutional Providers & Global Budgeting.* Institutional providers — including hospitals, skilled nursing facilities, and independent dialysis facilities — would negotiate an annual lump sum global operating budget with the regional director which would be paid on a quarterly basis.[93] The global operating budget would be based on:

---

[90] Medicare for All Act of 2022 §§ 301(b), 401(b)(1).
[91] Medicare for All Act of 2022 § 411.
[92] Medicare for All Act of 2022 § 611(b)(4).
[93] Medicare for All Act of 2022 §§ 611-615.

- the historical volume of services in the previous 3-year period and provider capacity,
- the actual expenditures as compared to other providers within the region and normative payment rates to be established,
- projected changes in volume and type of items and services to be furnished,
- employee wages,
- education and prevention programs, and
- other relevant factors and adjustments.

Each regional director would review institutional providers' performance on a quarterly basis and determine whether adjustments to the budget are needed, including additional funding needed for unanticipated care for individuals with complex medical needs or for changes in the market.

Providers would be able to request at any time interim adjustments of their global budget allocation if the provider incurs unanticipated costs or costs out of their control, including natural disasters, outbreaks of epidemics or infectious diseases; unexpected facility or equipment repairs or purchases; significant and unexpected increases in pharmaceutical or medical device prices; and unanticipated increases in complex or high-cost patients or care needs. Interim adjustments to provider global budgets would also be made for any reasonable increases in labor costs, including changes in collective bargaining agreements, prevailing wages, or local law.

- Individual Providers & Group Practices.[94]
    - *Fee Schedule.* Individual providers, including those in medical group practices, would be paid on a fee-for-service basis using a national fee schedule established by the Secretary. The fee schedule would consider the prevailing rates under Medicare, provider expertise, and the value of the items and services furnished. The bill establishes both a standardized documentation and review process of the relative values of physician services to determine appropriate fee payments and a physician consultation review board to review quality, cost effectiveness, and fair reimbursement of services and items delivered by physicians.

[94] Medicare for All Act of 2022 §§ 611-615.

- *Option for Salaried Payments.* However, as determined by the Secretary, certain group practices and other health care providers with agreements to provide health care services at a specific institutional provider may choose to be paid a salary through such institutional provider's global budget instead of on a fee-for-service basis.
- Addressing Health Inequities and Disparities.[95]
    - *Office of Health Equity.* The Office of Health Equity would be established within the Department of Health and Human Services to improve services in medically underserved areas and to address health disparities based on race, ethnicity, geography, Tribal affiliation, national origin, primary language use, English proficiency status, immigration status, length of stay in the U.S., age, disability, sex (including gender identity and sexual orientation), incarceration, homelessness, or other socioeconomic status.

      The Director of the Office of Health Equity would develop, coordinate, and promote policies to enhance health equity, including ensuring adequate public funding to address health disparities at the local and State levels and recommending training on cultural competency, increases in the diversity of the health care workforce, and programs to ensure sufficient levels of health care professionals and facilities to address health disparities.
- *Office of Primary Care.* The Office of Primary Care would be established within the Office of Health Equity to increase access to high-quality primary health care, particularly in medically underserved areas and for underserved populations, and to address health disparities with respect to race, ethnicity, national origin, primary language use, English proficiency status, length of stay in the U.S., age, disability, sex (including gender identity and sexual orientation), incarceration, homelessness, or other socioeconomic status.

  The Director of the Office of Primary Care would develop, coordinate, and promote policies on health professional education and training to address primary care health disparities; to increase primary health care practitioners, registered nurses, mid-level practitioners,

[95] Medicare for All Act of 2022 §§ 615-616.

and dentists; to recommend programs targeted towards Federally Qualified Health Centers, rural health centers, community health centers, and other community-based organizations; and on other programs to address primary care health inequities.

How Would the Single-Payer System Purchase Prescription Drugs?

The Secretary would negotiate prices for prescription drugs and establish a formulary system that encourages the use of generic medications to the greatest extent possible.[96]

How Would a Single-Payer System Contain Health Care Costs?

Studies have shown that Medicare for All would not only contain costs but would also save the country up to $5.1 trillion over 10 years.[97] Conservative estimates by the Mercatus Center found that the U.S. would save more than $2 trillion over a ten-year period under Medicare for All.[98] Specifically, the Medicare for All Act of 2022 contains costs and produces savings primarily by reducing administrative costs, negotiating prescription drug and medical device prices, and controlling provider payments.

- *Administrative Costs.* Under our current fragmented, multi-payer system, we spend about 31 percent of total health expenditures on administrative costs. This amounted to an estimated $1.1 trillion in 2017.[99] Implementing a single-payer system with a single,

---

[96] Medicare for All Act of 2022 § 614.

[97] Pollin, R. et al. "Economic Analysis of Medicare for All." Political Economy Research Institute, University of Massachusetts Amherst (Nov. 2018). Accessed May 9, 2022. https://www.peri.umass.edu/publication/item/1127-economic-analysis-of-medicare-for-all.

[98] Blahous, C. "The Costs of a National Single-Payer Healthcare System." Mercatus Working Paper. Mercatus Center, George Mason University: Arlington, VA (Jul. 2018). Accessed May 9, 2022. https://www.mercatus.org/system/files/blahous-costs-medicare-mercatus- working-paper-v1_1.pdf.

[99] Woolhandler, S., Himmelstein, D. "Single-Payer Reform: The Only Way to Fulfill the President's Pledge of More Coverage, Better Benefits, and Lower Costs." *Ann. Intern. Med.* (2017) 166(8): 587-588. According to the Centers for Medicare and Medicaid Services, national health expenditures was $3,492.1 billion in 2017. Centers for Medicare and Medicaid Services. "National Health Expenditure Accounts (2017)." U.S. Department of Health and Human Services. Accessed May 9, 2022. https://www.cms.gov/research-statistics-data-and-

comprehensive benefits plan would create uniformity in claims and billing processing. Insurer costs — such as costs associated with care denial and containment, marketing, profit, and executive compensation — would be eliminated. Health care providers would no longer need large billing departments nor have to spend time to manage numerous insurance cost-sharing schemes, collect unpaid bills from the uninsured and the underinsured, or obtain preauthorization for tests and treatments.

- *Prescription Drug and Medical Device Prices.* The Secretary would wield tremendous bargaining power by negotiating on behalf of the entire U.S. population. This would enable the Secretary to drive down costs for prescription drugs and medical devices.
- *Provider Payments.* As the single-payer, the Medicare for All Program would have the power to regulate provider payments. Payment inequities would also be addressed; some providers would see their reimbursement rates reduced[100] while others who are currently undervalued, such as primary care and mental health care professionals, would see their rates increased.
    - *Institutional providers* — Massive consolidation among private hospitals and other institutional providers, as well as the acquisition of physician practices, have enabled some health systems to charge exorbitant prices, while hospitals in rural and underserved areas close and funding for public hospitals dwindles. Under the Program, large conglomerate health systems would see their bargaining power and their ability to extract exorbitant reimbursement rates diminished, while safety-net hospitals would see reimbursement rates increase and funding stabilize.
    - *Health care professionals* — Rates also may change based on the type of medicine a physician or other health care professional practices. The bill addresses a pay inequity that undervalues the cognitive-based services that primary care physicians provide and overvalues procedure-based services that specialists tend to

---

systems/statistics-trends-and-reports/nationalhealthexpenddata/nationalhealthaccountshistorical.html.

100 As discussed above, reductions in reimbursement rates for the currently high-valued providers that may see decreases in rates would be offset by significant administrative and time savings for the provider.

provide[101] by establishing a review process of the relative values of physician services to review quality, cost effectiveness, and fair reimbursement of services and items delivered by physicians.[102]

How Would a Single-Payer System Be Financed?

Current U.S. expenditures provide sufficient funding for the Program, but they must be captured in a new way. Amounts equal to federal expenditures for programs that the bill sunsets — including Medicare, Medicaid, the State Children's Health Insurance Program, and the ACA marketplaces — would be deposited annually into a newly established Universal Medicare Trust Fund. These deposits would be adjusted annually for cost savings resulting from implementation of the Program and for changes in the consumer price index. Although the bill does not specify how the balance of the national expenditures would be financed, there are many options. These could include a corporate gross receipts tax, progressive personal income tax, financial transaction tax, and repealing the corporate tax cuts passed in 2017.[103]

Medicare for All Act of 2022: Ensuring Access to Care

The Medicare for All Act of 2022, which would establish the Medicare for All Program (Program) includes key design features to eliminate barriers to care that occur in our current health system and to ensure that new barriers to care are not created.

Ending Wait Times and Rationing due to Unaffordability

- Wait times and rationing occur today under our system of private insurance. Health insurers create financial and administrative barriers to care, including cost-sharing, deductibles, prior authorization, and

---

[101] Goodson, J. D. "Patient Protection and Affordable Care Act: Promise and Peril for Primary Care." *Ann Intern Med.* (2010), 152(11):742-744.
[102] Medicare for All Act of 2022 §§ 612-613.
[103] Medicare for All Act of 2022 § 701.

step therapy, to limit the financial risk to corporate returns. As a result, people delay seeking medical care or filling a prescription because they cannot afford it. Even those who have insurance delay care because they cannot afford the copayments, coinsurance, or deductibles.

- Because financial barriers imposed by premiums, deductibles, and cost-sharing would be eliminated under the Medicare for All Program, delays in care because of affordability, which are common in our current private insurance system and public programs, would no longer occur.

Emphasizing Primary Care and Prevention to Reduce Demand for Emergency or Specialist Care

Medicare for All emphasizes primary care and prevention rather than waiting to treat illnesses that must be addressed by a specialist or require hospitalization. With increased access to and use of primary and preventive care, people will be more likely to seek care before their health conditions become severe enough to require the high-cost acute, emergency, or specialty care that currently represents half of the country's health care spending.[104]

The bill would establish an Office of Primary Care that would focus on increasing the supply of primary care providers — for example, by paying for these providers' medical education — as well as evaluating payments to physicians, including primary care physicians. Doctors would be more likely to enter into primary or family care practices if they were not saddled with massive debt for their education and the gap between primary and specialty care reimbursement narrowed.

Creating Reliable Sources of Funding for Hospitals and Strengthening Our Safety-Net Health Care Institutions

- The Medicare for All Act of 2022's reimbursement and budget structures are designed to create reliable funding streams for hospitals

[104] *See* Agency for Healthcare Research and Quality. "Medical Expenditure Panel Survey, Total expenditures in millions by condition, United States, 2015." U.S. Department of Health and Human Services (2015).

and other institutional providers. Reimbursing hospitals through global budgeting aligns hospital payments with actual costs. Programming under the Office of Primary Care and Office of Health Equity would be targeted to increase staffing and to improve facility capacity in medically underserved and high social vulnerability index areas.

- Medicare for All would ensure that safety-net health care institutions would be sufficiently funded. Through transparent reimbursement negotiations, the Program would ensure that variations in provider prices are no longer exacerbating health and health care inequality. The Program's global budgeting and reimbursement structure is designed to create reliable and stable funding streams for hospitals and other institutional providers. The Office of Primary Care and Office of Health Equity would establish programs to ensure that safety-net hospitals and other providers in rural and urban underserved areas have sufficient resources and staffing to meet demand in their areas.

In the long-term, Medicare for All will more fairly and effectively distribute care across the system, funding and directing health care resources where they are needed most and where health inequities have been identified. The Program could use Office of Primary Care and Office of Health Equity funds to increase staffing and expand provider capacity in rural or underserved areas. Through global budgeting reviews and adjustments, regional directors can increase funding for hospitals with increases in patient care populations or that need resources to respond to new or emerging public health conditions.

Attracting Provider Participation by Capturing Demand in a Single Patient Pool under Medicare for All

- Medicare for All strongly encourages providers to participate in Medicare for All by capturing everyone in the pool of patients and by prohibiting private plans with duplicate coverage. In other words, the Program is designed to capture all health care demand (through comprehensive benefits and no cost-sharing). Operating as a nonparticipating provider would not be a suitable option for the vast majority of providers.

Prohibitions on Private Contracting to Prevent Tiered Access to Care

- As the Congressional Budget Office noted in its 2019 report on single-payer health system design, wait times may result if a single-payer system allows providers to provide private care or simultaneously see patients with substitutive private plans alongside public plan patients.[105] By limiting both substitutive private plans and private contracting, the Medicare for All Act of 2022 avoids these issues and stops providers from offering two tiers of services where individuals can pay to jump the queue ahead of Medicare for All enrollees.
- Medicare for All also prevents providers from creating tiered waiting lines for care by placing strict limits on when a participating provider can see non-Medicare for All patients and by prohibiting participating providers from entering into private contracts for covered services. If a provider furnishes covered services through a private contract, they will be ineligible to participate in the Medicare for All Program for one year.

Increasing Access to Health Care Professionals

- The Medicare for All Program directs resources into educating new health care professionals to enter into the system by including in the national budget a component for health professional education expenditures to cover costs associated with clinical education of new health care professionals.
- Under Medicare for All, precious time that doctor, nurses, and other health care providers currently spend on billing, coding, and interacting with health plans would be freed up, allowing providers to do more of what they do best — care for patients. Medicare for All would simplify the administrative process for doctors and other providers by having one payer.

---

105 Congressional Budget Office. "Key Design Components and Considerations for Establishing a Single-Pager Health Care System." CBO Publications (May 2019), pp. 13, 23.

Medicare for All Act of 2022: Eliminating Health and Health Care Disparities

Despite spending more on health care per capita than any other country in the world,[106] the United States has extreme health and health care disparities, including disparities related to race, ethnicity, income, gender, and location. The Medicare for All Act of 2022 addresses key contributing factors to health and health care disparities, including health care coverage, access to health care providers and facilities, linguistically and culturally competent care, and quality of care.[107]

The Medicare for All Act of 2022 would begin addressing health and health care disparities by providing universal health care coverage and improving health care access. Unlike our current market-driven system, the Medicare for All Act would ensure access to high quality, therapeutic health care for all individuals in every community in the United States, including rural and urban areas that are currently medically underserved. The Medicare for All Act provides comprehensive health care benefits to all without regard to the ability to pay and without premiums, deductibles, copayments, or other out-of-pocket costs.[108] This would remove the financial and administrative barriers to care created by private insurers seeking to extract profit at the cost of our health.

Currently, many Black, Indigenous, and people of color (BIPOC) and low-income communities face outdated and overcrowded hospitals and clinics, hospital closures, and staffing crises for nurses, doctors, psychologists, and other health care professionals. The Medicare for All Act of 2022 would ensure that our safety-net and critical access hospitals, both rural and urban, are sufficiently resourced and staffed so that all communities are able to promote good health and provide therapeutic care for everyone. Moreover, the Medicare for All Act contains provisions, discussed below, to ensure diversity

---

106 Organization for Economic Cooperation and Development. "Health at a Glance 2021." (2021). Accessed May 9, 2022. https://www.oecd- ilibrary.org/social-issues-migration-health/health-at-a-glance-2021_ae3016b9-en.

107 Ndugga, N., Artiga, S. "Disparities in Health and Health Care: 5 Key Questions and Answers." Kaiser Family foundation (May 11, 2021). Accessed May 9, 2022. https://www.kff.org/racial-equity-and-health-policy/issue-brief/disparities-in-health-and-health-care-5-key-question- and-answers/.

108 There is one exception that allows minimal cost-sharing. The Health and Human Services Secretary may impose copayments for non-preventive prescription medications totaling a maximum of $200 annually for individuals with a household income above 200 percent of the poverty line.

among health care professionals and improve cultural and linguistic competency across the health care workforce.

The sections below lay out the various provisions in the Medicare for All Act of 2022 that address health and health care disparities.

Non-Discrimination in Health Care Services

The Medicare for All Act of 2022 includes robust protections against discrimination by providers and non-discrimination in the provision of benefits, including prohibitions on discrimination based on "race, color, national origin, age, disability, marital status, citizenship status, primary language use, genetic conditions, previous or existing medical conditions, religion, or sex, including sex stereotyping, gender identity, sexual orientation, and pregnancy and related medical conditions[.]"[109]

Establishment of the Office of Health Equity

Section 615 would create the Office of Health Equity which would oversees monitoring, tracking, and availability of data regarding:

- the disproportionate burden of disease and death among people of color,[110]
- barriers to health,
- barriers to health care access,
- disparities in quality of care received, and
- disparities in utilization of care.

As the Office of Health Equity would "ensure coordination and collaboration across the programs and activities of the Department of Health

---

[109] Medicare for All Act of 2022 § 104.

[110] Section 615 of the Medicare for All Act of 2022 requires that data be disaggregated by race, major ethnic group, Tribal affiliation, national origin, primary language use, English proficiency status, immigration status, length of stay in the United States age, disability, sex (including gender identity and sexual orientation), incarceration, homelessness, geography, and socioeconomic status. The data also allows granular analysis across multiple identities categories to differentiate, for example, among various racial, ethnic, and Tribal groups broken down by sex or sexual orientation. Additionally, the bill provides public access to the data, strong privacy protections.

and Human Services with respect to ensuring health equity[,]" all of these issues can be addressed by the Medicare for All program as well as other health and social service programs within the Department of Health and Human Services (HHS).[111]

The Office of Health Equity would use the data it collects to establish policies to improve health equity. These policies include ensuring that there are sufficient health care providers and facilities, increasing cultural competency and diversity in the health care workforce, and providing the health care workforce training on implicit bias and ethics. Importantly, the Office of Health Equity would ensure that states and localities have sufficient public health funding to address health disparities.

The Medicare for All Act of 2022 would also establish an Office of Primary Health within the Office of Health Equity to focus on increasing "access to high-quality primary health care, particularly in underserved areas and for underserved populations"[112] as a critical step to addressing health disparities. To meet these goals, the Director of the Office of Primary Health would work with the HHS Secretary to develop policies regarding health professional education to increase the number of primary health care providers and to increase resources for health centers in underserved rural and urban areas.

National Health Budget and Funding Provisions

The Medicare for All Act provides a national health budget and funding provisions that would effectuate the policies and goals established by the Office of Health Equity.[113]

General Principles

- Allocated regionally, the national health budget includes funding for quality assessment; operating expenses; public health and prevention activities; health professional education; and capital expenses such as renovating facilities or building new ones or purchasing major equipment. Health and health care disparities would be considered in funding each of these components.

---

[111] Medicare for All Act of 2022 § 615.

[112] Medicare for All Act of 2022 § 616. Additional information on underserved areas and populations is discussed below.

[113] *See* Medicare for All of 2022 §§ 401, 502, 601.

- Funding would be provided based on regional needs as determined by data and other information provided by the Office of Health Equity[114] and state-based health care needs assessment reports created "in consultation with public health officials, clinicians, patients, and patient advocates[.]"[115] Funding allocation also would be based on "[d]ifferences in the health status of the populations of the different States, including income and racial characteristics, and other population health inequities[.]"[116]
- Funding would address ways to improve service to medically underserved areas and populations. Medically underserved areas are geographically defined areas (both rural and urban) with a shortage of primary care services. Medically underserved populations are sub-groups of people living within a geographic area that face cultural or linguistic barriers. Examples of a medically underserved population include people who are unhoused, low-income, Medicaid-eligible, Native American, or migrant farm workers.[117] Medically underserved areas and populations are based on their scores on the Index of Medical Underservice which is calculated based on four criteria: the ratio of providers to the population, the percentage of the population with income below the federal poverty level, the percentage of the population over the age of 65, and the infant mortality rate.[118]

Funding for Institutional Providers' Operating Expenses

- The Medicare for All Act of 2022 pays institutional health care providers such as hospitals and affiliated outpatient facilities, skilled nursing facilities, and dialysis centers through global operating budgets that are paid quarterly in a lump sum to cover employee wages and benefits, medical supplies, overhead, and health professional education but would exclude capital expenses such as

---

[114] In addition to the data collection requirements under Section 615, Sections 401 and 502 contain detailed reporting requirements on health and health care disparities based on race, ethnicity, gender, geography, and socioeconomic status so that funding can be directed where needed.

[115] Medicare for All Act of 2022 § 403(c)(1).

[116] Medicare for All Act of 2022 § 401(b)(2)(I).

[117] Health Resources and Services Administration. "Medically Underserved Areas and Populations (MUA/Ps)." U.S. Department of Health & Human Services (Last reviewed February 2021). Accessed May 9, 2022. https://bhw.hrsa.gov/shortage-designation/muap.

[118] Health Resources and Services Administration. "Scoring Shortage Designations." U.S. Department of Health & Human Services (Last reviewed December 2020). Accessed May 9, 2022. https://bhw.hrsa.gov/workforce-shortage-areas/shortage-designation/scoring.

renovating facilities or building new ones as well as purchasing major equipment.

- The Medicare for All bill prioritizes addressing health care disparities through the provider payment process. As one factor in determining the global budget payment, the Medicare for All Act includes "whether the provider is located in a high social vulnerability index community, zip code, op census track, or is a minority-service provider[.]"[119] It explicitly allows for adjustments to the lump-sum payments for "efforts to decrease health care disparities in rural or medically underserved areas"[120] (defined above). Payments for medically underserved areas or areas with high social vulnerability could include increased funding to hire more staff; pay compensation differentials to attract and retain health care professionals; extend operating hours; improve patient care, education, and prevention programs; or purchase additional medical supplies.

Funding of Provider Capital Expenses

Funding for capital expenses to purchase, lease, build, or renovate health care facilities or major equipment would be provided based on regional needs as determined by data provided by the Office of Health Equity[121] and state-based health care needs assessment reports created "in consultation with public health officials, clinicians, patients, and patient advocates[.]"[122]

Publicly-funded facilities — such as safety net hospitals and clinics — have been seriously underfunded leaving many BIPOC, low-income, and rural communities with overcrowded facilities or no facilities at all. Under the Medicare for All Act, funding for capital expenses would be allocated based on need — with the express aim of reducing, and ultimately eliminating, health care disparities — rather than on maximizing revenue. This creates a strong foundation for publicly funded health care facilities.

---

[119] Medicare for All Act of 2022 § 611(b)(2)(H). The CDC's social vulnerability index includes four themes: socioeconomic status, race/ethnicity/language, household composition, and housing/transportation. For more information, see: Centers for Disease Control and Prevention. "What is the CDC/ATSDR Social Vulnerability Index?" U.S. Department of Health & Human Services. (Last reviewed August 30, 2021). Accessed May 9, 2022. https://www.atsdr.cdc.gov/placeandhealth/svi/fact_sheet/fact_sheet.html.

[120] Medicare for All Act of 2022 § 611(b)(2)(G)(ii).

[121] In addition to the data collection requirements under Section 615, Sections 401 and 502 contain detailed reporting requirements on health and health care disparities based on race, ethnicity, gender, geography, and socioeconomic status so that funding can be directed where needed.

[122] Medicare for All Act of 2022 § 403(c)(1).

In contrast, current private funding for renovating or building new health care facilities and purchasing major equipment generally is based on whether, and how quickly, the expense will be recouped based on the revenue it generates. Thus, privately owned or funded organizations, even those that are not-for-profit, typically favor investing in affluent suburban and urban neighborhoods where people have more generous health plans and low numbers of uninsured people.

Funding for Health Professional Education

- The bill requires the HHS Secretary to allocate the budget in a way that "ensures that the health professional education expenditure component is sufficient to provide for the amount of health professional education expenditures sufficient to meet the need for covered health care services."
- Funding could be used to provide scholarships for health professionals, loan repayment in exchange for practicing in medically underserved areas or in areas with underserved populations or a shortage of health care professionals, and other programs.

Medicare for All Act of 2022: Global Budgets & Other Provider Reimbursements

Medicare for All: Putting Patient Care over Pocketbooks

The program outlined in the Medicare for All Act of 2022, takes several steps to ensure that providers can focus on patient care rather than on their pocketbooks.

- *Less Time on Billing, More Time for Patients.* Medicare for All would simplify the administrative process for doctors and other providers by having one payer. Precious time that doctors and other health care providers spend on billing, coding, and dealing with health plans would be freed up, allowing providers to do what they do best — care for patients.
- *Negotiating Lower Prices.* Under the Medicare for All Program, health care corporations would no longer be able to overcharge for their services. By leveraging its buying power as the single-payer for

health care, the Medicare for All Program would be able to negotiate better, fairer health care prices for everyone. Reimbursement rates for hospitals and doctors will be based on negotiations with the regional directors. Negotiations over health care prices would include prescription drug price negotiations.

- *Health Care Dollars No Longer Line Pockets.* The Medicare for All Program would bar Medicare for All providers from siphoning off health care dollars to line their pockets. The Medicare for All Act of 2022 does so through limits on executive pay and checks on incentives for both underutilization and overutilization. Importantly, provider reimbursements are structured to address health care disparities and to ensure that reimbursements go towards the provision of care.

Global Budgeting for Hospitals & Other Institutional Providers

Under the Medicare for All Act, each hospital and each institutional provider — including skilled nursing facilities, and independent dialysis facilities — will be paid through an institution-specific "global budget."

- *Negotiated Annually.* Each global budget would be negotiated annually between institutional providers and regional directors. Institutional providers would receive a fixed annual allowance, paid and reviewed quarterly, to fund operating expenses related to furnishing health care to Medicare for All enrollees. Major factors included in negotiations are historical volume and costs of care, projected changes in volume and type of care, and wages for all employees, including physicians that work directly for the hospitals. Capital expenditures for costs such as renovating facilities or building new ones would be funded separately.
- *Interim Adjustments.* At any time, an institutional provider can request adjustment to their global budget to account for unanticipated increases in costs, including natural disasters, emergent epidemic conditions or infectious disease outbreaks, unanticipated facility or equipment repairs, unanticipated increases in pharmaceutical or equipment prices, reasonable increases in labor costs, such as changes

to collective bargaining agreements, changes in law, or other emergent conditions.

- *Aligning Hospital Reimbursements with Actual Costs.* Global budgeting simplifies the reimbursement system so that payments more closely reflect the actual costs of providing health care to the population served by each hospital and institutional provider.[123] The global budgeting process would allow the Medicare for All program to ensure that providers get the appropriate funding for the health care services that their patients need — providers would be accountable for their spending and would no longer be able to overcharge.
- *Simplification of Hospital Reimbursements.* By eliminating the billing process, global budgets result in administrative simplicity and associated savings for hospitals and other institutional providers. Information necessary to predict annual global budgets — including financial cost data, case mix, and volume of services — is readily available and already captured by hospitals and other institutions.[124] Additionally, this information is already reported to the Centers for Medicare and Medicaid Services in Medicare cost reports.
- *Transparent and Accountable Spending.* Global budgets allow the public to track where our health care dollars are going and to ensure that rural hospitals and hospitals in underserved areas are getting the funding that they need. Providers must report all relevant data associated with operational costs and justify their spending during annual negotiations. With periodic audits and review, providers would be held accountable for their projected spending and the program could monitor whether the provider is meeting program goals and standards. Budget shortfalls, unexpected or emergent public health conditions, or other marginal cost differences between planned and actual health care spending can be addressed through budget adjustments year-over-year or through quarterly reviews.
- *Funding Certainty for Hospitals Serving Vulnerable Communities.* Global budgets can be a blessing to hospitals that serve rural or underserved communities and that currently have inconsistent or undependable funding streams. Global budgets would ensure that our

---

[123] Dredge, R. *Hospital Global Budgeting*. World Bank Health Nutrition and Population Discussion Paper. World Bank (2004), pp. 37-38.

[124] *Id.* at pp.18, 37-38.

safety-net hospitals that provide care to low-income, rural, and minority communities are sufficiently funded and resourced.

- *International Use of Hospital Global Budgeting.* Many countries with publicly-funded health care — Canada, Scotland, Wales, New Zealand, Australia, Denmark, Sweden, Switzerland, Norway, Iceland, Ireland, and Singapore — use global budgets as key components of their hospital payment methodologies.[125]

Payment Options for Doctors & Medical Group Practices

There are two payment options for doctors and doctor groups under the Medicare for All Act of 2022 — reimbursements based on the Medicare fee schedule or salaries based on negotiated global budgets. The Secretary of the U.S. Department of Health and Human Services would establish a national fee schedule in consultation with doctors and regional directors. Instead of payments based on the national fee schedule, individual providers and group practices could opt to receive salaries through an institutional provider's global budgeting process.

Medicare for All Act of 2022: Cost & Savings Analyses

The tables below summarize the findings from three major cost and savings analyses of national implementation of Medicare for All. The first study was conducted by the Congressional Budget Office (CBO).[126] The second study was conducted by Charles Blahous with the Mercatus Center of George Mason University.[127] The third study was conducted by Robert Pollin and his colleagues at the Political Economy Research Institute (PERI) of the

---

125 *See* Mossialos, E., Tikkanen, R. et al. (Eds.). "International Profiles of Health Care Systems, 2020." The Commonwealth Fund (Dec. 2020). Accessed May 10, 2022. https://www.commonwealthfund.org/sites/default/files/2020-12/International_Profiles_of_Health_Care_Systems_Dec2020.pdf; Wolfe, P., Moran, D. "Global Budgeting in OECD Countries." *Health Care Fin. Rev.* (1993) Vol 14:3.

126 CBO's Single-Payer Health Care Systems Team. "How CBO Analyzes the Costs of Proposals for Single-Payer HealthCare Systems That Are Based on Medicare's Fee-for-Service Program." Working Paper 2020-08. Congressional Budget Office (Dec. 2020). Accessed May 10, 2022. https://www.cbo.gov/publication/56811.

127 Blahous, C. "The Costs of a National Single-Payer Healthcare System." Mercatus Center, George Mason University (2018). Accessed May 10, 2022. https://www.mercatus.org/system/files/blahous-costs-medicare-mercatus-working-paper-v1_1.pdf.

University of Massachusetts Amherst.[128] These three studies contain the most rigorous methodologies for analyzing potential savings in addition to increases in cost that would result from implementation of Medicare for All. They all show that a Medicare for All program would produce significant savings over the status quo.

All three studies show that the savings produced by Medicare for All would exceed increases in cost resulting from universal health care coverage. Findings in Blahous' analysis demonstrate that Medicare for All could result in $2.1 trillion in savings over 10 years in National Health Expenditures (Table 1).[129] Pollin's analysis found that Medicare for All would result in $5.1 trillion in savings over ten years (Table 1).[130] Unfortunately, the CBO does not calculate savings for a 10-year period. The CBO projects 1-year savings of $317 billion in 2030, Blahous projects 1-year savings of $93 billion in 2022, and Pollin projects 1-year savings of $310 billion in 2017.

Table 2 shows increases and savings for a 1-year period based on the largest expenditure categories. The major driver of increased costs is increased utilization of health care when everyone is insured and cost-sharing is dramatically reduced. The major areas for savings result from reductions in administrative costs, payments to providers, and prescription drugs. The CBO study finds that there could be a $583 billion increase in costs as a result of increased health care utilization, but Medicare for All would also capture $900 billion in savings in administration and reduced payment rates for providers (Table 2).[131] Blahous' study demonstrates that although Medicare for All would increase health care demand by $435 billion, the program would also produce $528 billion in savings on administration, pharmaceutical payments, and provider rates (Table 2).[132] Pollin's findings show that although there could be, on the high-end, a $390 billion increase in costs as a result of an increase in health care utilization, Medicare for All would also capture $643 billion in savings in administration, pharmaceutical payments, and provider rates (Table 2).[133]

---

[128] Pollin, R. et al. "Economic Analysis of Medicare for All." Political Economy Research Institute (PERI), University of Massachusetts Amherst (2018). Accessed May 10, 2022. https://www.peri.umass.edu/publication/item/1127-economic-analysis-of-medicare-for-all.

[129] Blahous (2018) at p. 7 (Summing projected National Health Expenditures for 2022-2031 from Table 2).

[130] Pollin (2018) at p. 3, 125-26.

[131] CBO's Single-Payer Health Care Systems Team (2020).

[132] *See* Blahous (2018) at p. 4 (Table 1).

[133] *See* Pollin (2018) at pp. 40-44 (adjusting percentages to reflect percentage savings of national health expenditures).

A second, recently published CBO study found that, under a Medicare for All health care system, people would live longer and be more productive as their health improved and workers' wages would increase as employers shifted savings from money previously spent on health insurance to wages.[134] Furthermore, long-term supports and services benefits (LTSS) would reduce household out-of-pocket costs, increase wages for workers in providing LTSS care, and allow family members currently proving care to work more hours in their paid jobs.[135] Finally, the CBO study found that reducing administrative costs, which Table 2 shows as the single largest category of savings from Medicare for All, would shift financial resources to other sectors and increase productivity across the economy.[136]

Table 1. Projected savings in national health expenditures: CBO, Blahous, & Pollin

	CBO	Blahous	Pollin
Projected Savings MFA (10 Years) in National Health Expenditures	NA	$2.1 Trillion+	$5.1 Trillion*
Years	NA	2022-2031	2017-2026
Projected Savings MFA (First Year) in National Health Expenditures	$317 Billion^	$93 Billion++	$310 Billion
Year	2030	2022	2017

^ The CBO study analyzed five different single-payer scenarios that differed in the provider payment rates and cost-sharing requirements; one included the costs of long-term supports and services (LTSS). The numbers in the tables below come from combining Option 3, which had lower provider payment rates and lower cost-sharing, with the additional costs for LTSS provided in Option 5.

+ Calculated from Blahous' projected changes in health care spending between 2022 to 2031, in the aggregate, (decrease of $482 billion) summed with administrative cost savings, in the aggregate, for that same period ($1.572 trillion). *See* Blahous, at p. 7, in Table 2 for both figures.

++ Calculated from Blahous' projected changes in health care spending for 2022 ($10 billion) summed with administrative cost savings for 2022 ($83 billion). *See* Blahous, at p. 7, in Table 2 for both figures.

* The Pollin study used Health Consumption Expenditures and the CBO and Blahous studies used National Health Expenditures. To ensure compatibility in comparing the data, percentages from the Pollin Study were adjusted to reflect National Health Expenditures. *See* Pollin, p. 22, for explanation on use of Health Consumption Expenditures.

---

[134] Jaeger, N. "Economic Effects of Five Illustrative Single-Payer Health Care Systems." Working Paper 2022-02. Congressional Budget Office (Feb. 2022). Accessed May 10, 2022. https://www.cbo.gov/publication/57637.

[135] *Ibid.*

[136] *Ibid.*

Table 2. Major categories of projected increases and savings in national health expenditures: CBO, Blahous, & Pollin

	CBO^ (2030)	Blahous+ (2o22)	Pollin* (2017)
Increases in National Health Expenditures due to Increased Access to Health Care under Medicare for All			
Projected Increase in Utilization/Demand	$583 Billion	$435 Billion	$390 Billion
Percentage Increase in Utilization/Demand	8.79%	9.50%	11.73%*
Savings in National Health Expenditures due to Medicare for All			
Administrative Savings	$411 Billion	$83 Billion	$327 Billion
Percentage	5.69%	1.66%++	8.80%*
Reduced Provider Payment Rates	$489 Billion	$384 Billion	$102 Billion
Percentage	6.78%	7.68%++	2.74%*
Drug Savings	NA^^	$61 Billion	$214 Billion
Percentage	NA	1.22%++	5.77%*

^ The CBO study analyzed five different single-payer scenarios that differed in the provider payment rates and cost-sharing requirements; one included the costs of long-term supports and services (LTSS). The numbers in the tables below come from combining Option 3, which had lower provider payment rates and lower cost-sharing, with the additional costs for LTSS provided in Option 5.

^^ The CBO includes drug savings in the reduced provider payment rates.

+ *See* Blahous' projected increases in utilization/demand for 2022, at p. 4, Table 1.

++ Percentage calculations based on spending after introduction of Medicare for All, which includes Blahous' currently projected National Health Expenditures for 2022 ($4,562 billion), p. 7, Table 2, plus Blahous' projected increases in utilization/demand for 2022 ($435 billion), p. 4, Table 1.

* The Pollin study used Health Consumption Expenditures and the CBO and Blahous studies used National Health Expenditures. To ensure compatibility in comparing the data, percentages from the Pollin Study were adjusted to reflect National Health Expenditures. *See* Pollin, p. 22, for explanation on use of Health Consumption Expenditures.

** Projected National Health Expenditure savings in Table 1 are slightly different than total savings minus increases in Table 2 because of rounding in the Pollin Study.

Medicare for All Act of 2022: Canada, Taiwan & U.S. Comparison

Two international examples of single-payer programs — Canada's Medicare program and Taiwan's National Health Insurance program — are detailed below in comparison to U.S. health spending and costs (Table 1) and to the system design of the Medicare for All Act of 2022. The most recent year with health expenditure and administrative cost data from all three countries is 2017.

The single-payer health systems of Canada and Taiwan are most similar in design to the single-payer program proposed under the Medicare for All Act of 2022. Similar to the United States, Canada and Taiwan both have a mix of publicly and privately delivered health care.

Table 1. Health care spending & insurance administrative cost comparison: Canada, Taiwan & U.S. (2017)

	Canada	Taiwan	U.S.
Total Spending on Health, % of total national GDP (2017)	10.8%*	6.1%**	16.8%*
Mean Spending on health per capita, PPPUSD	$5,138*	$3,047**	$10,106*
Insurance administrative costs,*** by percentage	3.0% of total national health spending*	0.77% of NHI budget**	8.0% of total national health spending* 13% of private insurer spending** 7% of traditional Medicare and Medicare Advantage spending combined** 1.1% of traditional Medicare spending alone**

* Organization for Economic Cooperation and Development. "OECD Health Statistics 2021." OECD Stat (Updated Dec. 2021), available at http://www.oecd.org/els/health-systems/health-data.htm.

** Cheng, Tsung-Mei. "Health Care Spending in the US and Taiwan: A Response to *It's Still the Prices, Stupid, And a Tribute to Uwe Reinhardt*." *Health Affairs* (Feb. 2019), available at https://www.healthaffairs.org/do/10.1377/hblog20190206.305164/full/.

*** Health care providers also incur substantial billing and insurance administrative costs that are not included in these figures.

Table 2. Program design comparison: Canada, Taiwan & medicare for all act[137]

Design Feature	Canada	Taiwan	U.S.
Program Name	Medicare	National Health Insurance (NHI)	Medicare for All (MFA)
Level of Administration	Provincial or territorial government	National government	National government; regional subdivisions responsible for allocation of funds and negotiations with providers

[137] Information compiled from: Congressional Budget Office. "Key Design Components and Considerations for Establishing a Single-Payer Health Care System." CBO Publications (May 1, 2019), available at https://www.cbo.gov/system/files/2019-05/55150-singlepayer.pdf; and Mossialos, E., Tikkanen, R. et al. (Eds.). "International Profiles of Health Care Systems, 2020." The Commonwealth Fund (Dec. 2020). Accessed May 10, 2022. https://www.commonwealthfund.org/sites/default/files/2020-12/International_Profiles_of_Health_Care_Systems_Dec2020.pdf.

Table 2. (Continued)

Design Feature	Canada	Taiwan	U.S.
Program Name	Medicare	National Health Insurance (NHI)	Medicare for All (MFA)
Eligibility			
Universal coverage	Yes	Yes	Yes
Separate public programs for certain groups other than military	Yes	No	Yes. Although veterans and American Indians/Alaskan Natives may receive services through the Veterans Health Administration or Indian Health Services, respectively, they may also enroll in MFA.
Mandated Benefits Package			
Hospital and physicians' services	Yes	Yes	Yes
Outpatient prescription drugs	No	Yes	Yes
Long-Term Services and Supports (LTSS)	No	Has a "Long-Term Care 2.0" plan to fully cover comprehensive home-and community-based care under NHI by 2026. Home-based care programs are currently being rolled out to expand coverage.	Yes, with a prioritization of home-and community-based services.
Dental, vision, and mental health services	No	Yes. Also, includes Chinese medicine, and home nursing care.	Yes
Private Health Insurance			
Supplemental	Yes	Yes, plays a non-substantive role; used primarily as a cash benefit for private rooms, co-pays, etc., and not used for coverage of services with the exception of long-term care.	Permitted for services not overlapping with Medicare for All, which would be extremely limited given the comprehensive benefits of the program.

Design Feature	Canada	Taiwan	U.S.
Program Name	Medicare	National Health Insurance (NHI)	Medicare for All (MFA)
Private Health Insurance			
Substitutive	No	No	No
Other types of private insurance	No	No	No
Participating Provider Rules			
Balance billing allowed	No	No	No
Payments from private-pay patients for covered services	No	No	No
Hospitals			
Primary ownership	Mixed	Private	Private
Primary payment method	Global budget	FFS with overall hospital sector global budget	Global budget
Primary Care Physicians			
Primary employment	Private	Private	Private
Primary payment method	FFS	FFS with overall primary care global budget	FFS with option to elect salaried reimbursement through hospital global budgeting.
Outpatient Specialist Physicians			
Primary employment	Private	Private	Private
Primary payment method	FFS	Salary	FFS with option to elect salaried reimbursement through hospital global budgeting.

Hearing before the Committee on the Budget, United States Senate, "Medicare for All: Protecting Health, Saving Lives, Saving Money," Testimony by Abdul El-Sayed, MD, DPhil

Chairman Sanders, Ranking Member Graham, and members of the committee, thank you for the opportunity to testify before you today.

My name is Dr. Abdul El-Sayed, I trained as a physician and epidemiologist. I served the City of Detroit as Health Director between 2015 and 2017, where I was responsible for the basic health and welfare of nearly 700,000 Detroiters. I also lead the rebuilding of the Detroit Health Department after it had been privatized during municipal bankruptcy and financial takeover by the State of Michigan under the same system of emergency management that led to the Flint Water Crisis.

Today, I teach at the University of Michigan's Ford School of Public Policy, as well as American University's School of Public Affairs. I find myself shouldering the awkward responsibility of explaining the haphazard disfunction of American healthcare to some of the brightest young policy minds in the country. I watch my students faces crinkle when I explain how deductibles work — comparing them to having to pay $19.99 for each movie you watch on Netflix even though you already pay for your monthly subscription. Last year, my book on the very subject of this hearing, along with Dr. Micah Johnson, "Medicare for All: A Citizen's Guide" was published by Oxford University Press. I have given a copy to each of your offices.

Coverage and Costs

I want to start with the two most obvious problems in American healthcare:

1) *We fail to provide everyone health insurance coverage.*
2) *The cost of healthcare in America is spiraling upward.*

Coverage

We like to think of ourselves as "customers" of healthcare. But we are not. To understand why, let's review how being a "customer" actually works. Imagine you were to go to a farmer's market in search of some heirloom tomatoes. There are multiple varieties all at different prices.

Let's say you find a stall with some tomatoes you like. You ask the seller for the price. If that price is too high, you move on. But if it's fair, you purchase them. You tender payment — and you are now the proud owner of heirloom tomatoes.

That is a normal customer experience.

But that's not how we experience healthcare. Imagine I was to complain of chest pain during this hearing. I'd be exhibiting signs of a potentially deadly heart attack. I should hope that you would call 911. When the ambulance comes, I would have no choice as to where I was going—no choice of who would "sell" me healthcare. Indeed, I would need to be taken to the nearest hospital. Time is wasting.

When I arrive, I have no choice in the care I get or from whom I get it—I'm left at the mercy of the physicians assigned to provide me care. But there are several directions my care could go depending on the physician, the services provided at the hospital, and what they deem my pathology to be. No one every shares a price list for the care I will receive.

Afterwards, a bill is sent to my health insurer. My insurer is based in Michigan, while I would have had my heart attack in Washington, D.C., so I would have received out-of-network care. It is unclear exactly how much of the cost of my care they will pay. But it is May, and my family and I have been healthy this year. We have yet to pay down our deductible—the paywall in front of the health insurance my family pays a premium for every month. So, some of the cost would get pushed back to me. Either way, my insurance pays for my healthcare, and sends me a bill for whatever it will not cover.

Now compare this experience to the traditional "customer" experience I laid out at the farmer's market. I do not get to shop around between providers. I do not get to choose what product I want owing to the "information asymmetry"—the difference in knowledge between my provider and me. I am left to the provider to both tell me what I need and sell it to me. I am never asked what price I am willing to pay. It's assumed I'll pay whatever it costs considering I only have one heart that is priceless to me, a perfect example of what economists call "inelastic demand"; my demand for care does not change based on price. And finally, once I receive my care, I do not pay. Instead, a third-party insurer pays on my behalf and passes whatever it will not back on to me.

Rather than being the initiator and completer of a financial transaction, I am the reason a financial transaction between my insurer and provider has taken place. Ask yourself, in the traditional "customer" analogy: are we the customers … or the tomatoes?

Our profit-driven healthcare system renders our bodies into products, over which providing healthcare justifies financial transactions between major corporations. Healthcare is not a traditional market product because it violates so many of the requirements of market. We are not the ones who pay for our healthcare. We often receive healthcare in circumstances that preclude us from negotiating. We rely on our providers to both to tell us what we need and to sell it to us.

It's no wonder why "market-based healthcare" so obviously fails. If I were a customer, I would be free to walk away if the price is too expensive. That fact would force any seller to lower their prices if they wanted the sale. That's the power of negotiation in a true market—the fact that you do not *have to buy*. But in our system, no one can walk away. As a patient, I don't have time. As an insurer, the care has already been provided. So instead of keeping prices down, health insurance companies have realized that they can just pass more of their costs back onto us.

Premiums — what we pay every month for the privilege of "being insured" — have risen faster than wages and inflation over the past decade.[138] The median family premium is now $22,221 — nearly $6,000 of that is coming out of family, not employer, pockets.

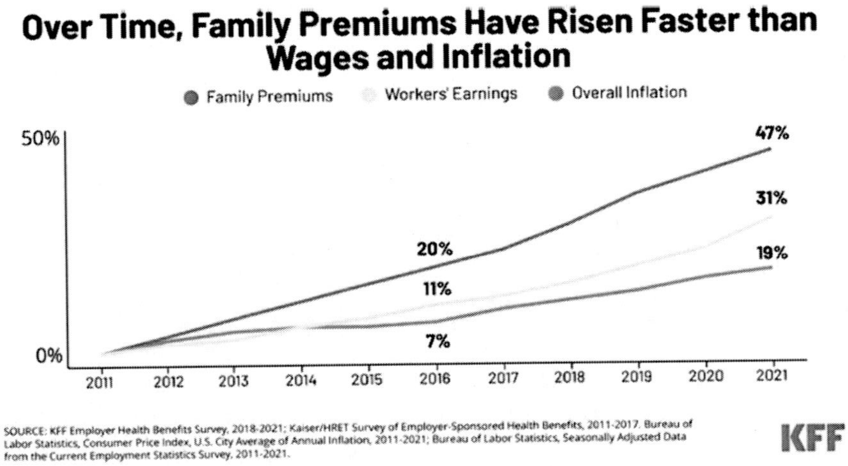

Considering that the median family earned about $80,000 in 2021, they spent 7.5 percent of their earnings on premiums. But that's not where the healthcare cost burden ends. Deductibles usually sit around $4,000 for private family plans.[139] That makes the annual cost of private health insurance nearly $10,000 per year, or 12.5 percent of the median family budget before taxes.

Out of pocket costs in the forms of deductibles and co-pays are not just financial costly, but they're also physically costly. Having to pay a deductible delays necessary healthcare. One study[140] found that high deductibles delayed treatment for breast cancer by nearly 9 months. Worse still, deductibles have more than doubled over the past decade.

---

138 Palosky C. "Average family premiums rose 4% this year to top $22,000; Employers boost mental health and telemedicine amid COVID-19 pandemic, benchmark KFF survey finds." *Kaiser Family Foundation.* November 10th, 2021. https://www.kff.org/health-costs/press-release/average-family-premiums-rose-4-this-year-to-top-22000/.

139 Kaiser Family Foundation. "2021 Employer Health Benefits Survey." November 10th, 2021. https://www.kff.org/report-section/ehbs-2021- section-7-employee-cost-sharing/.

140 J. Frank Wharam et al., "Vulnerable and Less Vulnerable Women in High-Deductible Health Plans Experienced Delayed Breast Cancer Care," *Health Affairs* 38, no. 3 (March 1, 2019): 408–15, https://doi.org/10.1377/hlthaff.2018.05026.

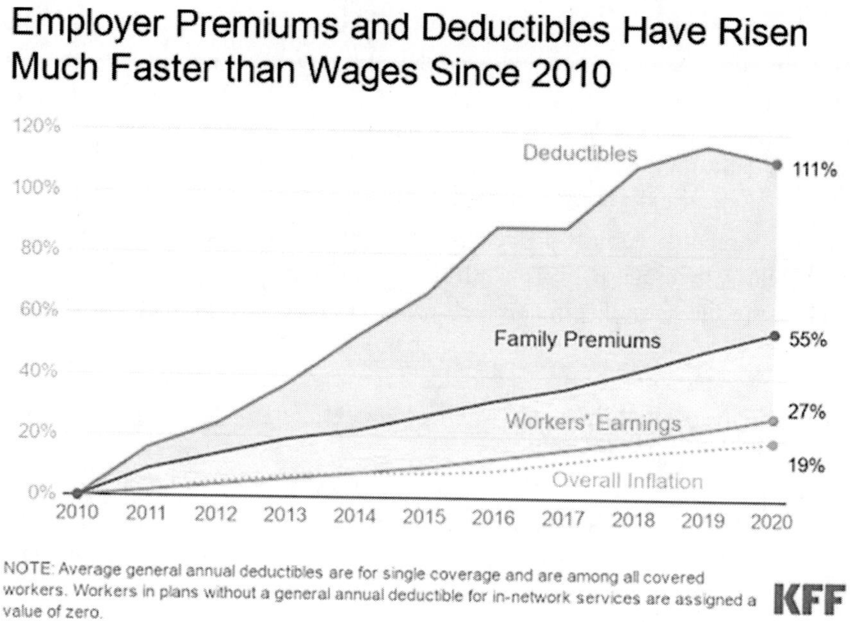

All of this contributes to the irony that the operative part of the word "insurance" is "sure." And the structure of our for-profit system leaves Americans increasingly *unsure* about their health insurance access. The nature of insurance coverage, itself, has changed. It's no wonder that nearly 44 percent of adults struggle to afford their care,[141] and 30 percent report rationing care because they cannot afford it.[142]

And that's for people *who are winning* in our for-profit healthcare system. These are the privately insured Americans who are routinely told that they have the "greatest healthcare in the world." What about those *who are losing* in our profit-driven system? That includes, of course, the uninsured of whom there remain 28 million according to the 2020 census.[143] That includes 9 percent of America's children.

---

[141] Barnes A. "112 million Amerians struggle to pay for health care: survey" *The Hill.* March 31st, 2022. https://thehill.com/changing-america/3012358-112-million-americans-struggle-to-pay-for-healthcare-report/.

[142] Picchi A. "Surge in Americans skipping medical care due to cost, Gallup says." *CBS News.* December 14th, 2021. https://www.cbsnews.com/news/health-care-costs-rising-americans/.

[143] Keisler-Starkey K, Bunch LN. "Health Insurance Coverage in the United States: 2020." *United States Census Bureau.* September 14th, 2021. https://www.census.gov/library/publications/2021/demo/p60-274.html.

It also includes about 87 million Americans enrolled in Medicaid,[144] our federally funded, state-operated health insurance program for low-income Americans. While Medicaid is a critical program, a lifeline for millions of Americans who cannot afford private health insurance, the program is only just that: a lifeline. Medicaid reimbursements, on average, are substantially lower[145] than private insurance reimbursements. And because healthcare providers are not required to accept Medicaid, beneficiaries are, in effect, second-class healthcare citizens. It is impossible to escape the fact that reimbursing the same healthcare services at a lower rate reflects an implicit lack of value of the body for which the healthcare is being provided. One study found that just a $10 increase in Medicaid reimbursements led to a 0.3 percent increase in the probability that a Medicaid beneficiary had seen a physician in the past two weeks.[146]

Because Americans of color are substantially more likely to be insured on Medicaid than their white counterparts, our tiered healthcare system is just another means by which our healthcare system assents to fundamental health inequities. Empirically, our system literally values Black bodies less than it does white ones.

Costs

We spend a whopping $12,530 per capita on healthcare[147] — more, by far, than any other country on Earth. Our neighbors just north spend less than half as much ($5,370). And the costs are rising faster than comparable countries, too.

---

[144] Corallo B, Moreno S. Analysis of recent national trends in Medicaid and CHIP enrollment. *Kaiser Family Foundation.* May 2nd, 2022. https://www.kff.org/coronavirus-covid-19/issue-brief/analysis-of-recent-national-trends-in-medicaid-and-chip-enrollment/#:~:text=After%20declines%20in%20enrollment%20from,steadily%20increase%20(Figure%201).

[145] Selden TM. "Differences between public and private hospital payment rates narrowed, 2012-16." *Health Affairs.* 2020: Volume 39: Issue 1. https://www.healthaffairs.org/doi/abs/10.1377/hlthaff.2019.00415?journalCode=hlthaff#_i10.

[146] National Bureau of Economic Research. "Increased Medicaid Reimbursement Rates Expanded Access to Care. *National Bureau of Economic Research Bulletin on Health.* 2019: Number 3. https://www.nber.org/bh-20193/increased-medicaid-reimbursement-rates-expand-access-care.

[147] NHE Fact Sheet. *Centers for Medicare & Medicaid Services.* Accessed May 11th, 2022. https://www.cms.gov/Research-Statistics-Data-and-Systems/Statistics-Trends-and-Reports/NationalHealthExpendData/NHE-Fact-Sheet.

Why do healthcare costs keep rising? Because corporations make money when they do. Healthcare providers make more when they bill more. Hospitals mergers and acquisitions continue to surge.[148] And as hospitals buy one another up in mergers and acquisitions, they eliminate their competition. One study found that hospital consolidation was associated with increased healthcare prices, often as high as 20 percent.[149]

You might expect health insurance companies have an incentive to negotiate healthcare costs downward on behalf of consumers, acting as a check on rising healthcare costs. But instead of negotiating these prices downward, insurers have leveraged cost-sharing mechanisms to pass rising costs back onto American families.

There are also the unintended consequences of the "80/20 rule" which required health insurance companies to spend at least 80 percent of their annual collected premiums on healthcare or return anything in excess back to beneficiaries in the form of a premium rebate. While it was intended to keep premiums low, it also removed the incentive health insurers had to negotiate down provider billing.[150] All of this illustrates the fundamental failure of assuming that negotiations over healthcare costs between profit-driven insurers and healthcare providers on behalf of the American public would do anything but maximize the profits of both of sets of corporations at the expense of the public.

The Pandemic Shows Us How America's Healthcare Failures Extend Well Beyond Incomplete Healthcare Coverage and Spiraling Costs

Now that I have discussed the most obvious problems with American healthcare, I want to expand the aperture. Though we often frame our healthcare discussion simply around coverage and cost, this framing

---

148 Japsen B. "Hospital mergers just keep getting bigger." *Forbes*. January 17th, 2022. https://www.forbes.com/sites/brucejapsen/2022/01/17/hospital-mergers-just-keep-getting-bigger/?sh=7968318975be.

149 Martin Gaynor and Robert Town, "The Impact of Hospital Consolidation—Update," Synthesis Project, Robert Wood Johnson Foundation, 2012, https://www.rwjf.org/content/dam/farm/reports/ issue_briefs/2012/rwjf73261.

150 Cicala S, Liever EM, Marone V. "Regulating Markups in US Health Insurance." *American Economic Journal: Applied Economics*. 2019: Volume 11: No. 4. Pages 71-104.

specifically excludes some of the most important issues facing health and healthcare in America.

To help us understand these, I want to take us back just two (albethey extraordinarily long) years, to early 2020. None of us will forget the horror of the first days of the pandemic that spring. We were facing a new virus with very little information about how it spread, how deadly it might be, and who was at highest risk. We had no vaccine nor any effective treatments. We were watching hospital wards fill up — their staff struggling without the ventilators or beds they needed to treat patients.

Frontline nurses, doctors, and hospital workers were doing all this without the basic personal protective equipment they needed to protect themselves and their patients from what was then called the "novel coronavirus." Indeed, this added to the already chronically poor working conditions for many healthcare workers—including unsustainable and unsafe staffing ratios, mandatory overtime, and vicious union-busting. Today, nurses are being forced to travel for more lucrative locum opportunities where they work alongside permanent colleagues who make far less for the same work — all this cementing a permanent staffing crisis in America's hospitals.

Desperate to "flatten the curve," mayors and governors around the country were forced to close schools and issue stay at home orders. We watched millions of Americans already teetering on the edge of financial insolvency lose their livelihoods. With their jobs, up to 27 million Americans also lost employer-sponsored health insurance during the pandemic.[151]

Meanwhile, local and state health departments, as well as the CDC, anemic after decades of disinvestment through the austerity of the Great Recession,[152] struggled under the load of the pandemic. Burnt out from the experience, a third of public health workers in a national survey say they are considering leaving the public health workforce in the next year.[153]

Despite the stress the pandemic put on hospitals around the country — and the desperate need that communities had for hospital beds — 21 hospitals

---

[151] Fronstin P, Woodbury, SA. "Update: How many Americans have lost jobs with employer health coverage during pandemic?" *Commonwealth Fund.* January 11th, 2021. https://www.commonwealthfund.org/blog/2021/update-how-many-americans-have-lost-jobs-employer-health-coverage-during-pandemic.

[152] Burnett S. "In years before outbreak, investment in public health fell." *AP News.* April 5th, 2020. https://apnews.com/article/health-ap-top-news-lansing-virus-outbreak-public-health-9960d22817a6402c7693bee74ad2b75d.

[153] De Beaumont Foundation. "Rising stress and burnout in public health. March 2022. https://debeaumont.org/wp-content/uploads/dlm_uploads/2022/03/Stress-and-Burnout-Brief_final.pdf.

shut down or ended service in the course of 2020 alone.[154] These hospitals are shutting down in disproportionally rural communities and in states that did not expand Medicaid. Millions of Americans are being forced to drive further and further for medical care, those distances posing serious obstacles in emergencies.

Hospitals, despite being gorged with patients, were being starved for cash flow. The pandemic forced them to cancel their most lucrative elective procedures to make way for COVID-19 patients. But it wasn't only shutdowns that robbed people of healthcare options; 2020 also featured 73 hospital mergers or acquisitions[155] that leave patients around the country with fewer choices for care. More than one in three (37 percent) of these deals involved a for-profit healthcare system, up from less than one in four (23 percent) in 2019.

Along with for-profit hospitals, guess what other industry had a banner year in 2020? The health insurance industry. Suddenly, they were flush with all the money they should have had to spend on elective procedures. UnitedHealth Group made $6.7 Billion in profits in the second quarter of 2020 — nearly double the $3.4 billion it made in the same quarter in 2019.

Where did they put that money? Well, 2020 was an election year — so they invested in making sure that nothing fundamentally changed about the nature of our healthcare system. They plowed that money back into our political process through everything from lobbying to electioneering. In the 2020 cycle, Blue Cross/Blue Shield—the biggest political spender among health insurers — spent $6,406,253 in political contributions. It also spent a whopping $49,879,310 lobbying. It was a key sponsor of the "Partnership for America's Healthcare Future,"[156] a lobbying group that ran millions of dollars in ads throughout the 2020 cycle to specifically target Medicare for All.

The pandemic has claimed nearly a million American lives. It's claimed millions more livelihoods. US life expectancy fell by several years — even more so among people of color — erasing a quarter century of growth.

This singular health catastrophe demonstrates so many of the other healthcare challenges in America in addition to coverage and cost.

---

[154] Ellison A. "21 hospital closures in 2020." *Becker's Hospital Review*. December 9th, 2020. https://www.beckershospitalreview.com/finance/21- hospital-closures-in-2020.html.

[155] King R. Kaufman Hall: Hospital industry made 79 deals in 2020, down from 92 in 2019. *Fierce Healthcare*. January 12th, 2021. https://www.fiercehealthcare.com/hospitals/kaufman-hall-hospital-industry-made-79-deals-2020-down-from-92-2019.

[156] Pear R. "Health care and insurance industries mobilize to kill 'Medicare for All.'" *The New York Times*. February 23rd, 2022. https://www.nytimes.com/2019/02/23/us/politics/medicare-for-all-lobbyists.html.

1) *American healthcare is precarious.* Employer sponsored insurance means that while you may have health insurance today, you could lose it for several reasons: losing a job, getting a new job, turning 26, getting married, getting divorced, or striking at work. Beyond that, in an America where we believe in the can-do entrepreneurial spirit, consider how many businesses are left unbuilt, career opportunities left unpursued for fear of losing health insurance.
2) *American consumers are losing healthcare choices.* The choice that Americans want in healthcare isn't which health insurer, but which doctor to see or what hospital to go to. But mergers and acquisitions, let alone hospital closures, are robbing Americans of the healthcare choices that matter most to them.
3) *Healthcare workers are being exploited.* The power of consolidating healthcare companies leaves healthcare workers—nurses, doctors, and other healthcare workers—at a disadvantage. When large hospital chains consolidate, workers are left with limited alternatives, reducing their ability to hold their employers accountable for unsafe staffing, forced overtime, and unsafe working conditions. They also fall prey to the well-documented reduction of pay due to what economists call "monopsony"—the ability of oligopolies to collude to suppress wages.[157]
4) *We are failing to invest in prevention and public health.* Our public health institutions were responding to the worst pandemic in modern history on shoestring budgets. But the continued defunding of public health does not align with Americans' preferences. If given the choice, most Americans would choose to stay healthy rather than pay for healthcare after they've already gotten sick. But our healthcare system rakes in trillions of dollars, nearly a fifth of our entire gross domestic product, to pay for *healthcare* while our national investment in public health—the means of keeping Americans healthy — remains minimal. We live far shorter lives than our counterparts in other high-income countries. Germany's life expectancy, for example, is more than four years longer than ours.[158]

---

[157] DePasquale C. "Hospital consolidation and monopsony power in the labor market for nurses." *Competition Policy International.* June 12th, 2020. https://www.competitionpolicyinternational.com/hospital-consolidation-and-monopsony-power-in-the-labor-market-for-nurses/.

[158] OECD Data. "Life expectancy at birth." Accessed May 11th, 2022. https://data.oecd.org/healthstat/life-expectancy-at-birth.htm.

Medicare for All: A Single Solution for All Our Healthcare Problems

Well-meaning people often attempt to explain why alternative proposals to Medicare for All could also provide universal coverage and reduce our healthcare costs. But as discussed, assuming that those are the only two problems we must solve hinges on a limited understanding of the full scope of America's healthcare challenges. When I introduce those challenges — the closing of rural hospitals, the expansion of for-profit healthcare through mergers and acquisitions that eliminate choice, the defunding of American public health, the exploitation of America's healthcare workforce, the tiered nature of our health insurance system that turns low-income Americans into second-class healthcare citizens — they propose Rube Goldberg add-on policies that render their proposals so complex as to be unworkable.

Medicare for All — a universal national health insurance program for everyone — is the most elegant, affordable, understandable, equitable solution to our myriad healthcare challenges.

Having enumerated a fuller scope of America's healthcare challenges, I want to map how Medicare for All would solve each of these.

Medicare for All Would Provide Universal Health Insurance Coverage

Medicare for All would offer the clearest pathway universal healthcare insurance coverage. Every single resident would have cradle-to-grave coverage. That coverage would insulate Americans from the escalating premiums, co-pays, and deductibles that leave even privately-insured Americans rationing, delaying, or forgoing healthcare right now.

Medicare for All would do away with second class healthcare citizenship. It would finally offer the equitable health insurance every single American deserves. Regardless of what you earn, the color of your skin, or wear you work, you would be entitled to the same coverage — that reimburses at the same rate — as everyone else.

This would save lives. A Yale study found that Medicare for All would save up to 68,000 lives every year.[159]

---

[159] Galvani AP, Parpia AS, Foster EM, Singer BH, Fitzpatrick MC. "Improving the prognosis of health care in the USA." *The Lancet.* 2020: Volume 395: Issue 10223. Pages 524-533. https://www.thelancet.com/journals/lancet/article/PIIS0140-6736(19)33019-3/fulltext#%20.

Medicare for All Is Durable

Turn 26, get a job, lose a job, get married, get divorced: none of these would cost you your health insurance under Medicare for All. Regardless of the nature of their employment, Americans would be secure in the knowledge that they would not lose their health insurance. Beyond the peace of mind, this would support America's economy as well: it could unleash the entrepreneurial spirit of Americans to start new businesses or explore new career opportunities without worrying about what it might mean should they or their families fall ill.

Medicare for All Would Slow the Hospital Mergers, Acquisitions, and Shutdowns That Rob American Consumers of Their Healthcare Choices

Mergers and acquisitions, let alone hospital closures, are robbing millions of Americans of the choice of what doctor to see or what hospital to go to. These deals are driven by non-transparent negotiations over reimbursement rates between hospitals and health insurers. Larger hospitals can leverage their size to negotiate better reimbursement rates than their competitors—allowing them to press their advantage and ultimately purchase their competitors. Meanwhile, hospitals in low-income or rural communities shut down because their communities lack density or people with private insurance, leaving residents with no healthcare options at all.

Under Medicare for All, there would be just a single insurer. Hospitals in similar catchment areas would be reimbursed at the same rate for the care they provide, barring larger hospitals from commanding better reimbursement rates simply for being larger. This allows smaller hospitals, as well as independent practices, to remain competitive, and offers consumers more choice.

Similarly, Medicare for All would keep rural hospitals open through "global payments" — rather than reimbursing for each unit of healthcare they provide, these hospitals would be paid in lump sum for the critical services they provide rural communities.

Medicare for All Empowers Healthcare Workers

Today, nurses are being exploited by consolidated healthcare systems, just as those systems are squeezing physicians out of their practices because they cannot command the same reimbursement rates. These systems dehumanize their employees and cheapen the provider-patient relationship. In curbing the power of these mammoth healthcare systems, Medicare for All empowers the people who *actually* provide America's healthcare, not the C-suite executives who manage their workplaces.

Medicare for All Aligns Incentives to Invest in Prevention and Public Health

Our disinvestment in prevention and public health is a function of the fact that prevention rarely makes financial sense in a system predicated on profits that accrue only after people fall ill. Indeed, many of the most important investments in prevention take decades to manifest. But because people transition between insurance providers so often during their lives—ultimately transitioning to Medicare after they turn 65 — an investment in prevention today is unlikely to save an insurer money in the long-term. Insurers have little incentive to invest in prevention that won't save them money.

Furthermore, the most important long-term investments in prevention and public health are structural interventions upon the "social determinants" of health, which are beyond the power of a single insurance company — these include rebuilding our decimated public health infrastructure, building walkable communities, addressing in-access to healthy foods, improving air and water quality, or investing in early childhood education.

Medicare for All aligns these incentives. In this system, there is no churn in insurance providers because every American is insured by the same entity throughout their entire lives. Every investment in prevention yields savings for the very same entity. And because the insurer is the federal government, rather than a corporation motivated by its profit margin, it has the power to act on those incentives to address the broader social determinants of health.

Medicare for All Would Reduce the Costs of Healthcare for Individuals, Families, and the Country and Expand the Economy

An authoritative report by the Congressional Budget Office,[160] which you will hear about in the second witness panel today, has demonstrated that Medicare for All would:

- Reduce household out-of-pocket costs
- Increase wages

---

[160] Nelson J. "Economic effects of five illustrative single-payer health care systems: Working Paper 2022-02" *Congressional Budget Office Working Paper.* February 23rd, 2022. https://www.cbo.gov/publication/57637.

- Improve the efficiency of the healthcare system and "economywide productivity"
- Increase labor productivity

Conclusion

Medicare for All saves lives. It saves money for families and the country. And it offers a sense of security that millions of Americans go without in our inhumane healthcare system. But opponents for Medicare for All continue to make the same fearmongering arguments opponents of national health insurance have been making for nearly a century.

They will tell you that Medicare for All would eliminate "healthcare choices," although Medicare for All is *critical* to addressing the consolidation that is, in fact, robbing Americans of the choices they *actually* care about: which doctor, clinic, or hospital at which to seek care.

They will say that Medicare for All is too expensive, that we cannot afford it. In fact, Medicare for All is the best way to protect Americans from the exorbitant — and rising — healthcare costs that force the median American family to pay 12.5 percent of their before-tax income for basic healthcare needs.

"But the free-market drives innovation!" they claim, even though healthcare providers would remain private under Medicare for All, and smaller, more innovative, providers would finally be able to leverage their innovation to compete with larger providers rather than get crushed by unfair reimbursement rates. Never mind the fact that the U.S. federal government is one of the most important funders of biomedical innovation in the world.

"What about rationing?" they'll ask, when in fact rising out-of-pocket costs are forcing Americans to ration, delay, or forgo their care every day in America under our current system.

They will tell you that more government is the problem, when in fact our private, for-profit health insurance system delivers mediocre healthcare outcomes despite being the world's most expensive healthcare system.

They will say Medicare for All is somehow "un-American," when what is truly un-American is staring at our broken healthcare system and the people it breaks along with it and choosing to look away.

But today, you are choosing to stare our broken healthcare system in its cruel, indifferent face. I commend you. And I hope that I have offered some insight into how and why it is so broken, and how Medicare for All is the solution to fix it.

Hearing before the United States Senate, Committee on the Budget on "Medicare for All: Protecting Health, Saving Lives, Saving Money," May 12, 2022, Chairman Bernie Sanders, Ranking Member Lindsey Graham, Testimony by Grace-Marie Turner, President, Galen Institute

Chairman Sanders, Ranking Member Graham and senators of the committee, thank you for the opportunity to testify today.

My name is Grace-Marie Turner, and I am president of the Galen Institute, a non-profit research organization focusing on patient-centered health policy. We concentrate on achieving affordable, quality health coverage and care for all Americans, especially the most vulnerable. I also have served as a member of the Advisory Board of the Agency for Healthcare Research and Quality, as a presidential appointee to the Medicaid Commission, and as a congressional appointee to the Long Term Care Commission.

Mr. Chairman, in calling this hearing today, you acknowledge the need to achieve universal coverage in the United States.

While there are different views on how to reach that goal, I believe there are important values we share in health reform:

- Everyone should be able to get health coverage to access the health care they need
- Coverage and care should be affordable
- We must guard the quality of care
- People should be able to see the physicians and other providers of their choice
- And perhaps most important, we must work to protect the most vulnerable and marginalized communities.

There is no question that Americans are frustrated with our current health care system. Millions remain uninsured, and coverage and care cost too much. Many are priced out of the market for health insurance. The costs of premiums can be prohibitive, especially for those who don't get subsidies. Many face deductibles that are so high they say they might as well be uninsured.

Those on public programs are often frustrated as well, including Medicaid recipients who often struggle to find physicians who can afford to take the program's low payment rates. Recipients can find it especially difficult to get appointments with specialists for more serious health problems. They deserve the dignity of being able to have coverage that gives them more options and choices of plans that meet their needs.

People are hurting, and they feel powerless against this system.

Health care has become a very big and lucrative business. Many patients feel they are simply cogs in our $4 trillion health sector with little power to impact choices of care or coverage.

Independent physicians are selling their practices and then find they now answer to more hospital executives and less to their patients. Some hospital systems have become virtual oligopolies, setting high prices and giving plans and purchasers little choice but to pay. Worse, because our health sector is so highly regulated, it relegates physicians and other health care professionals to checking bureaucratic boxes rather than spending more time listening to their patients.

These and other frustrations with the current system are generating interest in an alternative that would provide universal coverage for everyone, with no premiums, copayments, or deductibles, and the ability to choose any provider or hospital participating in the new system.

As I will document, a government-run system would have many if not more of the problems we experience today and would put even more health care decisions under the control of government, not doctors and patients.

Too Much Government

The high costs of health care in the United States compared to other developed countries and the number of Americans who remain uninsured are real and serious concerns that deserve attention.

The United States does not have a properly functioning market in the health sector. It does not respond to the needs of consumers and their demands for lower costs and more choices they are accustomed to receiving in other sectors of the economy.

The government is exerting greater and greater control over our health sector.

Wharton School Professor Mark Pauly, in a paper published by the American Enterprise Institute, has important findings about the controlling role that the federal government plays in our health sector today.[161] Pauly details how the federal government shapes a much larger share of spending than the portion it finances directly. He finds the share of "government-affected" spending in 2016 totaled nearly 80%—"not leaving much in the unfettered, market-based category."

The federal government finances nearly 55 percent of all "explicit and implicit" health spending, he reports—from Medicare, the federal share of Medicaid, and ACA subsidies, to tax preferences for employer-sponsored health insurance. But the federal government controls even more through regulations and mandates on other allegedly private plans.

The more government gets involved, the more that providers throughout the health sector are forced to respond to legislative and regulatory demands rather than the needs and preferences of patients. Some physicians, nurses, and other health professionals now contend that the mess can only be solved by having the government take over.

I would argue that the growing presence of government is a significant contributor to these problems. In the health sector, government officials, not the needs of consumers, increasingly determine what services can or must be covered, how much will be paid, and who is eligible to both deliver and receive these services. Third-party payment systems and the resulting lack of price and benefit transparency also lead to significant disruptions in the market. Physicians and other health care professionals say they are forced to spend more time complying with bureaucracy than in innovating to develop better care solutions for their patients.

Who Lacks Coverage?

In proposing a policy solution, it's important to begin by clearly defining the problem to be solved.

According to the Congressional Budget Office,[162] of the 29.8 million people who were uninsured in 2019, two-thirds were eligible for coverage but not enrolled—either in expanded Medicaid programs, traditional Medicaid or

---

[161] Mark Pauly, "Will Health Care's Immediate Future Look a Lot like the Recent Past?" American Enterprise Institute, June 7, 2019. https://www.aei.org/publication/health-cares-future-public-sector-funding-delivery- administration/.

[162] Congressional Budget Office, "Who Went Without Health Insurance in 2019, and Why?" September 2020. https://www.cbo.gov/publication/56504.

CHIP, subsidized coverage in the ACA marketplaces, or subsidized employer-based coverage.

Of the remaining third, the greatest number—an estimated four million—were not lawfully present in the U.S. and therefore need to be addressed separately through immigration/citizenship policy. Slightly more than 3 million of the uninsured had income below the federal poverty level and lived in states that did not expand Medicaid. The remaining 2.6 million had incomes too high to receive subsidies in the marketplace in 2019 but chose not to purchase coverage.

The chart below provides further detail:

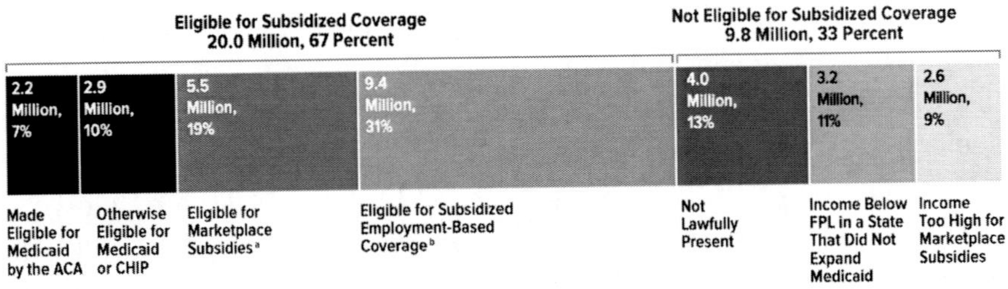

Source: Congressional Budget Office.

ACA = Affordable Care Act; CHIP = Children's Health Insurance Program; FPL = federal poverty level.

a. A small number of people in this group would technically be eligible for subsidies, but those subsidies would equal zero dollars.

b. A small number of people in this group were self-employed and could receive a subsidy by deducting their premiums from their federal income taxes.

Figure 1. Eligibility for Subsidized Coverage Among the Uninsured in 2019.

Most of the uninsured have *access* to health coverage. Uninsured rates continue to be higher in certain populations, including Latinos (18.3%) and Blacks (10.4%), people with incomes below the poverty level (17.2%), and residents of states that have not expanded Medicaid (17.6%), according to an HHS Assistant Secretary for Planning and Evaluation report on "Tracking Health Insurance Coverage in 2020-2021."[163]

Rather than dramatically expanding the role of government through Medicare for All or other new or expanded taxpayer-supported programs, I believe we need to target appropriate solutions to address the specific needs of those who are uninsured, focusing on those in marginalized communities.

---

163 https://aspe.hhs.gov/sites/default/files/documents/2fb03bb1527d26e3f270c65e2bfffc3a/tracking-insurance-coverage-2020-2021.pdf.

Coverage and COVID

Many experts had assumed there would be major losses of coverage during the economic shock of the COVID-19 pandemic, but the losses of coverage were much lower than expected.

A Heritage Foundation analysis found that *5.7 million more people had coverage* in December 2020—nearly a year into the pandemic—than were insured in December 2019.[164]

> Net enrollment in private coverage (group and non-group) decreased by 2 million individuals, or 1.2 percent, while enrollment in public coverage (Medicaid and the Children's Health Insurance Program) increased by 7.8 million individuals, or 10.9 percent. Furthermore, the analysis found that enrollment in individual market plans increased by 605,000 individuals (or 4.4 percent)—an increase that occurred before Congress increased ACA premium subsidies.

In 2021, Congress passed the American Rescue Plan Act (ARPA)[165], spending an estimated $90 billion to subsidize more people with more generous coverage through the ACA.

But most of that new spending is federal payments that are going to insurance companies on behalf of people who already had health insurance. Making the expanded ACA tax credits permanent will do little to help expand access to coverage to the uninsured, but it may well encourage even more people who have coverage today to switch to taxpayer-supported plans.

ARPA made the wealthiest people eligible for subsidized coverage and gave them the biggest average benefits. Those with incomes between 400-600% of the FPL receive average monthly ARPA subsidies of $213, a figure that is nearly seven times as high as the increased subsidy provided by ARPA to those with incomes less than 150 percent of the FPL, according to a paper by Heritage Senior Fellow Doug Badger.[166]

---

[164] Edmund Haislmaier, "COVID-19: Effects of the Response on Health Insurance Coverage in 2020," Heritage Foundation Issue Brief No. 6079, May 14, 2021, https://www.heritage.org/public-health/report/covid-19-effects-the-response-health-insurance-coverage-2020.

[165] https://www.congress.gov/117/plaws/publ2/PLAW-117publ2.pdf.

[166] Doug Badger, "Obamacare Subsidies: Six Reasons Congress Should Not Make Temporary Increases Permanent," The Heritage Foundation, May 26, 2021. https://www.heritage.org/health-care-reform/report/obamacare-subsidies-six-reasons-congress-should-not-make-temporary.

This is not the targeted solution we need.

The High Cost of Subsidized Coverage—for Patients

For the unsubsidized in 2021, the average exchange plan's annual premium plus deductible for a family of four was about $25,000—meaning that a family needed to spend about $25,000 before they received any real meaningful financial benefit from their insurance.[167]

In addition to the high cost, ACA plans tend to have narrow networks, excluding the best hospitals and doctors in local regions. The Goodman Institute surveyed ACA plans in Texas and found that none covers Houston's world-renowned MD Anderson Cancer Center, as just one example.

Galen Senior Fellow and Paragon Health Institute President Brian Blase testified recently before the House Education and Labor Committee about the costs of ACA coverage:[168]

> Rather than addressing underlying problems with the ACA that caused high premiums and deductibles and narrow plan networks, the American Rescue Plan Act (ARPA) further increased subsidies for this coverage. These subsidies have multiple problems, including being inflationary and inefficient. They push up prices and premiums, and they are a poor use of taxpayer dollars since much of the benefit accrues to higher-income people who are already insured.
>
> Due to these problems, the projected subsidy expansion in ARPA equates to about $17,000 each year per newly insured individual. The expanded subsidies will increase exchange enrollment but will do so by shifting more cost to the taxpayer. For example, an individual who faced a $600 monthly premium and qualified for a $500 subsidy and refused to purchase ACA coverage would likely enroll if an expanded subsidy covered the entire cost of the premium.

Chasing ever-rising health costs with more and more taxpayer dollars is not a sustainable solution.

---

[167] Davalon, "How Much Does Health Insurance Cost Without a Subsidy?" eHealth, January 21, 2022, https://www.ehealthinsurance.com/resources/affordable-care-act/much-health-insurance-cost-without-subsidy.

[168] https://edlabor.house.gov/imo/media/doc/BlaseBrianTestimony%20021722l.pdf.

Opinion Polling Swings

The Kaiser Family Foundation[169] regularly asks Americans about health policy issues as part of its Health Tracking Poll series. Its 2019 comprehensive survey found that 56% of Americans support a "national health plan, sometimes called Medicare for All" and an even larger 71% support the idea when told that it would "guarantee health insurance as a right for all Americans."

But then come the details. When the surveyors focused on the costs of a single-payer system, support for Medicare for All dropped below 40%. Support fell even further to 37% when they learned the plan would eliminate private health insurance and require people to pay more in taxes. And when they learned that some medical treatments and tests could be delayed, support dropped even further, to 26%.

More recent focus group testing has found that soaring inflation in our economy makes calls for more health spending and expansion of government programs "seem reckless, not compassionate."[170]

Can Government Manage Programs More Efficiently?

The government also doesn't have a terrific track record in efficiently managing massive complex programs. For example, a recent federal audit found eligibility errors for nearly one third of Medicaid enrollees. The audit examined a sample of 2,301 files of people enrolled under the ACA expansion authority, and eligibility review errors occurred in 29% of them, according to a review by Brian Blase.[171]

What does this cost taxpayers? "The federal government's improper Medicaid payments now exceed $100 billion a year," Blase reports. "This means that more than one-in-four dollars flowing out of Medicaid — our nation's third-largest government program — do not meet program rules. This

---

[169] "The Public On Next Steps For The ACA And Proposals To Expand Coverage," Ashley Kirzinger, Cailey Muñana, and Mollyann Brodie. Kaiser Family Foundation, Jan. 23, 2019. https://www.kff.org/health-reform/poll- finding/kff-health-tracking-poll-january-2019/.

[170] https://www.cahc.net/newsroom/2022/4/29/cahc-presents-to-house-education-and-labor-committee-to-advocate-for-a-new-small-business-health-care-platform.

[171] Brian Blase, "Mismanaging Medicaid, One Improper Payment at a Time," The Wall Street Journal, Feb. 3, 2022. https://www.wsj.com/articles/medicaid-health-care-benefits-eligibility-improper-waste-obamacare-expansion- 11643845321.

staggering failure doesn't just reduce health-care access for the truly eligible, it also harms taxpayers who fund it."[172]

A new paper also underscores how difficult it is for government to take the lead on innovation.

The National Taxpayers Union recently published an in-depth analysis[173] of the track record of the Center for Medicare and Medicaid Innovation, created as part of the Affordable Care Act with the promise that its demonstration projects would save tens of billions of dollars in Medicare.

The NTU paper shows how far CMMI is missing the mark in facilitating innovation and cost savings in programs as committed administrators and private sector participants crash into restrictive rules and regulation that limit their ability to achieve demonstrable results. Yet taxpayers still are spending $1 billion a year on this government program that is supposed to help us innovate our way out of high costs but which has little to show for the investment.

These studies provide further evidence that it would be extremely difficult to get health spending under control through regulation-bound government programs. The private sector is the answer, not expanded government programs.

Struggling to Achieve Promised Goals

I was in the gallery the night the House passed the Affordable Care Act in March of 2010 and heard Member after Member talk about the importance of passing the bill in order to "finally achieve universal coverage" and guarantee that everyone will be able to access quality, affordable care. Former President Obama promised repeatedly that people would be able to keep their doctors and their plans and that the typical American family's premiums would drop by $2,500 a year.

---

172 Brian Blase, "Medicaid is hemorrhaging $100B on Americans ineligible for the program," New York Post, Nov. 28, 2020. https://galen.org/2020/alarming-unlawful-medicaid-spending-brian-blase-in-ny-post/.

173 Pete Sepp, Andrew Lautz, Doug Badger, "Center for Medicare and Medicaid Innovation: 12 Years into the Game, Taxpayers Still Don't Know the Score," National Taxpayers Union, May 3, 2022. https://www.ntu.org/publications/detail/center-for-medicare-and-medicaid-innovation-12-years-into-the-game- taxpayers-still-dont-know-the-score.

Many Americans are frustrated that, 12 years later, our nation still is struggling to achieve these goals of access and affordability. They are understandably skeptical of new promises.

If You Like Your Plan…

As senators examine increasing the role of government—either through Medicare for All or derivatives, such as Medicare buy-in or a federal "public option"—we would fall further down the slippery slope where government control of our health sector would make private coverage less and less viable.

Former President Obama's promise that "If you like your plan, you can keep it" and "If you like your doctor, you can keep your doctor" was declared by PolitiFact to be The Lie of the Year in 2013.[174]

While the promises of Medicare for All sound utopian, what about the large portion of at least 173 million people don't want to give up their job-based insurance? What if 64 million seniors like their current Medicare and Medicare Advantage plans and don't want the program abolished and replaced? And what about union members who have made significant sacrifices in wages to earn their generous health benefit packages? Will they and others who like the coverage they have now be forced to pay significant new taxes to finance a government program that is inferior to the one they have now?

Medicare for All would mean that virtually everyone would lose the plan they have now in exchange for a single, government-run health plan. Employer coverage would end. Medicare as seniors know it would end. Medicaid, the single-largest publicly-supported health program in the country, would end. Medicare Advantage, the Medicare Prescription Drug Program, and the Children's' Health Insurance Program all would shut down.

"Free" health care would stimulate demand for health care while threatening its supply. It would lead to a shortage of doctors and hospital capacity, threatening both access to care and a decline in quality.

Americans could soon find themselves waiting in line for care and paying sharply increased taxes as federal indebtedness soars, putting at even greater risk future prosperity for our children and grandchildren.

---

174 https://www.politifact.com/truth-o-meter/article/2013/dec/12/lie-year-if-you-like-your-health-care-plan-keep-it/.

Congressional Budget Office Reports on Single-Payer

The Congressional Budget Office has produced a number of reports analyzing single-payer systems. The first, issued in 2019, evaluated key design elements and came to sobering conclusions.[175]

CBO found that establishing such a system would be a "major undertaking" that would be "complicated, challenging, and potentially disruptive" and that the "changes could significantly affect the overall U.S. economy." CBO says that "Setting payment rates equal to Medicare [fee-for-service] rates under a single-payer system would reduce the average payment rates most providers receive—often substantially."

Further, this would likely "reduce the amount of care supplied and could also reduce the quality of care." It says that "decreases in payment rates lead to a lower supply" and "fewer people might decide to enter the medical profession in the future. The number of hospitals and other health care facilities might also decline as a result of closures, and there might be less investment in new and existing facilities."

According to CBO, the government's low payment rates "could lead to a shortage of providers, longer wait times, and changes in the quality of care, especially if patient demand increased substantially."

Washington would assume the task of determining the list of covered benefits and updating it on an annual basis. This would inevitably lead to significant restrictions on access to care, including the long waiting lines and other barriers to timely care that we see in other countries with government-run health care systems and global budgets where demand outpaces supply. The most vulnerable patients would be the most severely impacted as they try to navigate a complex, bureaucratic system to get the care they need.

I am pleased you have invited the Honorable Phillip Swagel, CBO director, to testify today, likely focusing on recent CBO reports which describe the cost and economic effects of various single-payer models.[176,177] I also am

---

[175] Congressional Budget Office, "Key Design Components and Considerations for Establishing a Single-Payer Health Care System," May 2019. https://www.cbo.gov/system/files/2019-05/55150-singlepayer.pdf.

[176] Congressional Budget Office. "Economic Effects of Five Illustrative Single-Payer Health Care Systems." February, 2022. https://www.cbo.gov/system/files/2022-02/57637-Single-Payer-Systems.pdf.

[177] Congressional Budget Office. "How CBO Analyzes the Costs of Proposals for Single-Payer Health Care Systems That Are Based on Medicare's Fee-for-Service Program." December, 2020. https://www.cbo.gov/system/files/2020- 12/56811-Single-Payer.pdf.

pleased that Prof. Blahous is testifying today to address the CBO's analyses based upon his expertise as an economist.

The CBO, of course, acknowledges the incredible complexity of making assumptions and projections about sweeping changes impacting nearly one-fifth of our economy, calling it "an enormously complex endeavor," and acknowledging that "A high degree of uncertainty surrounds CBO's estimates."

The 2022 CBO report projects a number of positive outcomes, writing that "patients' cost sharing would generally be lower, more people would have insurance coverage, and there would be fewer restrictions on use of care and provider networks." But it also says: "Factors of a single-payer system that are explicitly not reflected in this paper's results include the effects of financing such a system and the system's effect on business dynamism, workers' job mobility, states' budgets and their policy response," which could be significant.

From my perspective regarding the impact on people and patients, the CBO assumes single-payer systems would:

- Reduce payment rates to physicians, hospitals, and other providers compared to private payers, the consequences of which I will address in a later section of my testimony
- Increase demand for health care, but this increase is expected to exceed the capacity to provide those services. "The increase in unmet demand would correspond to increased congestion in the health care system—including delays and forgone care—particularly under scenarios with lower cost sharing and lower payment rates," according to CBO.
- Increase taxable wages for employees that currently have health insurance through their workplace
- If labor taxes were increased to finance the single-payer system, it would reduce after-tax wages, hours worked, and unfortunately provide further incentives for workers to exit the workforce
- Result in the loss of at least 400,000 jobs in the insurance industry alone.

What Single-Payer and Global Budgets Would Mean to Patients

Disadvantaging the Most Vulnerable

Because just five percent of the population accounts for more than half of U.S. health care spending,[178] those who are sickest with the greatest health needs are most disadvantaged when the health system is under government control. Political leaders inevitably work to make sure the great majority of their constituents are at least satisfied with the system, even if it means restricting access to more expensive services to the smaller number with the greatest health needs.

Provider Shortages

Assigning Medicare rates to hospitals would entail payment rates that are roughly 40 percent lower than commercial rates, while physicians would be reimbursed at rates that are 30 percent lower than those paid by private insurers. These payment reductions would gradually grow larger over time for both. Medicare actuaries have warned that if Medicare payment rates contained in current law were put into place, many providers would face negative margins. That could mean that many physician practices and hospitals would be forced to close or significantly cut back on services. Some anticipate the new program would look more like mandatory Medicaid as a result.[179]

According to the Association of American Medical Colleges, even under our current health system, the U.S. will see a shortage of up to nearly 120,000 physicians by 2030.[180] The demand for physicians is expected to grow faster than the supply, and rural areas will be hit especially hard, according to the report.[181] The payment cuts envisioned under Medicare for All are likely to exacerbate this trend as more physicians close their practices or otherwise withdraw because the payment reductions will force many to close or curtail their practices.

---

[178] https://meps.ahrq.gov/data_files/publications/st497/stat497.pdf.

[179] Doug Badger, "Replacing Employer-Sponsored Health Insurance with Government-Financed Coverage: Considerations for Policymakers," Galen Institute, December 2018. https://galen.org/assets/Replacing-Empl-Spons-Insur-112618.pdf.

[180] https://news.aamc.org/press-releases/article/workforce_report_shortage_04112018/.

[181] Association of American Medical Colleges, "The Complexities of Physician Supply and Demand: Projections from 2017-2032," April 2019. https://aamc-black.global.ssl.fastly.net/production/media/filer_public/31/13/3113ee5c-a038-4c16-89af-294a69826650/2019_update_-_the_complexities_of_physician_supply_and_demand_-_projections_from_2017-2032.pdf.

Disruption of Current Coverage

I began my testimony talking about the very real problems and frustrations with health care in America, but any policy solution must also take into account what people value about the current system and assess the risks of such sweeping changes.

Today, 64 million people rely on Medicare for their health insurance coverage.[182] Seniors value Medicare, and many believe their access would be undermined if 268 million more Americans were competing with them for services from the same underpaid providers. Seniors have paid into the Medicare program throughout their working lives in order to have reliable access to medical care in their retirement years.

In 2021, 26 million Medicare beneficiaries, or about 42% of those eligible for the program, were enrolled in a Medicare Advantage plan.[183] Medicare For All would take away the private coverage that these 26 million seniors have voluntarily chosen under Medicare Advantage, and it would dramatically change the program for seniors in the traditional Medicare program as well, including outlawing private supplementary Medigap policies.

Medicare Advantage deploys private insurers to provide better access and better-coordinated care to seniors. The federal government simply is unable to develop creative programs to personalize care to the needs of individual patients—as we see Medicare Advantage and in other private plans today.[184]

Dramatic Federal Spending Increases

Using Medicare fee-for-service as a model for health reform risks incomprehensibly large deficit spending well into the future. I am pleased to share the witness table with Prof. Charles Blahous who has researched extensively the costs of a single-payer health care system.[185]

Restricted access to new medicines and other medical technologies also occurs in countries with government-centric health systems. In just one example, my organization published a report surveying access to new drugs in

---

[182] https://www.hhs.gov/sites/default/files/fy-2021-budget-in-brief.pdf.

[183] https://www.fiercehealthcare.com/payer/medicare-advantage-industry-s-hottest-market-2022-don-t-expect-to-change#:~:text=In%202021%2C%2026%20million%20Medicare,%2C%22%20the%20KFF%20analysts%20said.

[184] Avik Roy, "Medicare Advantage: A Platform for Affordable Health Reform," FREEOP, April 18, 2019. https://freopp.org/medicare-advantage-a-platform-for-affordable-health-reform-fbe31bf444f3.

[185] Charles Blahous, Statement before the U.S. House of Representatives Committee on Rules, April 30, 2019. https://docs.house.gov/meetings/RU/RU00/20190430/109356/HHRG-116-RU00-Wstate-BlahousC-20190430.pdf.

a number of countries with government-dominated health systems.[186] We found the French, for example, have access to only 48% of new drugs introduced between 2011 and 2018. Americans, by contrast, have access to 89% of those innovative medications. Nor is France an exception. The Swiss have access to only 48% of newly-developed drugs, the Belgians 43%, and the Dutch 56%.

Thwarting Innovation

The United States is a recognized leader in medical innovation. Over the past half century, the United States has been the birthplace of the majority of the world's biomedical innovations.[187] Our hospitals and physicians offer top quality care where Americans have access to the latest medical diagnostics. Americans are accustomed to better quality and access and are unlikely to be satisfied with restrictions and rationing and to stalling the innovation that continues to produce new and better treatments and medicines.

Recent studies have shown the impact that price control restrictions would have in the U.S.[188] that would cut spending on pharmaceutical research and development by hundreds of billions of dollars. Economic modeling estimates that show that price-control legislation would snuff out 56 new drugs—including 16 new cancer treatments—that would have otherwise been available to patients.[189]

Turning the Clock Backward

In our increasingly complex health care system, many patients are bewildered when faced with a health challenge. Significant progress has been made in developing coordinated care to provide patients with an integrated network of physicians, from primary and specialty care to lab services, pharmaceutical benefits, and hospital services.

---

[186] Doug Badger, "Examination of International Drug Pricing Policies in Selected Countries Shows Prevalent Government Control over Pricing and Restrictions on Access," Galen Institute, March 5, 2019. https://galen.org/2019/examination-of-international-drug-pricing-policies-in-selected-countries-shows-prevalent-government-control-over-pricing-and-restrictions-on-access/.

[187] https://www.americanactionforum.org/weekly-checkup/new-drug-patents-country/.

[188] Peter Pitts, "Rejuvenating American Healthcare," Journal of Commercial Biology, May 2022. http://www.commercialbiotechnology.com/index.php/jcb/article/view/1018.

[189] https://vitaltransformation.com/2019/11/international-reference-pricing-under-h-r-3-would-devastate-the-emerging-biotechnology-sector-leading-to-56-fewer-new-medicines-coming-to-market-over-10-years/.

In addition to improving the quality and effectiveness of health care, providing personalized care is more cost effective and humane. Putting government in charge of our health sector would turn back the clock on the progress we are making to move away from Medicare's 1965-model fee-for-service system. Government rules and payment policies would stifle the movement toward personalized care.

Administrative Costs

Medicare for All advocates say the administrative savings would help fill the funding gap. But the new single-payer system still would require many of the same administrative functions in any insurance system. Physicians, hospitals, labs and other service providers would have to be approved and payment rates set. The government would need documentation that approved services were actually provided, providers would have to be paid, and there would be an even greater need for safeguards against fraud and abuse.

Merrill Matthews of the Institute for Policy Innovation and colleagues analyzed Medicare administrative costs vs those of private insurers.[190] He found that an apples to apples comparison showed little administrative savings between Medicare and private payers when, for example, services such as the costs that other government agencies perform, such as collecting premium revenue, are considered.

Employer-Sponsored Health Insurance: A Central Pillar in Our Health Sector

In our multi-payer health sector, employer-sponsored health insurance (ESI) is the single-largest conveyer of health coverage in America. As such, it is worth taking a deeper dive into this program and its central role in our health sector—including supporting public health programs that too often pay less than the cost of providing care.

---

[190] Merrill Matthews, "Medicare's Hidden Administrative Costs," Council for Affordable Health Insurance, January 10, 2006. http://mforall.net/files/CAHI_Medicare_Admin_Final_Publication.pdf.

The great majority of Americans who receive health coverage through the workplace, either as an employee, retiree, or dependent,[191] highly value their coverage—coverage that would be eliminated under Medicare for All.

Employers know that high quality health coverage leads to better health outcomes and a healthier workforce. They offered prescription drug coverage for many years before Medicare was created. They innovate in offering preventive and wellness services because they know that addressing health issues before they become a crisis can minimize costs and lead to better outcomes. Employers continue to outpace public programs in the management of chronic illness, price transparency, and the availability of health savings accounts and other innovations to increase health care choices and reduce costs.

Employers and employees both have a vested interest in getting the best value for their health care dollars to obtain the highest quality care and coverage at the lowest cost.

Most large firms offer coverage to their employees (99 percent of all firms with more than 200 employees offer health coverage). Sixty-seven percent of firms with 10 to 100 employees offer health coverage to their workers, but just 30 percent of employers with fewer than 50 employees offer coverage.

These companies want to provide coverage to their workers. According to a July 2021 survey of small businesses:[192]

- 37% said they felt they couldn't expand their workforce because of the cost of health coverage for workers.
- 47% said they felt their company would lose out on the best workers if they couldn't offer competitive benefits.
- 60% said they limited healthcare benefit options because of high costs.
- 59% said they felt they couldn't compete with the benefit offerings at larger companies.

The smaller the firm, the less likely they are to offer coverage. Small businesses need the option to get the economies of scale that larger businesses

---

[191] U.S. Census Bureau, Health Insurance Coverage in the United States: 2020. Chart: Number and Percentage of People by Health Insurance Coverage Status and Type: 2018 to 2020. https://www.census.gov/library/publications/2021/demo/p60-274.html.

[192] Council for Affordable Health Coverage, letter to Affordability Task Force, February 4, 2022.

enjoy by pooling together through Association Health Plans, which I discuss later in my testimony.

Senior Fellow Doug Badger provides much more detail about the importance of employer-based health insurance in a paper he wrote for the Galen Institute, "Replacing Employer-Sponsored Health Insurance with Government-Financed Coverage: Considerations for Policymakers."[193] He explained the crucial role that higher-paying private plans, primarily employer-sponsored insurance (ESI) that covers half of Americans, play in financing the U.S. health care system:

> Replacing our admittedly inelegant health care financing system with single payer is not like swapping U.S. customary units for metric measurements. It could have profound and unforeseeable consequences on the capacity of doctors, hospitals and other providers to deliver quality care.
>
> Displacements, even if temporary, carry potentially grave consequences. Planting a new financing system requires uprooting another, one that has grown, adapted and evolved over decades. Policymakers should carefully weigh the risks of scuttling an employer-based system that provides health security to the majority of Americans and that largely finances public programs that provide coverage to others…
>
> Shifting people with ESI to a federally financed program that pays Medicare rates [has great] potential for adverse consequences.
>
> Table 6 shows 2016 payments to hospitals by private insurers, Medicare and Medicaid and what those payments would have been—holding utilization constant—if all hospitals had been paid at Medicare rates.

Table 6. 2016 payments to hospitals

	PHI	*Medicare*	*Medicaid*	*Total*
Current Law	$426.7	$267.5	$189.8	$884.0
M4A	$255.5	$267.5	$187.9	$710.9
Change	-$171.9	$0	-$1.9	-$173.1
Source: NHE, Table 7 and MedPAC				

[193] Doug Badger, "Replacing Employer-Sponsored Health Insurance with Government-Financed Coverage: Considerations for Policymakers," Galen Institute, December 2018. https://galen.org/assets/Replacing-Empl-Spons-Insur-112618.pdf.

> [T]his table compares hospital financing in 2016 with what it would have been had Medicare rates applied to Medicare and private health insurance (PHI, which includes ESI). Assuming that utilization remained unchanged, hospitals would have received a total of $173.1 billion less in 2016 from the three major sources of revenue had Medicare reimbursement rates applied.
>
> One might argue that hospitals could absorb a 40 percent reduction in payments on behalf of privately insured patients through greater efficiencies. It is also worth considering, however, that the rates paid by private insurers—predominantly through ESI—may be helping preserve access to medical care for those enrolled in public programs…
>
> [H]ospitals have consistently run negative margins on their Medicare patients. That margin in 2016 was -9.6%. Since Medicaid payments are only slightly higher than Medicare (and a smaller source of funds), it is likely that the combined Medicare-Medicaid margins are very close to that negative margin. Putting all Americans on the Medicare payment scale would worsen those margins by sharply reducing reimbursement rates for services provided to those who currently have private insurance.

We can see, by driving just a short distance from Capitol Hill, the impact of these low payment rates on hospitals.

Nearby Providence Hospital ended its acute care services in 2018. Founded in 1861, it had been the city's oldest continuously operated hospital, serving some of the District's poorest residents. At least half of its patients were on Medicaid.

And Providence is far from alone. In downtown Philadelphia, Hahnemann University Hospital announced in 2019 that the hospital would close for good in August. A majority of the more than fifty thousand patients that the hospital treated each year had publicly funded medical insurance or none at all. Other hospital closures in that city have followed: Brandywine Hospital in Chester County and Jennersville Hospital in West Grove. These are just a few of the growing list of urban medical centers sinking in red ink.

Medicare and Medicaid, which account for more than sixty per cent of all U.S. hospital care, often pay less than the cost of treatment. According to an analysis by the American Hospital Association, in 2018 Medicare and Medicaid underpaid the cost of care by a combined $76.6 billion.

As is too often the case, those with the lowest incomes and the greatest health care needs are impacted most. If these hospitals were forced to close because they became overly reliant on payments from Medicare and Medicaid, what will that mean for the health care system overall if the private plans cease to exist and are replaced by Medicare for All?

Alternative Government-Centered Reform Options

Single-Payer and the States

Some have suggested that the movement to a federal single-payer system can start with state-based single-payer programs. But in Colorado, in the Chairman's state of Vermont, and most recently in California, attempts have failed to develop single-payer systems.

Colorado voters rejected a single-payer initiative in 2016 by a four to one margin, with residents especially concerned about the high taxes that would be required to finance it and about losing the coverage they have now to the uncertainties of the new system.

In Vermont, officials worked feverishly to design a single-payer system but found that the costs of the program would be prohibitive and that the higher taxes required would seriously damage the economy.

And California, which has veto-proof legislative majorities and a willing governor, recently shelved a single-payer bill because costs and tax levies would have been prohibitive.[194] AB 1400 would have all but eliminated private health coverage and replaced it with a centralized state-run financing system known as CalCare. The program was estimated to cost between $314 billion and $391 billion *a year*, requiring major tax increases in the already highly taxed state.

Public Option

Others have suggested creating a national "public option" government insurance plan to compete with private insurers. We have recent experience with a similar program— Consumer Oriented and Operated Plans—co-ops created through Affordable Care Act financing.[195]

The ACA set aside $6 billion to fund these entities but continued to cut back funding as Congress soon saw the programs floundering. The co-ops were founded on the idealistic belief that community members could band together to create health insurance companies that would be member-driven,

---

[194] "California's Single-Payer Bill Dies," Politico, January 31, 2022. https://www.politico.com/news/2022/01/31/californias-single-payer-bill-dies-00003924.

[195] https://galen.org/2015/obamacare-co-ops-cause-celebre-or-costly-conundrum-2/.

service-oriented insurance co-ops and would not have to answer to shareholders or turn a profit.

But the 23 co-ops that were created had significant start-up costs, no experiential data upon which to set premiums, generally had to pay extra to lease physician and hospital networks, and had few people in the companies and none on their boards with insurance experience. The idealism has quickly faded.

Medicare Buy-In

Still others suggest a Medicare Buy-In approach.

It is hard to see what problem Medicare Buy-in would solve. If early retirees were able to buy into the Medicare program and pay their full share, the cost would be an estimated $1,111 per person.[196] For many, that would be prohibitively expensive, possibly requiring yet another federal program to provide taxpayer-financed subsidies.

When government officials are making decisions about what services will be covered, how much providers will be paid, and how much citizens must pay in mandatory federal taxes, consumers will have even fewer choices and less control than they do today. Medicare for All surely will pay providers less, reduce access to new technologies, stifle innovation, and result in much higher tax burdens. Other proposals to expand government control would only be smaller steps to the same outcomes. I believe there is a better path to achieve the goals I outlined at the beginning of my testimony.

A Path to Patient-Centered Reform

Americans are concerned about a range of health policy issues, and their attentions have shifted since the Covid era. Better health, health security, and secure coverage are more important than ever.

---

[196] Medicare premiums are community rated, and they don't vary by age. A disabled 40 year old disabled beneficiary pays the same premium as a 90 year old. The monthly premium for Part A is $437. Part B is $135.50, but 75 percent is subsidized. The full, unsubsidized premium would thus be $542. The average Part D premium is $33. Eliminating the subsidy would raise that to $132. Thus, without government subsidies, the monthly premium for Medicare would be $1,111. Source for A and B premiums: https://www.cms.gov/newsroom/fact-sheets/2019-medicare-parts-b-premiums-and-deductibles Source for D premiums: https://www.mymedicarematters.org/costs/part-d/.

Better Options

I would like to commend Ranking Member Graham for his hard work in developing proposals to unleash the innovation and energy that have been pent up in our health sector, returning power to doctors and patients. The Ranking Member has provided ideas and guidance for the work of 82 health policy leaders and organizations in the Health Policy Consensus Group to develop the Health Care Choices proposal.[197]

Our proposal contains 35 specific policy recommendations organized around the idea of choice and competition to provide every American an opportunity to get affordable health care and coverage. It would begin to help states' revive their individual and small group health insurance markets that have been so damaged by the ACA. The plan would increase the number of people with health insurance and lower the cost of coverage by up to 25% without any new taxpayer spending.[198] Choice and competition are the centerpiece of the plan, not more top-down, government-managed centralized programs.

The plan would provide states with resources to assist people who need help in purchasing health insurance, especially those with pre-existing conditions, and it would empower states with new flexibility to create more affordable options for coverage. It would redirect resources to the states coupled with new incentives to better meet the needs of their citizens by providing more flexible health care and coverage arrangements and more effective assistance to those who most need help.

The Health Care Choices proposal we have been proud to work on with Sen. Graham would get the federal government out of the business of micro-managing the individual and small group health insurance markets.

Government has created tens of thousands of pages of regulations that rule our health sector in its clumsy and misguided effort to overhaul the market, as I have described in my testimony. It has driven up costs, reduced choices, and made it harder for sick people to get care—all while giving a blank check from taxpayers to health insurers, hospitals, and other big health care businesses.

Health care is too local and personal for a one-size-fits-all approach to work. Here is what the Health Care Choices plan would do…

---

[197] https://healthcarechoices2020.org.

[198] https://www.healthcarechoices2020.org/wp-content/uploads/2020/10/The-Health-Care-Choices-Proposal-Score.pdf.

1) Give patients personal, individual, portable coverage with patients and doctors, not government bureaucrats, in control of health care decisions.
2) Offer a wide variety of competing plans with transparency in pricing and benefits. The coverage would be secure and portable to give people and families protection.
3) Modeling[199] has shown that premiums would fall by up to one third—and even more for young people.
4) More people would be able to own and keep health insurance because premiums would be more affordable.
5) The Health Care Choices proposal would do a better job of taking care of people with pre-existing conditions with focused resources, unlike the Affordable Care Act.

Many of the problems with health care and costs are *because* of big government intervention so we don't need *more* of it.

The Health Care Choices plan contains many other provisions to lower costs and enhance access to modern coverage arrangements like Health Savings Accounts plus ways to create much greater price transparency so newly empowered consumers can get better value in their health spending.

We believe the Health Care Choices Plan would give states more power to make sure their healthy residents can get and keep affordable health coverage and that their most vulnerable citizens have better options for care.

The magic of individual choice and competition that is transformative in the rest of our economy also can work in health care to produce an explosion of options for care and coverage. But first we need to free up innovators and states to allow more affordable consumer-focused solutions.

There is more information about the proposal at www.HealthCareChoices2020.org, where we explain our vision of how states would be empowered to free up their health care markets to provide many more choices of plans and innovative options for more affordable care.

* * *

199 *Ibid.* [https://www.healthcarechoices2020.org/wp-content/uploads/2020/10/The-Health-Care-Choices-Proposal- Score.pdf].

In addition to this legislative proposal, the Trump administration led with regulatory changes that also open the door for more choices and competition in the health sector. Several examples:

Association Health Plans

After the passage of the ACA, smaller employers found it increasingly difficult and costly to offer health insurance to their workers. The Trump administration created new options for smaller and medium-sized firms through its new Association Health Plans rule.

The rule took effect in the fall of 2018 and was off to a successful start. *The Washington Post* reported that: "Chambers of commerce and trade associations have launched more than two dozen of these 'association health plans' in 13 states in the seven months since the Labor Department finalized new rules making it easier for small businesses to band together to buy health coverage in the same way large employers do. And there are initial signs the plans are offering generous benefits and premiums lower than can be found in the Obamacare marketplaces."[200]

There have been some criticisms that these plans might not be offering the same protections as ACA-compliant plans. But a 2019 by Kev Coleman, a former analyst at the insurance information website HealthPocket, found that they were offering benefits comparable to most workplace plans, without any discrimination against patients with preexisting conditions.[201] "We're not seeing skinny plans," he said.

Expanded access to Association Health Plans has been stuck in court since March 2019.

Short-Term Limited Duration Plans

The Trump administration finalized a rule to expand access to short-term, limited-duration plans to give Americans access to health insurance coverage that better fits their needs. The Obama Administration had limited the policies to three months of coverage and prohibited their renewal. Under the new rule,

---

[200] Paige Winfield Cunningham, "The Health 202: Association health plans expanded under Trump look promising so far," January 30, 2019, *The Washington Post.* https://www.washingtonpost.com/news/powerpost/paloma/the-health-202/2019/01/30/the-health-202-association-health-plans-expanded-under-trump-look-promising-so-far/5c50ba751b326b29c3778d05/?noredirect=on&utm_term=.6435676a70d4.

[201] Kev Coleman, "First Phase of New Association Health Plans Reveal Promising Trends," Association Health Plan News, January 2019. https://www.associationhealthplans.com/reports/new-ahp-study/.

these plans can be offered for up to 364 days and renewed for up to 36 months, subject to state regulation.

Short-term plans[202] are helpful to people with gaps in employment, to early retirees who no longer have employer-sponsored health insurance and need bridge coverage before they qualify for Medicare, people between jobs, young people who no longer have coverage from their parents and are working in the gig economy, people who are leaving the workforce temporarily to attend school or training programs, and entrepreneurs starting new businesses, among others. Premiums for short-term health plans typically are less than half those of ACA plans.

The administration's rule also extended consumer protections. Under the Obama administration's previous 2016 rule, people could lose their coverage after three months if they acquired a medical condition during the three-month period. By extending the contract period, people can be protected from losing their coverage if they fall ill.

The plans are not required to cover the comprehensive list of benefits required by the ACA, and education is important to help consumers understand how they differ from ACA-compliant plans.

Several states limit their residents' access to STLD plans, but in so doing, they deny them what may be their only realistic option for coverage.[203]

A White House Council of Economic Advisers (CEA) report on "Deregulating Health Insurance Markets: Value to Market Participants"[204] provides important data showing the positive impact of this consumer-friendly health policy change.

While some say that STLD plans are "junk" insurance that sabotages the ACA, the CEA report provides solid evidence that consumers will benefit, both in expanded coverage and lower costs. CEA estimated that this policy option, together with other deregulatory reforms, could generate benefits to Americans worth an estimated $450 billion over the next 10 years.

---

202 https://www.federalregister.gov/documents/2018/08/03/2018-16568/short-term-limited-duration-insurance.

203 Doug Badger and Whitney Jones, "Five Steps Policymakers Can Take to Permit the Sale and Renewal of Affordable Alternatives to Obamacare Policies," The Heritage Foundation, April 26, 2018. https://www.heritage.org/health-care-reform/report/five-steps-policymakers-can-take-permit-the-sale-and-renewal- affordable.

204 Council of Economic Advisers, "Deregulating Health Insurance Markets: Value to Market Participants," February 2019. https://www.whitehouse.gov/wp-content/uploads/2019/02/Deregulating-Health-Insurance-Markets- FINAL.pdf.

Health Reimbursement Arrangements

The administration also finalized a rule to enhance employer and employee options through Health Reimbursement Arrangements (HRAs). HRAs are tax-preferred, notional accounts that employers use to reimburse employee medical expenses. The Obama administration issued rules that prohibited people from using their HRA to purchase individual market coverage. Many workers who are offered health coverage at work do not participate in their employer plans, often because of costs, and therefore are more likely to be uninsured.

In 2019, the Departments of HHS, Labor, and the Treasury issued a final rule permitting employers to offer HRAs that reimburse individual market premiums. Through these individual coverage HRAs, employees use tax-preferred employer contributions to buy coverage in the individual market that works best for them. The projection in the final rule indicated that 800,000 employers would offer individual coverage HRAs later this decade with 11 million people enrolled in the individual market with these HRAs.

During the comment period on the proposed rule, the Galen Institute submitted public comments encouraging the administration to take the rule one step further by allowing spouses to integrate HRA funds to obtain a family plan.[205] We argue that current law would allow the integration of HRAs with group health plans sponsored by the employer of a spouse.[206]

As an example, consider that one spouse is offered health insurance at work. The employer may allow the plan to be extended to cover the family but only if the employee pays the full extra costs, which may be prohibitive for this lower-income worker.

If the other spouse's employer offers an HRA contribution, that employee could use the funds to buy into the first spouse's plan. This working couple could benefit from the ability to combine the HRA funds and obtain a family health insurance plan.

We encourage Congress to consider legislation to expand this new funding option to expand insurance coverage options and portability of health insurance.

---

[205] https://galen.org/2019/increasing-access-to-health-insurance-for-working-families/.

[206] Doug Badger and Grace-Marie Turner, "Give Working Families A Break," *RealClearHealth*, January 7, 2019. https://www.realclearhealth.com/articles/2019/01/07/give_working_families_a_break_110856.html.

State Innovations

The solution is more, not fewer, choices. States have much more experience than the federal government in overseeing health insurance markets and greater flexibility to meet the needs of their residents.

One part of the ACA provides an option for State Innovation Waivers to allow states to reallocate existing resources to take better care of those with pre-existing conditions, for example.

States that have used early waiver authority to create risk-mitigation programs have seen in many cases dramatic results with no new federal spending.

Doug Badger and Ed Haislmaier of Heritage explain how early targeted waivers granted to states helped them to better manage patients with chronic and pre-existing conditions.[207]

"Several states have successfully used a waiver to change market conditions sufficiently that premiums fell for individual health insurance while still protecting the ability of people with high health care costs to access care," they write.

After a waiver reform in Alaska, premiums for the lowest-cost Bronze plans fell by 39 percent in 2018, they report. Oregon showed similar results in 2018, with premiums for the lowest-cost Bronze plans falling by 5 percent. Premiums for the highest-cost Bronze plans plunged by 20 percent. In Minnesota, the third state with an approved waiver, premiums dropped in both 2018 and 2019. Average premium for ACA coverage in 2019 will be lower for every Minnesota insurer than they were in 2017. Four other states have had waivers approved for 2019: Maryland, Maine, New Jersey, and Wisconsin.[208] Georgia currently has an innovative waiver pending with the Biden administration.

According to the Heritage paper, "States repurpose a portion of federal money that would otherwise have been paid to insurers as premium subsidies, supplement this federal money with non-federal sources, and then use the resulting pool of money to pay medical claims for policyholders who incur high medical bills. Since this process would reduce premiums, it also would

---

[207] Doug Badger, Ed Haislmaier, "State Innovation: The Key to Affordable Health Care Choices," The Heritage Foundation, September 27, 2018. https://www.heritage.org/health-care-reform/report/state-innovation-the-key- affordable-health-care-coverage-choices.

[208] Grace-Marie Turner, Doug Badger, "Several States Have Found Ways To Mitigate Obamacare's Damage To Their Health Insurance Markets," *Forbes*, October 3, 2018. https://www.forbes.com/sites/gracemarieturner/2018/10/03/several-states-have-found-ways-to-mitigate-obamacares- damage-to-their-health-insurance-markets/#56d1b71730da.

reduce federal premium subsidies, making it budget neutral to the federal government."

States are employing various risk mitigation strategies to finance coverage for those with high health costs, repurposing federal money to pay medical bills for residents in poor health. By separately subsidizing those with the highest health costs, they can lower premiums for individual health insurance, and the lower premiums also mean increased enrollment.

This offers states flexibility through new Section 1332 guidance to tailor solutions to the needs of their residents.

A few states have found a key to undoing some of Obamacare's damage to their individual health insurance markets by redirecting some federal funding to better help sick people. These states are providing separate assistance to those with the highest health costs, thereby reducing premiums and increasing enrollment for healthy people driven out of the market by soaring costs.

In a paper published by The Heritage Foundation, scholars Doug Badger and Ed Haislmaier detail how several states have successfully used Obamacare's Section 1332 waiver authority to begin to revive their non-group health insurance markets with better risk-mitigation strategies.

They explain in "State Innovation: The Key to Affordable Health Insurance Choices"[209] that Obamacare's rigid and centralized federal regulation of the nongroup market has driven premiums up, choices down, and forced millions of people out of the individual health insurance market.

Section 1332 of the Affordable Care Act permits states to seek waivers from certain federal health insurance requirements if they believe they can do a better job as long as their program doesn't cost the federal government more money. But the rules the Obama administration subsequently issued were so strict that they make it very difficult for states to get approval for the broader innovative reform proposals envisioned by the provision's authors.

Alaska, Minnesota, and Oregon received waivers from the Trump administration for targeted reform initiatives that have been successful in lowering premiums for individual health insurance by separately subsidizing those with the highest health costs. And the lower premiums also mean increased enrollment.

According to the paper:

---

[209] "State Innovation: The Key to Affordable Health Care Coverage Choices," by Doug Badger and Ed Haislmaier, The Heritage Foundation, September 27, 2018. https://www.heritage.org/health-care-reform/report/state-innovation-the-key-affordable-health-care-coverage-choices.

"Alaska was the first state to obtain a section 1332 waiver to implement this type of approach. The state sought a waiver of Obamacare's 'single-risk-pool' requirement, under which people who are likely to file large medical claims must be pooled with those who might never see a doctor. This Obamacare mandate had touched off a vicious cycle, in which insurers charge ever higher premiums, repelling the healthiest customers but not the sickest, resulting in premiums that are increasingly affordable only to those who receive federal subsidies.

"Alaska instead proposed to move customers with one of 33 medical conditions into a separate pool. Their medical claims would be funded in part by a portion of federal premium-subsidy payments diverted to the pool. Non-federal funding sources include ceded premiums (meaning, in the case of an enrollee whose claims costs the insurer transfers to the pool, the insurer must also transfer to the pool some portion of the premium it received from that enrollee), state assessments on insurers, and state general fund contributions. Based on an actuarial analysis commissioned by Alaska in support of its waiver application, the state concluded that it would reduce premiums and increase enrollment in the individual market at no additional cost to the federal government."

The analysis was correct. After the waiver reform in Alaska, premiums for the lowest-cost Bronze plans fell by 39 percent in 2018.

Oregon showed similar results in 2018, with premiums for the lowest-cost Bronze plans falling by 5 percent. Premiums for the highest-cost Bronze plans plunged by 20 percent. In Minnesota, the third state with an approved waiver, premiums dropped in both 2018 and 2019. Average premium for Obamacare coverage in 2019 were lower for every Minnesota insurer than they were in 2017.

Four other states had waivers approved for 2019: Maryland, Maine, New Jersey, and Wisconsin. Insurers in Maryland had sought 2019 premium increases averaging over 30 percent. Insurers filed those rate requests before the federal government approved Maryland's waiver application. After receiving approval, Maryland announced that 2019 rates would drop by more than 13 percent. Instead of a 30 percent premium hike, Maryland consumers will pay 13 percent less, on average, than they did in 2018.

Waivers alone, however, are not enough. Congress should enact legislation to empower states to establish consumer-centered approaches that reduce health care costs and increase choices with the Health Care Choices proposal.[210]

The proposal would rely on states to devise even more creative ways to provide help for the sick as well as those needing assistance in purchasing health coverage. The Health Care Choices plan would repeal Obamacare's federal entitlements to premium assistance and Medicaid expansion and replace them with formula grants to the states so they can set up consumer-centered programs.

Instead of asking Washington's permission for some limited flexibility, states would use federal resources to finance approaches that best serve the needs of their residents. The limited experience of redirecting funds toward risk mitigation shows that states can and should be leading on health reform.

The Health Policy Consensus Group, a project of the Galen Institute, submitted public comments to HHS regarding the Section 1332 State Relief and Empowerment waiver program, encouraging codification of the 2018 Guidance regarding the waivers:

> Section 1332 of the Affordable Care Act (ACA) permits the Secretary of Health and Human Services (HHS) and the Secretary of the Treasury to approve a state's proposal to waive specific provisions of the ACA, provided the proposal meets certain requirements. The "State Relief and Empowerment Waivers" guidance issued in the Federal Register (83 FR 53575) (hereinafter referred to as the "2018 Guidance") superseded previous guidance published on December 16, 2015, in the Federal Register (80 FR 78131). We strongly support CMS's proposal to codify the agency's 2018 Guidance into federal regulation.

John McDonough, a Harvard professor who served as a senior advisor to the U.S. Senate Committee on Health, Education, Labor, and Pensions from 2008 through 2010 when the ACA was debated and enacted, in 2014 wrote:[211]

> "Section 1332 of Title I of the Affordable Care Act offers to state governments the ability to waive significant portions of the ACA, including requirements related to qualified health plans, health benefit exchanges, cost sharing, and refundable tax credits. It permits state

---

[210] "Health Care Choices 20/20: A vision for consumer-directed health reform," Health Policy Consensus Group, September 2021. http://www.healthcarechoices2020.org.

[211] John E. McDonough, "Wyden's Waiver: State Innovation on Steroids," Journal of Health Politics, Policy, and Law (2014) 39(5): 1099-1111.

governments to obtain funding that otherwise would have gone to residents and businesses through the ACA and to use those funds to establish, beginning in 2017, an alternative health reform framework within statutory limits."

Unfortunately, the 2015 Guidance served to restrict states' ability to utilize 1332 waivers to improve their health insurance markets by tightening the statutory "guardrails" that must be satisfied for waiver approval. Three of these guardrails pertain to the number of people with coverage as well as the affordability of that coverage and nature of that coverage. The fourth guardrail requires that the waiver not increase the federal deficit.

This 2015 guidance was far more restrictive than the statutory requirements and virtually nullified states' ability to innovate through section 1332.

As a result of the restrictive guidance and approach, only one state submitted and had a 1332 waiver approved prior to January 1, 2017.

Fortunately, the 2018 Guidance offers both an interpretation of the guardrails that makes 1332 waivers more useful for states as well as an interpretation that is more consistent with the statute. By codifying the 2018 Guidance, the Departments will further the intended aim of 1332 waivers to promote state policy innovation in designing programs that expand options, lower costs, and promote coverage without increasing the federal deficit…

Twelve states received 1332 waivers since 2017 in addition to three states with waivers approved in 2017. States with approved 1332 waivers have generally experienced positive results. A June 2020 CMS analysis of the effect of 1332 waivers found that premiums were an average of 17.7 percent lower during the 2020 plan year in the 12 states that had approved 1332 waivers in place than they would have been without those waivers.[212]

In 2020, another three states secured 1332 waivers. Consumers have thus benefited from 1332 waivers that are consistent with the existing guardrails.

These programs could be models for future health reform, devolving power away from centralized federal programs to states and ultimately to consumers in a market catering to their needs rather than to Washington's bureaucracy.

---

[212] CCIIO Data Brief Series, "State Relief and Empowerment Waivers: State-based Reinsurance Programs, June 2020. https://www.cms.gov/CCIIO/Programs-and-Initiatives/State-Innovation-Waivers/Downloads/1332-Data- Brief-June2020.pdf.

* * *

I would like to recount the experience of "Janet," a patient in Colorado who wrote to us about her experience with a government program that was her only option for coverage.[213] Her story encapsulates for me the problems with federal government control over health care.

Janet reported to us:

> "In 1999, I was diagnosed with Hepatitis C, which made me ineligible for insurance, (denied for pre-existing conditions)," she said. "I live in Colorado, and they had a high-risk pool that covered people like me. I applied for that and was accepted.
>
> "My premiums in 2010 were $275/month with a total out of pocket of $2,500. [While I was on] this plan, my liver failed, and I needed a liver transplant. It was approved without a question. My $600,000 transplant was covered 100% with a $2,500 out of pocket maximum!"

When Obamacare went into effect in 2014, Colorado's high-risk pool was closed. "I was forced into the regular marketplace that everyone was telling me was a good thing because I couldn't get denied. I think my first year on that policy, my premiums were in the $450 range—which I thought wasn't too terrible, but still more than I had been paying.

> "The thing I noticed from the start was that instead of full coverage, almost everything I needed was denied, which threw me into the world of having to appeal (sometimes several times) to get the basic care I needed.
>
> "Since then, my premiums skyrocketed. In 2017, I paid $735 a month with total out-of-pocket costs of $5,500. In 2018, my premiums went up to $1,100 a month with a deductible of $6,300. Once I hit that mark, I'm covered 80%.
>
> "Further, none of my anti-rejection meds are on the formulary of my insurance. If I could not afford them, my body would most certainly reject my liver, causing another liver transplant that would not be covered 100%.
>
> "I have to spend $19,500 before my insurance pays anything, and it doesn't cover all my prescription costs. My old plan was almost a third of what I have to pay now.

---

[213] See www.HealthCareChoices2020.org testimonials.

"I have many friends and work associates in the same boat as me. Many of them are doing without insurance and are betting that they won't need more than what they can afford to pay out of pocket. I cannot do that, because if something happened and I needed another transplant, it would bankrupt my family."

Janet received coverage under the ACA but said her access to care was inferior to the state high-risk pool coverage she had before—but with much higher costs for her coverage. The current system is not working for Janet and others like her in receiving the care she needs. Americans want more, not fewer, choices in health coverage, and Medicare for All would put them all on a single government program.

Conclusion

The Galen Institute is non-partisan, and we welcome the opportunity to work with health policy colleagues on both sides of the aisle. We seek out colleagues and legislators who are open to our ideas on patient-centered health reforms that would rely on competition and choice to produce better, more affordable health care and coverage options.

Thank you for inviting me to offer this perspective. I look forward to your questions and would welcome the opportunity to work to with you to achieve the goals of better access to more affordable coverage and better protection for the vulnerable.

Statement of Charles P. Blahous[214], before the U.S. Senate Committee on the Budget, May 12, 2022

Thank you, Chairman Sanders, Ranking Member Graham, and all of the members of the committee. I appreciate this opportunity to testify on the federal budget costs of enacting Medicare for All (M4A).

My testimony is based largely on research I published in 2018 to estimate the federal cost of enacting Medicare for All. Let me begin with a few caveats

214 Charles P. Blahous holds the J. Fish and Lillian F. Smith Chair at the Mercatus Center at George Mason University, where he is also Senior Research Strategist. He is also a Visiting Fellow with the Hoover Institution at Stanford University.

before summarizing these estimates and the assumptions that underlay them. The first caveat is that while there are many similarities between various bills to enact M4A, there are also important differences between them, and thus any estimates developed for one particular bill will not apply exactly to a different one. My 2018 study analyzed one specific bill introduced by Chairman Sanders in 2017, which differed in several important particulars from subsequently introduced M4A bills. That study represents the only comprehensive cost estimate I have developed, and thus I can offer only approximate guidance as to the likely budgetary effects of legislation introduced more recently.

Second, the narrow purpose of my research was to estimate the federal budget costs of enacting M4A. It was not to opine on whether M4A would be good or bad policy, nor did it engage various important value judgments or difficult health policy calls that must be made in the course of any comprehensive healthcare legislation. While the study (as well as this testimony) does describe possible effects of various policy decisions associated with implementing M4A, it does so only to illuminate how the budgetary estimates might be affected by them, and not to presume particular value judgments that are appropriately the prerogative of lawmakers.

Third, although various incarnations of these proposals have titles that include the phrase "Medicare for All," the federal healthcare systems they would establish differ from current Medicare in fundamental ways. Instead of extending the current Medicare program to the population as a whole, these bills would move all Americans, including seniors currently on Medicare, into a new system offering different (mostly more generous) benefits, while doing away with many of Medicare's current financing mechanisms such as patient deductibles and copays. I have not attempted to analyze an expansion of eligibility for traditional Medicare. Nor have I analyzed any of the various proposals to allow new participants to buy into the current Medicare program.

Fourth, a number of things have changed since my study was performed. Other bills have subsequently been introduced that differ in important particulars from the provisions I analyzed. Other legislation has subsequently been enacted that would directly affect my estimates if I were to redo them. Baseline projections for national health expenditures have also changed, as they always do. And importantly, we now have the benefit of other important published analyses, including work by the Congressional Budget Office (CBO), which models certain important effects that I could not. Later in my testimony, I will attempt to summarize how this newer information might affect a future recalculation of my estimates.

Cost Estimates

Let me first summarize the findings of my 2018 study before proceeding to discuss how its results differ from what an updated study might find. My study found that the additional federal costs of enacting Medicare for All would likely be somewhere in the range of $32.6-$38.8 trillion over its first ten years of full implementation, which at the time the study was conducted would have been 2022-2031. The $32.6 trillion projection was presented in the paper as a lower-bound estimate, representing an unlikely scenario in which the provisions of M4A that are intended to lower costs all produced the full amount of their potential savings, without regard for any accompanying adverse effects this might have on healthcare access, timeliness or quality. Alternatively, if after M4A's enactment, historical patterns of federal government behavior remained more consistent with past practice, the new federal costs would be closer to $38.8 trillion over the first ten years.

We have no experience with enacting permanent federal cost increases of this magnitude, which renders these numbers especially difficult for many people to conceptualize. To provide context, the study translated them into a share of GDP. The $32.6 trillion estimate equated to an addition to federal budget costs of roughly 10.7% of GDP in 2022, gradually increasing to 12.7% of GDP in 2031, and growing further afterward. If instead, new federal costs were $38.8 trillion over ten years, federal obligations would be increased by 12.6% in 2022 and by 15.1% in 2031, also growing larger over subsequent time. To illustrate the qualitative size of the cost increase, the study noted that even under the lower-bound estimate of $32.6 trillion, a doubling of all currently projected federal individual and corporate income taxes would be insufficient to finance the added federal costs of enacting M4A.

Table 1. Projected federal cost increases under M4A

Scenario	New Federal Costs, 2022-31 ($T)	New Federal Costs, 2022 (% of GDP)	New Federal Costs, 2031 (% of GDP)
Lower-bound estimate	$32.6 T	10.7%	12.7%
Estimate assuming continuity in provider + drug payments	$38.8 T	12.6%	15.1%

The estimates in the preceding table do not reflect the total federal costs of M4A, but rather just its addition to federal costs above and beyond currently projected federal healthcare spending and tax subsidies, which include

Medicare, Medicaid, the tax subsidy for employer-sponsored health insurance, Affordable Care Act exchange subsidies, and other health programs. Total projected health cost obligations under M4A were estimated to be substantially higher than the net cost increases shown in Table 1, somewhere within the range of $54.6 trillion and $60.7 trillion over the first ten years. Under the lower-bound estimate, federal spending on M4A alone would be 20.8% of GDP by 2031. For reference, 20.8% of GDP is more than all federal spending as a percentage of GDP as recently as 2018.[215] Further, these figures did not account for all national health-related spending under M4A, as for example they excluded long-term care spending that would remain the responsibilities of individuals and state governments.

Factors Affecting the Cost Estimates

The vast majority of new federal costs under M4A would result from the federal government's assuming responsibility for most national health spending currently financed by other entities, including private insurance, state and local governments, and individuals. By itself, and before considering possible offsetting savings, M4A's expansion of coverage combined with shifting from privately-financed to federally-financed insurance would not only cause federal budget obligations to increase, but national health expenditures as well. This increase occurs partially because of increased expenditures on health services for the currently uninsured, and partially because of M4A's coverage of some services not now covered by traditional Medicare, such as dental, vision and hearing benefits. Additional expenditure increases would also occur because M4A would offer first-dollar coverage of individuals' health services, unlike traditional Medicare and most current private insurance. It is well established in the economics literature that the more of an individual's health services that are covered by insurance, the more they tend to consume, irrespective of the services' efficacy or value. M4A's first-dollar coverage of health services would therefore fuel substantial additional demand.

M4A seeks to offset these additional costs through various means. One is through the replacement of private health insurance by a federally-administered system that sponsors intend to have lower administrative costs.

---

215 Congressional Budget Office, "Historical Budget Data," Feb. 2021, https://www.cbo.gov/data/budget-economic-data#2.

My study adopted an aggressive assumption that over half of the administrative costs currently borne by private insurance would be eliminated. These assumed administrative cost savings would offset roughly 4% of the additional federal costs arising from the federal government's becoming the financier of nearly all US healthcare. For another comparison, these assumed administrative cost savings would offset roughly 28% of the additional national health spending expected to arise from increased health service demand under M4A. In other words, health insurance administrative costs would be lowered, but these savings would offset only a fraction of the additional national health expenditures projected as a result of M4A's expanded and enhanced coverage.

Another means by which the M4A legislation I analyzed would attempt to contain costs is by having the Secretary of Health and Human Services negotiate drug prices with a particular emphasis on replacing brand-name medications with less expensive generics. To understand how cost projections are affected by such features, it is important to distinguish between potential savings and likely savings. There are hard limits on the potential savings that can arise from such a provision because prescription drugs accounted (at the time of my study) for just 10 percent of total national health expenditures, and generics already made up 85 percent of all prescription drugs sold. Nevertheless, my lower-bound estimates employed aggressive assumptions for prescription drug cost savings, specifically an immediate 12 percent reduction in prescription drug expenditures, without attempting to model potential adverse effects of this reduction on the pharmaceutical industry or the pace of innovation.

History provides reason for skepticism that this level of savings would be achieved. Historically the federal government has tended to prioritize health benefits for those dependent on federal programs over the interests of taxpayers in restraining cost growth. Though it is theoretically possible that under M4A the federal government would switch its emphasis from allowing patients full access to the fruits of pharmaceutical and other healthcare innovation, to protecting the interests of taxpayers through cost containment, the political economy incentives under M4A make this unlikely. Under M4A, the lack of deductibles, copayments and cost-sharing would largely eliminate consumer (and thus voter) direct sensitivity to healthcare prices, including drug prices. Moreover, the established national tendency to favor access to pharmaceutical innovation and development over cost containment has likely become even more entrenched during the ongoing pandemic. Dramatic drug price savings under M4A should therefore be considered an aspirational goal rather than the basis for an intermediate cost projection. This is one of multiple reasons why my study found that actual costs under M4A would likely exceed the lower-bound projection scenario.

The most significant variable affecting M4A cost projections is that of provider payment rates. The study's lower-bound projection assumed that all provider payment rates would immediately be set to Medicare rates, which for inpatient hospital services were roughly 40% lower than private insurance rates over the time window in the study. Several earlier studies had assumed higher payment rates than this would be required, because Medicare payment rates were substantially below providers' reported costs of providing services. The CMS Medicare actuary, for example, projected at the time of the study that 80% of hospitals would experience negative margins in the near term when treating Medicare patients, a situation M4A would extend to the population as a whole. See Figures 1 and 2, reproduced from a memorandum from the CMS Medicare actuary's office.[216]

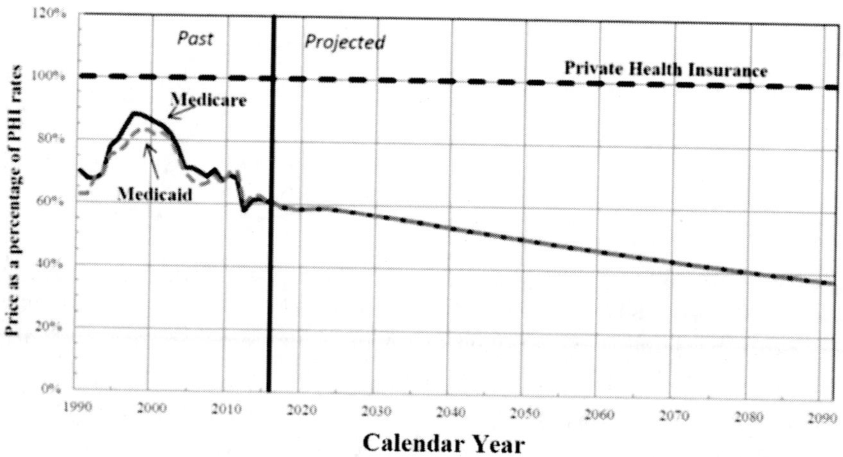

Figure 1. CMS Medicare Actuary Comparisons of Inpatient Hospital Payment Rates.

[216] The figures shown here are reproduced from CMS Office of the Actuary, "Projected Medicare Expenditures under an Illustrative Scenario with Alternative Payment Updates to Medicare Providers," https://www.cms.gov/Research-Statistics-Data-and-Systems/Statistics-Trends-and-Reports/ReportsTrustFunds/Downloads/2018TRAlternativeScenario.pdf. These figures from the 2018 memorandum were chosen for inclusion in this testimony because they illustrate data cited in the study. CMS has more recently published updates of these figures that are qualitatively similar. See https://www.cms.gov/files/document/illustrative-alternative-scenario-2021.pdf.

We do not know how providers would respond to payment reductions of this magnitude for treatments now covered by private insurance, concurrent with a simultaneous increase in patient demand for health services under M4A. It was clearly likely that there would be some disruptions in the availability, timeliness and quality of healthcare services, but my 2018 study did not attempt to model the extent to which the supply of healthcare services may be insufficient to meet expanded demand under M4A.

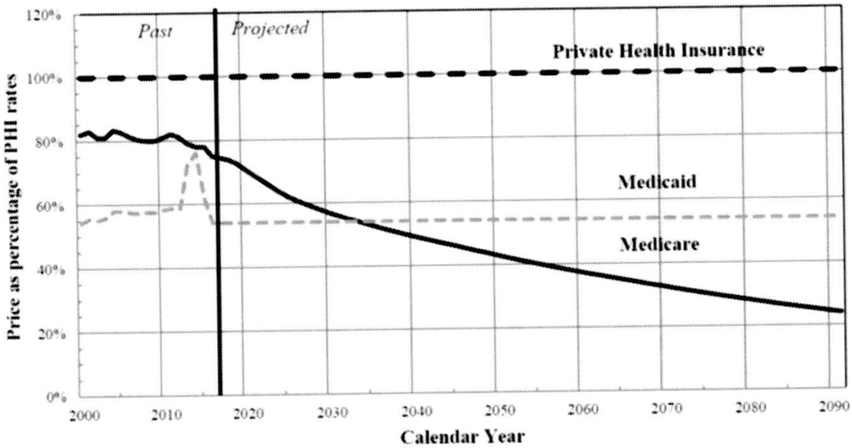

Figure 2. CMS Medicare Actuary Comparisons of Physician Payment Rates.

The study's lower-bound estimates assumed the universal and immediate application of Medicare payment rates. Throughout recent history, lawmakers have repeatedly balked at applying payment reductions that are far smaller, less sudden, and applicable to a lesser number of payments, than this assumption. For example, lawmakers began annual overrides of the Medicare physician payment Sustainable Growth Rate formula when the pending cuts were just 4-5% and applied only to Medicare treatments. By contrast, inpatient hospital service payment cuts M4A would start at over 40% in the lower-bound projection scenario and apply to the larger number of treatments now covered by private insurance.

Table 2 summarizes how the 2018 M4A cost estimates were affected by these various assumptions.

Table 2. Effect of various assumptions upon M4A cost projections

Scenario	Additional Federal Costs, 2022-2031 ($T)
= Added federal costs from coverage increase	= $40.368 T
-Administrative cost savings	-$1.572 T
= Estimate assuming administrative savings	= $38.797 T
-Potential drug cost savings	-$0.846 T
= Estimate assuming drug and admin. savings	= $37.950 T
-Lowering provider payments to Medicare rates	-$5.307 T
= Lower-bound estimate	= $32.644 T

Other Contemporaneous Perspectives on Federal Costs

An occasional question about such estimates is whether they reflect a particular policy viewpoint or instead reflect broader agreement among experts as to the likely costs of M4A. The answer is that cost estimates produced by experts from a wide range of policy perspectives and affiliations arrived at roughly the same results as my study, after adjusting for different years estimated, as well as assumptions regarding provider payment rates, drug prices, and whether long-term services and supports (LTSS) are included. The following table translates my 2018 estimates into what they would have been for M4A's implementation during 2017-2026, as assumed in studies published by the Urban Institute, the Center for Health and Economy, and Emory University professor Ken Thorpe.

Table 3. Alternative estimates for added federal costs under M4A, if effective 2017-2026

Estimate	New Federal Costs over 2017-2026 ($T)
Center for Health and Economy, Alternative Estimate	$40.2
Blahous (w/o provider cuts or drug savings)	$29.5
Urban Institute (w/o LTSS benefit)	$29.1
Blahous (w/drug savings, w/o provider cuts)	$28.9
Center for Health and Economy, Primary Estimate	$27.3
Blahous (w/provider cuts & drug savings)	$25.2
Thorpe	$24.7

As Table 3 shows, my 2018 estimates are generally within the range of those produced by other experts, the differences between them largely attributable to differences in key assumptions. The Urban Institute study produced an estimate of $32.0 trillion, which included LTSS coverage.

Adjusting for the fact that the 2017 bill I studied did not include this coverage brings the Urban Institute's estimate down within the range of my own. My lower-bound estimate was generally smaller than those of other experts because it assumed the immediate imposition of Medicare provider payment rates, which are lower than the payment rates the other studies all assumed would be the minimum necessary. The Thorpe study estimated higher total national health spending than mine, while mine assumed the federal government would pay for a higher percentage of the whole. In general, however, the estimates are qualitatively similar regardless of who made them, providing the same general picture of the scale of federal government expansion M4A would bring about.

How Future Estimates Might Change in Light of Recent Information

As noted earlier, I have not performed a comprehensive cost re-estimate since my 2018 study was performed. However, there are multiple reasons why an updated version of my study would likely produce somewhat different estimates. We now have additional information that was not available to me at the time of my study, including a comprehensive report from CBO in December of 2020.

The CBO report modeled five options for creating a national single-payer healthcare system along the lines of M4A, projecting the new federal costs of each option in a single year (2030). Only one of these options, option 5, resembled current proposals for M4A, which generally include LTSS coverage. CBO found that option 5 would increase federal costs by $3.00 trillion in 2030 alone, as well as increasing national health expenditures (NHE). CBO's options 1 and 2 are less relevant to the M4A discussion because they are for models with significant patient cost-sharing, at cross purposes with the stated policy goals of most M4A advocates and sponsors. Options 3 and 4 also differ from current M4A proposals in omitting long-term care benefits, but are nevertheless useful for predicting how my own previous estimates (which also omitted long-term care costs) might change in light of more recent information. Table 4 compares key assumptions and results from CBO's options 3 and 4 to my own.

As Table 4 shows, there are substantial differences between CBO's estimates and mine, even between scenarios (such as CBO's Option 4 and my study's "maintain provider payments" scenario) where key underlying payment rate assumptions are in the same general range. This raises the question as to why CBO's estimates differ so much from mine (and by extension, from those of the Urban Institute, the Center for Health and Economy, and Thorpe). In an effort to answer this question, I grouped the sources of projection differences into four broad categories depicted in Figure 3.

Table 4. Alternative payment assumptions and results

Scenario	Key Assumptions	New Federal Costs in 2030 ($T)
Blahous lower-bound	No LTSS benefits, Medicare payment rates, 12% drug price cuts	$3.97
CBO Option 3	No LTSS benefits, hospitals at 123% of Medicare payment rates, physicians at 111% of Medicare rates, 30% drug price cuts	$1.77
CBO Option 4	No LTSS benefits, hospitals at 142% of Medicare payment rates, physicians at 120% of Medicare rates, 7% drug price cuts	$2.40
Blahous drug price cuts only	No LTSS benefits, current-law hospital/physician payment rates, 12% drug price cuts	$4.63
Blahous, no provider payment or drug price cuts	No LTSS benefits, current-law hospital/physician payment rates, no drug price cuts	$4.73

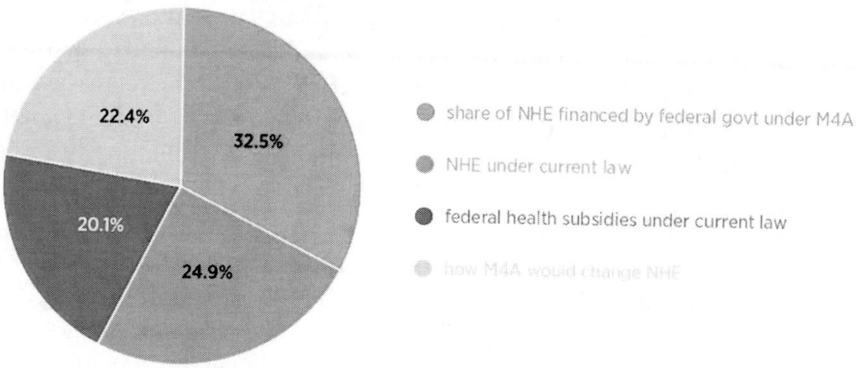

Note: M4A = Medicare for All; NHE = national health expenditures.
Source: Author's calculations based on data from CBO's Single-Payer Health Care Systems Team, "How CBO Analyzes the Costs," cross-referenced with Blahous, "Costs of a National Single-Payer Health Care System."

Figure 3. Differences between CBO Option 4 and Blahous Maintain-Provider-Payments Scenario.

As Figure 3 shows, the largest differences between my estimates and CBO's are unrelated to M4A's effect on national health costs. The largest share of difference (32.5%) pertains to different estimates of the share of national healthcare that would be financed by the federal government, instead of continuing to be financed by others, including state and local governments, philanthropies, and individuals out of pocket (for example, on LTSS and prescription drugs). CBO also estimated something I did not; the amount of healthcare services that would continue to be provided by physicians and other providers who opt out of the M4A system. While I believe that some of these various categories of healthcare spending are likely to be absorbed or crowded out by M4A, I also believe CBO is correct to conclude that substantial amounts of this care would continue to be paid for by Americans outside of the M4A system.

The second largest category of difference (24.9%) involves downward movement of the current-law baseline projections for NHE. After my study was published, the Centers for Medicare and Medicaid (CMS) lowered their NHE projections somewhat. Additionally, CBO derived its own estimates for NHE that were somewhat lower than CMS's. Each of these two effects (CMS's downward revisions and CBO's additional adjustments) reduces the cost estimates in roughly equal measure. Hence, were I to repeat my study using CMS projections again, it is reasonable to estimate that I would incorporate roughly half of this category of differences into my revisions.

The smallest category of difference (20.1%) involves alternative calculations of federal healthcare subsidies under current law. A substantial portion of this difference is rooted in legislative events subsequent to the publication of my study, such as the repeal of the so-called "Cadillac plan tax," medical device tax and other health insurance taxes, thereby increasing net federal health subsidies under current law. Accordingly, if my study were to be updated, a substantial portion of these changes would need to be incorporated.

Perhaps surprisingly, alternative views of the likely effects of M4A on national health spending account for only 22.4% of the difference between my federal cost estimates from CBO's. Though relatively small, these differences are likely to be of strong interest to policy makers, because they pertain to whether M4A decelerates national health spending growth or accelerates it still further, and because they also pertain to whether patients receive the care they seek. CBO's cost estimates here are lower than mine because they a) assume lower administrative costs and b) find that a substantial amount of healthcare sought under M4A would simply be denied.

CBO's report acknowledges that it assumes lower administrative costs under M4A than other studies do, as well as lower than in other U.S. public insurance systems and single payer systems abroad. CBO devotes substantial space to explaining its lower estimates. CBO projects an administrative cost rate for M4A of between 1.5%-1.8%, whereas other studies' estimates have ranged from 4.7%-6.0%, existing single-payer systems internationally generally range from 2%-3%, and current Medicare/Medicaid's are roughly 8%. While I commend CBO for the thoroughness and rigor of their administrative cost derivations, and while M4A has the potential to further reduce administrative costs below my 2018 assumptions, CBO's assumptions go further than I feel comfortable adopting. We must remember important factors in play here, for example that other nations have not generally achieved administrative cost rates that low despite many years of experience, and also that current Medicare serves an older population with higher average healthcare costs than M4A would, meaning that M4A could not achieve administrative cost rates below current Medicare fee-for-service's 2.3 percent unless M4A's administrative costs per capita were dramatically lower.

Perhaps the most striking difference between my study and CBO's is that CBO modeled the amount of care that would be denied under M4A, whereas I lacked the capacity to model this phenomenon and implicitly assumed that the supply of healthcare services would expand to meet additional demand, while cautioning that this might not happen. Our respective estimates of increased healthcare demand in 2030 were remarkably similar ($684 billion in my study vs. $661 billion in CBO's Option 4), but CBO found that $254 billion of this new demand for healthcare would simply go unmet. In its Option 3 (the option that attempts to slow the growth of health spending by more stringently restricting provider payments), CBO found that the majority of additional demand ($319 billion out of $591 billion) would go unmet. In other words, Americans would be promised more healthcare, but the majority of these promises would go unfulfilled.

CBO's assumptions of large administrative cost reductions become especially important in this context. CBO's model assumes that health providers under M4A will be able to dramatically reduce their time spent on administrative tasks, and that this time saved will be converted to additional supply of healthcare. However, the numbers become daunting if we shift our perspective from what I would regard as aggressively optimistic to prudently optimistic.

For example, CBO projects that 80% of the time nurses spend on administrative tasks would be eliminated by M4A. If we simply assume that

M4A does half as well – that is, reducing nurses' administrative duties by 40% rather than 80% --and combine this with assumptions of Medicare-level payment rates, as well as CBO's reasonable and well-studied assumptions regarding the prevalence of opt-outs, provider supply responses to payment cuts, and the ability of health providers and drug manufacturers to expand supply in response to demand – then we find that almost all of the additional health services promised by M4A would fail to materialize. Only $96 billion of a projected $684 billion in healthcare demand increase – or 14% -would be met, whereas an overwhelming 86% would be denied. Moreover, $81 billion of the supply increase that would occur would consist entirely of prescription drugs: by contrast, over 97% of the additional physician and hospital services sought under M4A wouldn't be delivered. In this scenario, it would be no exaggeration to say that M4A would increase eligibility and demand for additional healthcare, while in practice denying the promised additional access almost completely.

These findings are not only of concern from a health policy perspective, they carry important implications for the potential costs of M4A. For example, the provider payment rates assumed in my study's lower-bound projection scenario are more clearly unrealistic if they would lead to 97% of the new demand for hospital and physician services under M4A being denied. Lawmakers are highly unlikely to tolerate such a situation after national investment in the promise of universal access to healthcare. The CBO report therefore enables us to say with increased certainty that the higher-payment scenarios in my study are far more probable than my lower-bound projections.

The CBO report also indicates that M4A bills introduced in Congress would almost certainly add to, rather than subtract from, the problem of rising national health expenditures. Option 5, the option that most closely tracks proposed legislation, would increase NHE under CBO's analysis. Option 4, which subtracts the long-term care benefits of existing bills, would also add to NHE even if as little as 11 percent of CBO's projected reduction in administrative costs failed to materialize. These NHE increases would be larger if lawmakers deemed the projected denials of care to be unacceptable, and relaxed scheduled provider payment cuts in an effort to alleviate them.

Although I cannot attach precise numbers to a hypothetical update of my analysis in light of the CBO report, I will try to give a sense of how the numbers might move if such an analysis were attempted. The provider payment rate assumptions in my lower-bound scenario (resulting in a $32.6 trillion federal cost projection over ten years in my 2018 study) have appeared more unrealistic since my study was performed, and this scenario should probably be discarded on the grounds of being too implausible. The payment rate assumptions underlying my $38.8 trillion estimate are more plausible, and an updated estimate could reasonably be fashioned via revisions to them. The largest factor increasing this cost projection would be the inclusion of LTSS benefits contained in current bills to establish M4A. Offsetting this would be factors reducing the projected cost, with the largest factors likely to be, in order: changes in the current-law federal baseline since my study was performed; care projected to be denied under M4A; a larger estimate of private entities', states', localities', and individuals' continuing roles in financing care; changes in baseline projections for NHE; and lower administrative costs than previously assumed. Taking all these factors in combination, it is reasonable to guess that a revised estimate of the ten-year cost of this scenario would be closer to $31 trillion rather than $39 trillion, if applied to the same hypothetical years as my previous study. If $31 trillion were indeed the number, this would again exceed what could be financed by doubling all currently projected individual and corporate income taxes.

Despite the projected federal cost likely being lower in a hypothetical future study than in my previous study, this projection scenario would still show a net increase in NHE because the expansion of benefits to include LTSS, dental, vision and hearing, as well as the increase in patient demand resulting from more expansive insurance coverage, would together increase costs by more than administrative cost savings and outright denials of care would reduce them. Only if provider payments and drug prices were cut substantially would we expect this projection to produce a net reduction in NHE. Note that these findings would be broadly consistent with CBO estimates for Option 5, which show a net increase in NHE. Although my methods would still feature some differences with CBO's, the incorporation of many of CBO's inputs including updated estimates of federal health subsidies under current law, current-law NHE projections, and modeling of supply limitations, would likely bring my federal cost estimates within 20 percent of CBO's parallel estimates, even before payment rate changes are considered.

My study focused on federal cost projections under M4A, in part because such cost estimates play a key role in Congress's legislative procedures and are thus critical information for lawmakers. Many have correctly noted, as also described earlier in this testimony, that the vast majority of these projected costs are not new to the US economy as a whole, are currently being shouldered by others, and would be shifted to the federal government under M4A. Lawmakers should be cognizant that just as with other major national expenditures such as what Americans spend on food or housing, the fact that we are already bearing most of these costs does not necessarily imply that the federal government would find it easy or even practicable to assume them, nor does it necessarily suggest that the federal government can readily provide these goods and services free of charge to every American while satisfying their diverse needs and preferences. While total national health spending is an important piece of policy information, federal lawmakers considering M4A would not be able to avoid the central question of how to finance its costs to the federal budget.

I hope this information is useful to committee members as Congress considers the various implications of enacting M4A legislation.

Testimony: A Single-Payer Health Care System That Is Based on Medicare's Fee-for-Service Program, Phillip L. Swagel, Director, before the Committee on the Budget, United States Senate, May 12, 2022

Chairman Sanders, Ranking Member Graham, and Members of the Committee, thank you for inviting me to today's hearing. There are various ways to achieve near-universal health insurance coverage using some form of automatic coverage.[217] A single-payer system is one approach, and it could be implemented in different ways.[218]

Today, I will discuss how single-payer health care systems based on the Medicare fee-for-service program would affect our nation's health care and budget and its economy. The Congressional Budget Office has analyzed five options in detail among many possibilities.[219] Those options illustrate the effects of differences in providers' payment rates, patients' cost sharing, and the system's coverage of long-term services and supports. The system proposed by Chairman Sanders in S. 1129, the Medicare for All Act of 2019,

---

[217] See Congressional Budget Office, *Policies to Achieve Near-Universal Health Insurance Coverage* (October 2020), www.cbo.gov/publication/56620.

[218] See Congressional Budget Office, *Key Design Components and Considerations for Establishing a Single-Payer Health Care System* (May 2019), www.cbo.gov/publication/55150.

[219] See CBO's Single-Payer Health Care Systems Team, *How CBO Analyzes the Costs of Proposals for Single-Payer Health Care Systems That Are Based on Medicare's Fee-for-Service Program*, Working Paper 2020-08 (Congressional Budget Office, December 2020), www.cbo.gov/publication/56811.

is like the options in some ways and different in others; CBO has not analyzed S. 1129.

Effects on Health Care and the Budget

For the single-payer options analyzed, CBO found the following effects relative to what would occur under current law:

- Federal subsidies for health care in 2030 would be significantly larger, with the increases in subsidies ranging from $1.5 trillion to $3.0 trillion.
- National health expenditures would change by amounts ranging from a decrease of $0.7 trillion to an increase of $0.3 trillion depending on the system's design features. The most important factors tending to reduce national health expenditures are lower payment rates for providers and reductions in payers' administrative spending. The most important factor tending to increase those expenditures is increased use of care—especially if long-term services and supports are a covered benefit.
- Health insurance coverage would increase, as virtually all U.S. residents would be enrolled in the system.
- The total amount of out-of-pocket costs would be smaller.
- The supply of personal health care—that is, medical services and goods provided to individuals—would increase because of fewer restrictions on utilization, less money and time spent by providers on administration, and providers' responses to increased demand for care. The amount of care used would rise, and in that sense, overall access to care would be greater.
- The increase in demand for personal health care would exceed the increase in supply, resulting in greater unmet demand than the amount under current law. Those effects on overall access to care and unmet demand would occur simultaneously because people would use more care and would have used even more if it were supplied. The increase in unmet demand would correspond to increased congestion in the health care system, including delays and forgone care.

Differences in payment rates for health care could have large effects. To illustrate the potential size of such effects, CBO estimated the outcomes for single-payer systems under scenarios in which payment rates differed and the other specifications remained the same. In the higher-rate scenario, the average payment rates for health care providers under the single-payer system would be close to the average of the rates that the agency projects for all payers in 2030 under current law. In the lower-rate scenario, rates would be 13 percent lower for hospitals and 7 percent lower for physicians, on average. Also, prices for prescription drugs would be 23 percent lower, on average. The differences between the scenarios were related to the differences between payment rates for private insurers and for Medicare and Medicaid under current law. Relative to what would occur under the higher-rate scenario, the outcomes under the lower-rate scenario would be as follows:

- Federal subsidies for health care would be 12 percent lower.
- National health expenditures would be 9 percent lower.
- The supply of personal health care would be
- 2 percent lower, with the demand for such care roughly unchanged.
- As a result, the demand for personal health care that was not met would increase by 2 percentage points.

In the long term, payments lower than those projected under current law might cause fewer people to enter health care professions and fewer new drugs to be developed. If providers were unable to adjust to slower growth in payment rates by operating more efficiently and remaining financially viable, they could cease to operate, possibly leading to greater congestion in the health care system. Although effects in the long term are especially hard to predict, I want to emphasize that all of CBO's estimates of the effects of a single-payer system are inherently uncertain.

Effects on the Economy

Turning to the economic effects, I will describe the outcomes under the five options CBO analyzed if the system was financed by either a payroll tax or an income tax—and the estimates differ depending on the type of tax.[220] CBO made these projections:

---

[220] See Jaeger Nelson, *Economic Effects of Five Illustrative Single-Payer Health Care Systems*, Working Paper 2022-02 (Congressional Budget Office, February 2022), www.cbo.gov/publication/57637.

- Gross domestic product (GDP) would be approximately 1 percent to 10 percent lower by 2030 than the amount projected under current law, and aggregate nonhealth consumption per capita would change by amounts ranging from an increase of 3 percent to a decline of 7 percent.
- Lifetime nonhealth consumption would rise among lower-income households and decline among higherincome households relative to the levels under current law, and the number of lifetime hours people choose to work would be lower for most households across the income distribution.

The net reductions in GDP would occur primarily because of the effects of increased taxes on labor and capital income. Taxes on labor income reduce after-tax wages, so they reduce the return on each additional hour worked. They also lower people's expected future income, which creates an incentive to work more to make up for their lost after-tax income. On average, the former effect is greater than the latter in CBO's assessment; therefore, higher labor taxes tend to reduce the number of hours worked in the economy. Higher taxes on capital income, such as dividends and capital gains, lower the average after-tax rate of return on private wealth holdings (or the return on investment), which reduces the incentive to save and invest and leads to reductions in the capital stock. Those effects lead, in turn, to lower income.

If the system was financed through other types of taxes, government borrowing, or reductions in other types of government spending, the net effect on the economy and the distributional implications would be different. Perpetually financing any of the single-payer systems CBO analyzed through increased borrowing—without a corresponding increase in revenues or a reduction in other spending at some point in the future—would be unsustainable.

In addition to the effects of its financing, a single-payer system would have the following economic effects:

- The composition of workers' labor compensation would change because employers would no longer provide health care benefits and would pass along the savings to employees, increasing their taxable wages.

- Households' health insurance premiums would be eliminated, and their out-of-pocket health care costs would decline.
- Because administrative expenses in the health care sector would decline, productive resources for other sectors would be freed up and would ultimately increase economywide productivity.
- Reduced payment rates would cause providers to find ways of providing care with fewer resources. Some of the reduction in payment rates would initially lower wages for workers in the health care sector and throughout the supply chain. In the long run, that effect on wages would diminish as labor markets adjusted.
- Longevity and labor productivity would increase as people's health outcomes improved.
- Long-term services and supports, if included in the system, would further reduce out-of-pocket spending, provide payments for care that is currently unpaid, increase wages among workers providing care, and allow some unpaid caregivers to increase the hours they work at their primary occupation.

This testimony summarizes information provided in two of the Congressional Budget Office's working papers: How CBO Analyzes the Costs of Proposals for Single-Payer Health Care Systems That Are Based on Medicare's Fee-for-Service Program and Economic Effects of Five Illustrative Single-Payer Health Care Systems. In keeping with CBO's mandate to provide objective, impartial analysis, neither the working papers nor this testimony makes any recommendations.

The testimony was reviewed by Leigh Angres, Alice Burns, Chad Chirico, Carrie Colla, Devrim Demirel, Berna Demiralp, Mark Doms, Noelia Duchovny, Theresa Gullo, Tamara Hayford, Grace Hwang, Deborah Kilroe, John Kitchen, Jeffrey Kling, Leo Lex, Paul Masi, Sarah Masi, John McClelland, Alexandra Minicozzi, Eamon Molloy, Jaeger Nelson, Karen Stockley, Robert Sunshine, Emily Vreeland, Jeffrey Werling, and Chapin White. John Skeen was the editor. The testimony is available on CBO's website at www.cbo.gov/publication/57973.

Phillip L. Swagel
Director

Responses to Written Questions of Senator Van Hollen to Adam Gaffney, MD, MPH

Question: I believe that one of the great promises of a Medicare for All system is that it would ensure accessible, quality health care for everyone. Currently, Americans are truly struggling to access affordable health care, even when they have insurance. Whether it's private insurance, Medicaid, or Medicare, our entire system puts the burden on individuals to find out if they are eligible, to enroll, in some cases to submit income data, to compare plans, and after all is said and done- and you receive your insurance card in the mail- you then have to seek a provider that accepts that specific insurance plan. However, for Americans that suffer from chronic conditions, disabilities, behavioral and mental health issues, cancer, or anything that requires any kind of specialized care, the burdens of seeking an in-network provider are constant barriers to health care. And, seeking an in-network provider is not an easy endeavor- especially when we have a severe shortage of specialty physicians and behavioral health providers.

Last month, in Maryland, the Baltimore Sun ran the story of seven-year-old Lily Williams who has coverage under Maryland's state Medicaid program. She was getting access to therapy for a genetic condition that causes developmental and speech delays, when suddenly her provider left the Medicaid network. They left over reimbursement issues with the insurance group running the state's Medicaid claims process. Now, rather than focusing on caring for Lily and her twin brother, Lily's mom works as much as possible to ensure that she can cover the health costs for Lily's therapies under a private plan that of course comes at a significant higher cost.

Dr. Gaffney, last year I introduced the Easy Enrollment in Health Care Act, which if passed would use data from filed tax returns to automatically enroll people in health insurance if they are eligible for free coverage via Medicaid or ACA subsidies. However, it's clear that even when people are enrolled in affordable plans, our system fails to guarantee that they will have access to the providers they need.

From your perspective as a specialist provider, how would Medicare for All improve the management of care and health outcomes of our most vulnerable communities, specifically, low-income communities, and children with chronic conditions or disabilities?

Answer: Thank you for your important question. As you describe, lack of access to needed providers, narrow insurance networks, administrative barriers, expensive premiums, "churn" in and out of insurance plans, and burdensome out-of-pocket costs remain grave problems in American healthcare, particularly for the chronically ill and even for those with insurance. In a recent study, colleagues and I estimated that the number of underinsured children — whether because of inadequate coverage of services, costs, or providers — has been on the rise in recent years, hitting 18 million in 2019. For such underinsured children, as your example of Lily illustrates, healthcare imposes a heavy burden on families in time, money, and stress. Moreover, for the chronically ill, having to periodically change medications to a new formulary, or transition all of one's providers to a new insurance network each year is not merely inconvenient: it is medically disruptive and potentially hazardous.

Medicare for All would improve care and outcomes for such patients in several important respects. First, it would ensure not just that coverage is universal, but seamless — which is to say, no gaps or interruptions in coverage in childhood or adulthood. Second, Medicare for All would include virtually all doctors and hospitals, more akin to traditional Medicare and much different than most private insurance, managed Medicaid, or Medicare Advantage plans. This is particularly important for children with complex medical needs, who often require the services of multiple specialists and tertiary medical centers. Third, the provision of full coverage under Medicare for All, achieved in some other nations, would mean that American families are no longer burdened with copays, deductibles, or coinsurance. Such out-of-pocket payments are particularly punishing for those with low incomes, or the medically ill who require costly specialist care and medications. For these patients, such "cost-sharing" functions as a tariff on illness. Fourth, by unburdening physicians from much of the administrative busywork engendered by our current complex financing system, Medicare for All would increase the time that specialists can spend caring for their medically complex patients. Together, these changes could improve care for patients, free families from fear about the costs of illness, and improve quality of practice for physicians.

Responses to Written Questions of Senator Van Hollen to Bonnie Castillo, RN

Question: Ms. Castillo, I know that the National Nurses Union is a strong champion of Medicare for All. It's not surprising that our frontline workers would endorse a system that guarantees everyone health coverage without the worry of a hospital visit turning into crippling debt. Afterall, the number one reason people file for bankruptcy in this country is medical debt. The poor outcomes we see for Americans managing chronic conditions reflect the barriers that people face to attaining health insurance coupled with the very real fear of going into debt. As you pointed out in your testimony, it was clear by the overflow of ICU patients during the peak Covid-19 period that our health care system has failed them.

A Medicare for All type system could ensure easy, simple, access to all doctors and for all patients. It would ensure that no one has to ration their insulin or delay treatment due to not being able to afford the cost-sharing set by insurance companies. It means a system focused on preventative medicine and comprehensive care. I do believe that Medicare for All is the system we should be working towards.

Ms. Castillo, we know that it's likely that we may continue to experience surges of deadly illness from Covid-19 variants or from a new virus altogether. **From your perspective, what are the consequences of failing to improve our health care infrastructure? Is the status quo sustainable for patients, providers, and specifically the nurse workforce?**

Answer: The status quo of our fragmented, for-profit health care system is wholly unsustainable for patients and caregivers alike, and certainly for nurses, who are always at the bedside, providing direct patient care. Because access to health care is based on ability to pay, patients simply do not get the care they need. In the context of a global pandemic, inequitable access to care harms the health of everyone. If we don't fundamentally change our current profit-driven system, the U.S. will be unable to provide the care that patients will need in years to come and health disparities will worsen. Tens of millions of working families will still worry about losing their health insurance if they lose their jobs. Millions with insurance will still not get the care they need because they cannot afford the deductibles or copayments. Hospital corporations will continue to short staff, close hospitals that produce low returns, and ration personal protective equipment and other medical supplies. In short, health care and the health of our patients will continue to get worse under the status quo. That's why we need Medicare for All.

Patients are constantly being forced to choose between getting the care they need and paying their bills. Half of U.S. adults surveyed in December 2021 said they put off or skipped some sort of health care due to cost.[1] Moreover, health care corporations that are driven to maximize revenue engage in strategic corporate consolidation and hospital closure tactics that result in unequal distribution of our health care infrastructure, with health care deserts in less affluent areas and hyper concentration of services for patient populations that can capture higher reimbursement rates from private payers. As a result, many patients don't have access to the providers and facilities they need, particularly for low-income communities, communities of color, and rural areas. As of June 30, 2022, the Health Resources and Services Administration reported that94.8 million people in the U.S. live in a primary care Health Professional Shortage Area and 152.2 million live in a mental health Professional Shortage Area.[2]

[1] Kearney, A. et al. "Americans' Challenges with Health Care Costs." Kaiser Family Foundation (Dec. 2021). https://www.kff.org/health-costs/issue-brief/americans-challenges-with-health-care-costs/.

[2] Health Resources and Services Administration, Bureau of Health Workforce. "Designated Health Professional Shortage Areas Statistics." U.S. Department of Health and Human Services (June 30, 2022). https://data.hrsa.gov/Default/GenerateHPSAQuarterlyReport.

When patients are unable to get the care they need, conditions that could have been managed more readily if they were seen quicker develop into conditions that not only are more severe than they could have been but are also more expensive to treat. In the worst-case scenario, this inability to get necessary care results in death: 34 million people in this country as of 2019 personally knew somebody, either a friend or family member, who died because they weren't able to afford necessary treatment.[3]

Meanwhile, our current health care system also does a disservice to nurses, doctors, and other health care professionals who provide hands-on patient care. For example, doctors and nurses are increasingly spending less and less time with their patients because they are forced to navigate an increasingly complicated multi-payer system of private insurance. Two-thirds of a given doctor's time is spent on paperwork rather than patient care.[4] One study estimates that nurses and medical assistants in the U.S. spend 20.6 hours per physician per week on administrative tasks related to health plans.[5]

For nurses, the consequences of our inhumane health care system can be found in the employer-manufactured nurse staffing crisis. Despite industry claims, there is no shortage of registered nurses (RNs), and a 2017 U.S. Health and Human Services report on the supply and demand of the nursing workforce from 2014 to 2030 makes clear that except for a handful of states, there are sufficient numbers of registered nurses to meet the needs of the country's patients.[6] Additionally, based on the best available data, there are 4.4 million licensed RNs and 3.3 million employed RNs, a surplus of 1.1 million licensed RNs.[7] There is, however, a shortage of nurses willing to work in unsafe and dehumanizing conditions that many of our employers have increasingly subjected us to in the pursuit of greater profits, conditions that predated, but only have gotten worse during, the pandemic. Corporate greed, budget cuts, a lack of adequate support staff, and moral distress are responsible for an employer-manufactured staffing crisis.

In an attempt to minimize labor costs, hospitals are unwilling to hire sufficient nurses and other health care workers, and instead are increasingly trying to make nurses and other health care workers do more with less.[8] Hospitals are intentionally failing to maintain a robust pool of nurses from which to draw when scheduling shifts. From the experience of NNU members, hospitals often cancel or "call off" nurses who are scheduled to work on a daily contract basis, will send nurses home who have reported for their scheduled

---

[3] "34 Million Americans Know of Family Member or Friend Who Died in the Last 5 Years After Being Unableto Afford Treatment." West Health-Gallup (Nov. 12, 2019). https://www.westhealth.org/press-release/34-millionamericans-know-of-family-member-or-friend-who-died-in-the-last-5-years-after-being-unable-to-afford-treatment/.

[4] Sinsky, C. et al. "Allocation of Physician Time in Ambulatory Practice: A Time and Motion Study in 4 Specialties." *Annals of Inter Med* (Dec. 2016). https://www.acpjournals.org/doi/10.7326/M16-0961?url_ver=Z39.88-2003&rfr_id=ori:rid:crossref.org&rfr_dat=cr_pub%20%200pubmed.

[5] Morra, D. et al. "U.S. Physician Practices Spend Nearly Four Times as Much Money Interacting with Health Plans and Payers Than Do Their Canadian Counterparts." *Health Affairs* (Aug. 3, 2011). https://www.commonwealthfund.org/publications/journal-article/2011/aug/us-physician-practices-spend-nearlyfour-times-much-money.

[6] Health Resources and Services Administration. "National and Regional Supply and Demand Projections of the Nursing Workforce: 2014-2030." U.S. Department of Health and Human Services (2017). https://bhw.hrsa.gov/sites/default/files/bureau-health-workforce/data-research/nchwa-hrsa-nursing-report.pdf.

[7] National Council of State Boards of Nursing. 2022, Jun 2. Active RN Licenses. A Profile of Nursing Licensure in the U.S. https://www.ncsbn.org/6161.htm U.S. Bureau of Labor Statistics. 2022, Mar 31. May 2021 National Occupational Employment and Wage Estimates. U.S. Department of Labor. https://www.bls.gov/oes/current/oes_nat.htm

[8] National Nurses United. "Protecting Our Front Line: Ending the Shortage of Good Nursing Jobs and the Industry-created Unsafe Staffing Crisis." National Nurses United (Dec. 2021). https://www.nationalnursesunited.org/sites/default/files/nnu/documents/1121_StaffingCrisis_ProtectingOurFrontLine_Report_FINAL.pdf

shifts, are not hiring or are extremely slow to hire for open positions, and will cancel contracts with travel or agency nurses.

During the Covid-19 pandemic, hospitals rejected nurses' advice to prepare and plan for predictable staffing needs, including hiring and training more nurses, and cross-training current staff nurses to work in critical care departments. Instead, hospitals cut and laid off staff from units that had temporarily low patient census, and canceled RN traveler contracts. Again, the industry was shortsightedly looking for immediate ways to cut costs and boost profits instead of planning for patient and public health needs. Hospital employers' actions and inaction have resulted in a lack of critical care staff to respond to the Covid-19 pandemic.[9]

As a result of hospital employers' shortsighted profit-driven decisions, the nursing workforce experiences high levels of moral distress. Nurses are exhausted and approaching their limits. Piecemeal reforms, however, won't solve the problems of unaffordable care, inequitable distribution of our health care infrastructure, and intentional understaffing, which result from our current system of profit- driven health care. Instead, we need to transform our health care system away from one that prioritizes profits and into one that prioritizes patient care and healing. Failing to do so will mean more patients will get sick and die without the ability to get the care they need, and providers will continue to struggle. The only people who stand to benefit from this health care system are health care executives and shareholders. A move to Medicare for All will ensure that patients can get the care they need when they need it, doctors are free to spend their time on care rather than paperwork, and nurses can care for patients at the bedside with adequate support and resources.

National Nurses United also has written more about the issue of the industry-created nurse staffing crisis and our proposals to address it, which includes Medicare for All, in our December 2021 report, "Protecting Our Front Line: Ending the Shortage of Good Nursing Jobs and the Industry-created Unsafe Staffing Crisis."

Question: Maryland is a unique state in that our hospitals are under a global budget system similar to the one you described in your testimony and now included in the Senate proposal of Medicare for All. During the height of the pandemic when other hospitals around the country saw grim revenue losses over the lack of elective surgeries, Maryland hospitals had a consistent cash flow coming in from pre-set annual budgets. This helped our hospitals stay open while at least 21 hospitals in other states closed during the first year of the pandemic.

Ms. Castillo, can you elaborate further on how scaling up regional budget systems as described in Medicare for All would support not just the financial stability of hospitals but how they could improve conditions for the people that work there and the patients they see?

Answer: If we had Medicare for All before this pandemic started, hospitals would have been better prepared to respond because the reimbursement and funding structure ensures that all health care facilities, including hospitals that provide a safety-net for rural and underserved areas would be fully funded and resourced. For years, hospital corporations have relied on "just-in-time" models for staffing and supply. In most of the country hospitals did not hire enough nurses for regular patient care pre-pandemic and did not have supplies for public health emergencies. Through the global budgeting payment mechanism in the Medicare for All

---

[9] See also National Nurses United. "Deadly Shame: Redressing the Devaluation of Registered Nurse Labor Through Pandemic Equity." National Nurses United (Dec. 2020). https://www.nationalnursesunited.org/campaign/deadly-shame-report

Act, hospitals would be required to have mandatory minimum nurse staffing levels and to have one-year supplies of PPE and critical medical supplies. This would have made the pandemic response much safer for patients and for workers.

Similar to Maryland's hospital global budgeting model, the Medicare for All Act would adopt annualized global budgeting for each hospital and health care facility, which would be administered regionally through the Medicare for All program. Hospital global budgeting would stabilize funding for rural and safety-net facilities and provide the ability to adjust global budgets as circumstances change or emergent public health events, like a global pandemic, arise. Global budgets would be tailored to the health care needs of each hospital's patient population and account for factors including historic volume of services, actual expenditures, wages, maximum capacity, maintenance, and protected changes in level or kinds of services. Importantly, hospital global budgets would include funding for safe nurse staffing ratios and funding to maintain a one-year supply of personal protective equipment and other supplies to ensure hospitals are prepared for the next public health emergency. Like in Maryland, the hospital global budgeting structure in the Medicare for All Act offers a level of financial stability and predictability, with appropriate flexibility to adjust budgets when unpredictable need arises, that our current health care system does not provide and cannot afford.

Importantly, hospital global budgets under Medicare for All would help address the crisis of rural and safety-net hospital closures afflicting the nation. Stabilizing their funding source will help ensure that rural hospitals, as well as critical safety net hospitals in other medically underserved areas, can stay open and continue to provide necessary care.

Shifting from a fragmented multi-payer system of insurance to hospital global budgeting under Medicare for All will also help cut down on hospitals' administrative costs. Medicare for All would eliminate point-of-service charges, balance billing, and other forms of cost-sharing and insurance administration, resulting in massive administrative savings for hospitals and other providers. Nurses and other health care workers also stand to benefit immensely from the transition to institutional global budgets under Medicare for All. Nurses and other health care staff are constantly having to spend more and more time focused on billing and paperwork, leaving less time for direct patient care. Streamlining the care delivery process and reducing the need for administrative bureaucracy by fully paying for services with global budgets will reduce the amount of time away from the bedside that nurses and other care providers need to spend on paperwork and other billing practices. Global budgets also provide the ability to guarantee that money is available for certain workplace protections for health care providers. For example, in S. 4204, hospital global budgets would include the funding necessary to hire and train nurse staffing required to meet mandatory minimum safe nurse-to-patient ratios. Hospital global budgeting under S. 4204 would also include the funding required to maintain equipment stockpiles, PPE, and other expenses necessary to keep the workplace safe.

In summary, hospitals, providers, and patients all stand to benefit from implementing a system of global budgeting as called for by the Medicare for All Act. Hospitals reap the benefit of certainty and predictability in their revenues, and rural and safety net hospitals will have a level of stability they do not enjoy under our current profit-driven system. Health care professionals will benefit from less administrative work and more time to provide patient care. Patients will benefit from elimination of payment at the point of service, well-resourced hospitals regardless of their geographic location, and health care providers able to devote more of their time to patient care.

Responses to Written Questions of Senator Van Hollen to Abdul El-Sayed, MD, DPhil

Question: Dr. El-Sayed, about half of all Americans have employer-based private health insurance. However, despite the premiums that are deducted from employee paychecks, copays made at the doctor's office, and the deductibles billed for other services, insurance companies can still refuse to pay for diagnostic exams, treatments, prescription drugs, etc. As you are aware, insurance companies set up prior authorization requirements where physicians are constantly having to fill-out paper work and spend hours on the phone convincing insurance companies to cover prescribed services or drugs for patients. And for patients, this means not receiving the care that they need in a timely fashion and poorer health outcomes.

Similarly, I've heard from constituents who desperately wish they could take the medications as prescribed and recommended by their doctors. Yet, insurance companies often decide they will only cover a medication if the patient first follows a step-therapy protocol of trying a drug or series of alternative drugs before receiving coverage for the one initially medically prescribed. We all know that these fail first protocols have very little to do with patient safety but everything to do with profit seeking by insurance companies.

I share the frustration of many Americans who've been turned down coverage for something they have already paid for. Our system is broken, and we must do more to center patient care and health above all else.

Dr. El Sayed, can you explain which provisions of Medicare for All would protect Americans from experiencing similar cost-savings tactics used by insurance companies that impede adequate coverage for prescription drugs and services?

Answer: Thank you for this important question. And I'm deeply saddened to hear about these experiences your constituents report. I have also heard similar stories from the people whom I served as Health Director in Detroit. Insurance companies engage in these pernicious rationing and gatekeeping practices because every dollar that they spend in actual healthcare—what they call a "medical loss— is a dollar that they don't get to keep as profit. Indeed, it's a function of their profit motive that they do this. Under Medicare for All, every single American would be insured by the federal government, which, of course, does not have a profit motive—meaning that this kind of insurance-driven gatekeeping would no longer occur. The best indication of this is that today's Medicare program does not engage in these kinds of practices.

Responses to Written Questions of Senator Chris Van Hollen to Phillip Swagel, Ph.D.

Question: A concern of mine when it comes to transitioning into a single-payer Medicare for All system is how do we ensure our medical providers, physicians, specialists, and nurses are treated fairly in terms of their pay and reimbursement rates.

Dr. Swagel, in your analysis of single-payer-models and specifically the model that most reflects this Medicare for All bill, would our medical providers still receive the same levels of compensation they receive now or similar?

Answer: Under the Congressional Budget Office's illustrative options for a single-payer system, the compensation that health care professionals receive could be more or less than under current law depending on the policy specifications and the type of provider. In its analysis, CBO considered a higher payment-rate scenario and a lower payment-rate scenario:

In the higher scenario, the average payment rates for hospitals and physicians would be similar to the average of the rates that CBO projects for all payers (including government programs and private insurers) under current law.

In the lower scenario, hospitals and physicians would be paid lower rates, on average, than CBO projects for all payers under current law (in 2030, 13 percent lower for hospitals and 7 percent lower for physicians). The rates in both scenarios would be higher than what Medicare or Medicaid pays but considerably lower than what private insurers pay under current law. In both scenarios, providers would be paid using a system that closely resembles Medicare's fee-for-service system. Variation in payment rates among different types of providers would more closely resemble the variation in Medicare than in private insurance or other public plans.

The rates in both scenarios would be higher than what Medicare or Medicaid pays but considerably lower than what private insurers pay under current law. In both scenarios, providers would be paid using a system that closely resembles Medicare's fee-for-service system. Variation in payment rates among different types of providers would more closely resemble the variation in Medicare than in private insurance or other public plans.

The rates in both scenarios would be higher than what Medicare or Medicaid pays but considerably lower than what private insurers pay under current law. In both scenarios, providers would be paid using a system that closely resembles Medicare's fee-for-service system. Variation in payment rates among different types of providers would more closely resemble the variation in Medicare than in private insurance or other public plans.

S. 1129, as introduced in the 116th Congress, does not specify the rates that would be paid, so it is unclear whether those rates would be closer to the higher payment-rate scenario, the lower payment-rate scenario, or outside that range. In general, lower payment rates for providers would push down costs to the federal government and the health care system but would also reduce the average compensation of health care professionals.

Besides the policy specified for payment rates, a provider's characteristics and its compensation under current law could determine whether the payments it receives would increase or decrease. For instance, under the higher payment-rate scenario CBO examined, hospitals that serve relatively more people with private insurance would see their payment rates fall, on average, whereas those that serve relatively more people with Medicare or Medicaid coverage would see their average payment rates rise. That outcome would occur because rates paid by private insurers are generally higher than the rates paid by Medicare and Medicaid. Additionally, a single-payer system that established a more uniform payment rate would cause some providers (such as certain high-cost specialists) to receive smaller payments than they would receive under current law, whereas other providers (such as certain low-cost general practitioners) would see larger payments.

The compensation of health care professionals accounts for a large share of the costs of producing health care services and would tend to rise or fall with the rates paid by the single-payer system.

Question: I am a strong supporter of allowing the government to negotiate drug prices with drug companies. It makes no sense that we restrict ourselves from being able to help our constituents afford their prescriptions. I've supported provisions to allow for drug negotiations in President Biden's Build Back Better agenda, and I support this provision in Medicare for All legislation.

Currently, Americans pay two to three times more for prescription drugs than people in other countries for the same drugs and up to 10 times as much for insulin. Last year, the CBO analysis of the Elijah E. Cummings Lower Drug Costs Now Act, showed that allowing price negotiation in Medicare would reduce drug prices by 57% to 75%; and that when coupled with limiting drug price increases to the rate of inflation, the government would save $160 billion over a decade.

Dr. Swagel, do you have any estimates on the savings price negotiation generates under the Medicare for All system?

Answer: In its analysis of illustrative options for a single-payer system, CBO projected that spending on retail prescription drugs (prescription medicines that people purchase at pharmacies or by mail order) under current law would be $574 billion in 2030. In the higher payment-rate scenario, prices for prescription drugs would be 6 percent lower than under current law—which equates to a reduction of $34 billion in total spending on retail prescription drugs for the quantity purchased under current law; in the lower payment-rate scenario, prices would be 28 percent lower than under current law—for a reduction in spending of $161 billion.[1] CBO did not quantify reductions in spending on prescription drugs administered in a facility, such as a hospital outpatient department.

CBO assumed that the single-payer system would begin providing health insurance coverage in 2025. For brand-name retail prescription drugs already on the market in 2025, under the higher payment-rate scenario, CBO assumed that prices would be set equal to the average of the prices projected for all payers under current law in 2025 and that they would increase at the rate of the consumer price index for all urban consumers (CPI-U) plus 4 percentage points. Under the lower payment-rate scenario, CBO assumed that prices for retail prescription drugs in 2025 would be set at the average of net prices paid by Medicare Part D and Medicaid and that those prices would grow at the rate of increase in the CPI-U.

CBO anticipates that, under the illustrative options for a single-payer system, the federal government could restrain the average launch prices of brand-name drugs introduced after 2025 by using various tools. Those tools could include price-setting based on comparative-effectiveness analyses (which identify which treatment works best for improving health) or cost-effectiveness analyses (which compare the cost of a treatment with the number of additional quality-adjusted years of life it provides).

CBO did not specify the process that would yield the prices assumed under the higher and lower payment-rate scenarios. Exclusion from the single-payer system's formulary (its list of covered drugs) is one possible tool to restrain drug prices. The authority to impose a tax if a manufacturer did not agree to the single-payer

[1] See CBO's Single-Payer Health Care Systems Team, How CBO Analyzes the Costs of Proposals for Single-Payer Health Care Systems That Are Based on Medicare's Fee-for-Service Program, Working Paper 2020-08 (Congressional Budget Office, December 2020), www.cbo.gov/publication/56811.

system's price would have the same effect if the tax was high enough to cause the manufacturer to lose money on sales of the drug in the United States.

S. 1129, as introduced in the 116th Congress, specifies that the Secretary of Health and Human Services would negotiate the prices paid for prescription drugs, establish a formulary, and "promulgate rules regarding the use of off-formulary medications." It is unclear whether the prices resulting from that process would fall closer to the higher payment-rate scenario, the lower payment-rate scenario, or outside that range. In general, the prices paid for prescription drugs under a single-payer system would depend crucially on how the Secretary determined whether a negotiation was successful and what the consequences of an unsuccessful negotiation would be.

PUBLIC CITIZEN 50 YEARS

Statement for the record of

Eagan Kemp

Health Care Policy Advocate, Public Citizen

for the

U.S. Senate

Committee on the Budget

Medicare for All: Protecting Health, Saving Lives, Saving Money

May 12, 2022

We appreciate the opportunity to submit this statement for the record on this vitally important issue. And thank you for holding this historic hearing on Medicare for All. Public Citizen is a national non-profit organization with more than 500,000 members and supporters across the country. We represent the public interest through legislative and administrative advocacy, litigation, research, and public education on a broad range of issues including ensuring access to health care. Pertinent to this hearing, Public Citizen has supported the creation of a single-payer health care system since our founding in 1971. Our health care system currently fails to meet the needs of the American people, while a Medicare for All system would guarantee coverage to everyone in the United States. Despite the successes of the Affordable Care Act (ACA) in expanding access to coverage, more than 30 million Americans remain uninsured and tens of millions more are underinsured, meaning they are unable to afford the care they need despite having health insurance.[1]

As the first hearing on Medicare for All in the Senate, this historic hearing will provide an opportunity for the Committee to explore both the historic and emerging challenges of our current health care system and how Medicare for All would address them. Our fragmented health care system, including private, employer-sponsored insurance, left us unprepared for COVID-19 and showed just how little our health care system is focused on health. Medicare for All would finally bring a rational approach to health care and would make patients' wellbeing the focus instead of profit. By taking the most popular part of our health care system, Medicare, improving it and expanding it to everyone in the U.S., we can finally guarantee that everyone in the country can get the care they need when they need it.

I. THE COVID-19 PANDEMIC FURTHER HIGHLIGHTED THE NEED FOR MEDICARE FOR ALL

1. The Private Insurance System Hindered Access to Care

The cardinal sin of our health care system is that it puts profits over people and corporations over communities. At the start of the COVID-19 pandemic, approximately 87 million Americans were uninsured or underinsured.[2] While this placed the health of millions of Americans at risk in normal times, the risks were even higher during a pandemic.

The COVID-19 pandemic showed just how greedy private insurers are, as they were reporting record profits because they were paying out far less in claims due to millions of Americans delaying care.[3] This disparity highlights just how little value insurers are bringing to the health care system despite how much they cost consumers and the health care system in general. And insurers continue to focus on their profits, even as Americans continue to struggle to get the care they need. For example, the Centers for Medicare and Medicaid Services (CMS) had to recently step in to stop insurers from denying claims for COVID-19 testing, as well as to increase compliance with COVID-19 relief legislation that required that plans cover

[1] Sarah R. Collins, Munira Z. Gunja, and Michelle M. Doty, The Commonwealth Fund, How Well Does Insurance Coverage Protect Consumers from Health Care Costs? — Findings from the Commonwealth Fund Biennial Health Insurance Survey, 2016, at 1 (October 2017), https://bit.ly/2D3WbG5.
[2] The Commonwealth Fund, Health Insurance Coverage Eight Years After The ACA, 5 (2019), https://bit.ly/3rFsrVJ.
[3] Reed Abelson, *Major U.S. Health Insurers Report Big Profits, Benefiting From the Pandemic*, The New York Times (August 5, 2020), https://nyti.ms/3bC26C5.

such tests without cost sharing.[4] If people aren't getting tested out of fear about the cost, it may increase the spread of COVID-19 and keep the pandemic going longer than it would with adequate testing and treatment.

2. Employer-Sponsored Insurance Failed at the Worst Possible Time

Another absurdity of our system, where more than half of all Americans depend on insurance provided through their job, was also laid bare by COVID-19 pandemic. Americans are always at risk of losing coverage through job loss, especially during an economic downturn and catastrophically so during a downturn caused by a global pandemic. Around 22 million Americans lost their job due to the first wave of COVID-19, meaning millions also lost their insurance during a global pandemic.[5]

Compounding the overall uninsured and underinsured rates is that many industries deemed to be essential—and thus are unable to be done from home—have among the highest uninsured rates for their employees. A Public Citizen analysis found high rates of uninsured workers across several industries deemed essential.[6] Prior to the pandemic, more than half of all agricultural workers were uninsured, while around one in four workers across construction, home care, and restaurant workers lacked insurance.

Even before COVID-19, paying for health insurance coverage for their workforces was a huge burden for employers, hurting their competitiveness. If an employer does not provide insurance to its employees, it may struggle to attract and retain top-level talent. And if an employer does choose to provide health insurance, the rising annual costs may mean fewer wage increases, less generous plans, cuts to other benefits or perhaps even challenges to their ability to stay in business.

Small businesses – which have been hit hard by COVID-19 – were already facing particular challenges providing health insurance on top of those faced by other companies. Because of their size and the lack of economies of scale, small businesses often struggle to afford insurance for their employees. They face a significant disadvantage when negotiating with insurers and end up paying higher prices than larger companies. For example, one study found that employers with fewer than 10 employees face premiums nearly 20% higher, for the same benefits, than those paid by large businesses, and employers with 10 to 25 employees can expect to pay around 10% more.[7]

II. MEDICARE FOR ALL WOULD ENSURE GUARANTEED ACCESS TO NEEDED CARE

1. Medicare for All Would Guarantee Comprehensive Benefits

Medicare for All offers the most comprehensive benefits of any health reform proposal and builds those benefits on a strong, existing foundation. By improving Medicare and expanding it to everyone in the

[4] Nick Paul Taylor, *CMS Moves to Stop COVID-19 Testing Denials, Cost Sharing in Private Plans*, MedTech Dive (March 1, 2021), https://bit.ly/3t352Oe.
[5] Jonathan Ponciano, *It Could Take 4 Years to Recover The 22 Million Jobs Lost During Covid-19 Pandemic, Moody's Warns*, FORBES (November 30, 2020), https://bit.ly/3rGvY5U.
[6] Public Citizen, Holes in the Safety Net, 1 (October 2020), https://bit.ly/3rF6s16.
[7] Claire Martin, *In the Health Law, an Open Door for Entrepreneurs*, The New York Times (November 23, 2013), https://nyti.ms/2O463R5.

United States, Medicare for All would finally allow everyone in America to access the care they need, when they need it. Studies have shown that Medicare patients have consistent access to care, with more than 95 percent reporting having a usual source of care, such as a doctor's office or primary care clinic.[8] Around 90 percent of Medicare beneficiaries reported that they were able to schedule timely appointments for primary and specialty care.[9] Seniors with Medicare were more likely than adults age 50-64 with private insurance to report that they had never had to wait longer than they wanted for a routine care appointment.[10]

Expanding access to medically necessary care, including preventive services, would reduce the incidence of many preventable diseases and allow earlier treatment for a variety of illnesses. This, in turn, would reduce both personal and system-wide spending on treating preventable illnesses and would allow treatment of illnesses at earlier stages, when they are cheaper and easier to treat. Far too many Americans are unable to get the care they need because they are uninsured or underinsured. By eliminating out-of-pocket costs, Medicare for All would ensure access to needed care for everyone in the United States. Studies have found that out-of-pocket costs cause consumers to decrease their use of potentially important health care.[11]

Medicare for All would also improve provider choice for all Americans by allowing people to choose their doctor and hospital, as every provider and hospital would be "in-network." Currently, Americans must spend inordinate amounts of time figuring out which providers are in-network versus out-of-network. For example, more than one-third of Medicare Advantage enrollees have to deal with narrow networks—defined as including less than 30 percent of physicians in a given county.[12]

Medicare for All would also guarantee access to vision and dental services, which many Americans, including seniors, struggle to afford. Lack of access to dental services can put Americans at risk for infection, decreased quality of life, and difficulty eating. Low-income seniors were particularly likely to not have had a dental visit, with only around one in four having done so in the past year, compared to nearly 75 percent of beneficiaries with higher incomes.[13] Seniors also struggled to access vision services, with over 40 percent of Medicare beneficiaries with vision impairment reporting they had not received an eye exam in the past year and, among people who did receive care, beneficiaries reported paying around 60 percent of the cost of vision services out of pocket.[14]

2. Medicare for All Would Provide Access to Long-term Care

Another important benefit of Medicare for All is that it would also ensure access to long-term care for everyone in the U.S. This would improve patients' quality of life while also bringing down the cost of

---

[8] Cristina Boccuti, Christina Swoope, Anthony Damico and Patricia Neuman, Kaiser Family Foundation, Medicare Patients' Access to Physicians: A Synthesis of the Evidence, at 2 (December 2013), https://bit.ly/2D6KFtl.
[9] *Id.* at 3.
[10] *Id.*
[11] Zarek C. Brot-Goldberg, et al,, *What does a Deductible Do? The Impact of Cost-Sharing on Health Care Prices, Quantities, and Spending Dynamics*, 132 The Quarterly Journal of Economics 1261-1318, 1261 (2017).
[12] Gretchen Jacobson, et al., Kaiser Family Foundation, Medicare Advantage: How Robust Are Plans' Physician Networks?, at 4 (October 2017), https://bit.ly/2D7l4Ri.
[13] *Id.*
[14] Amber Willink, Cathy Schoen, and Karen Davis, Commonwealth Fund, How Medicare Could Provide Dental, Vision, and Hearing Care for Beneficiaries, at 1 (January 2018), https://bit.ly/31iryWl.

care, as more people would be able to receive care in their homes instead of in expensive institutions, like nursing homes. Medicare for All would ensure that beneficiaries could be served in the setting of their choice with the services they need. And by providing more care through long-term home and community-based services, Medicare for All could save money compared to institutional care, given that a year of care in a nursing home costs more than twice as much as having a home health aide for a year and five times as much as a year of care through adult health day care.[15]

Improving the efficiency of our long-term care is crucial because around 70 percent of people over 65 will require at least some long-term care in their lifetimes.[16] Given our changing demographics—by 2030 all baby boomers will be 65 or older and by 2035 Americans age 65 and older will outnumber the number of children under 18 for the first time in U.S. history—we must ensure that we are providing access to needed long-term care in the most humane and efficient way possible.[17] Medicare for All would meet both of these goals and begin the crucial transition from the institutional bias of our current long-term care system to a system that serves patients in the setting and community of their choice.

3. **Medicare for All Would Protect Patients**

Our for-profit health care system does a better job protecting investors than it does protecting patients. Nearly one in four Americans reported skipping a health care appointment due to the cost, a number more than double the average across comparable countries.[18] For lower-income Americans, than number was even higher, with more than 40 percent reporting having unmet health care needs due to cost—meaning not going to the doctor; skipping a test, treatment or follow up; or not filling a prescription or skipping doses.[19] Another study found that the U.S. ranked worst out of 16 industrialized countries for deaths that could be prevented with proper medical care.[20]

And when Americans seek care, many face medical debt or bankruptcy. A survey by the Consumer Financial Protection Bureau found that medical debt was the most common reason for debt collection calls in the United States.[21] Nearly 60 percent of consumers who were contacted about debt collection were contacted due to outstanding medical debt.

Even Americans with insurance may have difficulty paying their medical bills. The percentage of working-age adults with insurance through their job who were underinsured—meaning they face such

---

[15] ERICA L. REAVES AND MARYBETH MUSUMECI, KAISER FAMILY FOUNDATION, MEDICAID AND LONG-TERM SERVICES AND SUPPORTS: A PRIMER, at 3 (December 2015), https://bit.ly/2CAzEPY.

[16] Emily Gurnon, *The Staggering Prices of Long-Term Care 2017*, FORBES (September 26, 2017), https://bit.ly/2W5hFZp.

[17] Press Release, U.S. Census Bureau, *Older People Projected to Outnumber Children for First Time in U.S. History* (Sep. 6, 2018), https://bit.ly/2p8zoOY.

[18] Irene Papanicolas, Liana R. Woskie and Ashish K. Jha, *Health Care Spending in the United States and Other High-Income Countries*, 319 JOURNAL OF THE AMERICAN MEDICAL ASSOCIATION 1024-1039, 1037 (2018).

[19] *Id.*

[20] Ellen Nolte and Martin McKee, *Variations in amenable mortality—Trends in 16 high-income nations*, 103 HEALTH POLICY 47-52, 49 (2011).

[21] CONSUMER FINANCIAL PROTECTION BUREAU (CFPB), CONSUMER EXPERIENCES WITH DEBT COLLECTION: FINDINGS FROM THE CFPB'S SURVEY OF CONSUMER VIEWS ON DEBT, at 21 (January 2017), https://bit.ly/2ODIkk5.

excessive out-of-pocket costs that they cannot afford to use their coverage—rose from 10 percent in 2003 to 25 percent in 2016.[22]

Rising out-of-pocket costs, such as co-pays and deductibles, contribute to many Americans facing challenges affording the care they need. Further, a recent survey found that middle-income Americans with private insurance were the most likely to report increases in their out-of-pocket costs.[23] By eliminating out-of-pocket costs, Medicare for All would ensure access to needed care for everyone in the United States.

III. MEDICARE FOR ALL WOULD CONTROL HEALTH CARE COSTS AND REDUCE WASTEFUL SPENDING

1. Medicare for All Would Reduce Overall Health Care Spending

In the United States, we spend $4.1 trillion, or more than $12,530 per person, on health care annually—a staggering sum—a great deal of which is wasted or unnecessary.[24] As a country, we spend far more on health care than other comparably wealthy nations. Our public spending on health care, per capita, alone is higher than what nearly all other wealthy countries pay, per capita, for their *entire* health care systems. This is all the more remarkable because all of these countries, unlike the United States, provide universal coverage to their residents. Despite this excessive spending, the United States has the worst health outcomes compared to similar countries.[25]

Numerous studies have analyzed the prospective effectiveness of single-payer plans nationally and at the state level.[26] Most of these studies found considerable savings, to varying degrees. These findings are supported by the experiences of countries that already have universal health care and provide care more efficiently than the United States.[27] A recent study found that Medicare for All could save nearly 20 percent versus our current system, with the largest sources of savings being increased administrative

---

[22]A person in the study was considered underinsured if they had out-of-pocket cost, excluding premiums, over the prior 12 months were 10 percent or more of household income (or 5 percent of household income for households making less than 200 percent of the federal poverty level) or if their deductibles was 5 percent or more of their household income. Sarah R. Collins, Munira Z. Gunja, and Michelle M. Doty, The Commonwealth Fund, How Well Does Insurance Coverage Protect Consumers from Health Care Costs? — Findings from the Commonwealth Fund Biennial Health Insurance Survey, 2016, at 1 (October 2017), https://bit.ly/2D3WbG5.
Rich Daly, *Narrow Networks Spread From ACA Plans to Employers*, HMFA (December 5, 2017), https://bit.ly/2O6GLSo.
Stephen Miller, *Employers May Adopt 'Narrow Networks' of Health Care Providers*, SHRM (January 10, 2017), https://bit.ly/2ikrVLi.

[23]Nearly sixty percent of respondents with private insurance responded that their out-of-pocket health care spending had increased, compared with 51 percent of the uninsured, 46 percent for Medicare, 43 percent for Medicaid and 39 percent for VA & TRICARE.
Ipsos, Health Care Experience Study, at 3 (April 2018), https://bit.ly/2TjlRpr.

[24]Centers for Medicare and Medicaid Services, National Health Expenditures 2020 Highlights, at 1 (December 2021), https://go.cms.gov/3wiaslq.

[25]Irene Papanicolas, Liana R. Woskie and Ashish K. Jha, *Health Care Spending in the United States and Other High-Income Countries*, 319 Journal of the American Medical Association 1024-1039, 1024 (2018).

[26]See *e.g.*, *Listing of Single Payer Studies*, Healthcare-NOW, https://bit.ly/2yplxwr (viewed May 20, 2019).

[27]Irene Papanicolas, Liana R. Woskie and Ashish K. Jha, *Health Care Spending in the United States and Other High-Income Countries*, 319 Journal of the American Medical Association 1024-1039, 1024 (2018).

efficiency and significantly lower pharmaceutical prices.[28] Another recent estimate found that simplified administration under Medicare for All would save the U.S. more than $500 billion a year.[29]

Medicare for All would create enough savings that even a significant increase in the number of people covered by Medicare, including tens of millions of Americans who are currently uninsured, and amount of care provided, as Medicare for All would mean previously underinsured Americans would finally be able to afford health care, would be more than offset.[30] These savings would be achieved by reducing administrative waste and through harnessing the federal government's negotiating power to bring down the price of care, including setting global budgets for institutions.

2. Medicare for All Would Reduce Wasteful Spending on Administration

In the 1980s our nation's health care spending was much more in line with similar countries, before rapidly rising over the last few decades.[31] Increased administrative costs are one of the key reasons that overall health care costs have risen sharply over the past 40 years. The United States has the highest rate of administrative health care costs among wealthy countries.[32] Excessive administrative spending is wasteful because it contributes nothing to treating patients or improving health outcomes. Under our fragmented system, around one-third of U.S. health care dollars are spent on administrative functions, including insurance company overhead; administrative costs of hospitals, practitioners, nursing homes and other providers; and costs incurred by employers in managing their workers' benefits.[33]

Costs relating to managing health insurance are a major factor behind rising administrative costs. Private insurers spend around 12 percent of their annual budgets on administration.[34] Traditional Medicare is much more efficient, spending only around two percent on administrative costs.[35] Higher administrative costs for hospitals also contribute to our excessive spending. If our hospital administrative spending were brought in line with more efficient countries, the U.S. could save more than $150 billion each year on hospital spending alone.[36]

---

[28]Robert Pollin, et al, Political Economy Research Institute, Economic Analysis of Medicare for All, at 66 (November 2018), https://bit.ly/2E6AhCw.
[29]Steffie Woolhandler and David U. Himmelstein, *Single-Payer Reform: The Only Way to Fulfill the President's Pledge of More Coverage, Better Benefits, and Lower Costs*, 166 Annals of Internal Medicine 587-588, 588 (2017).
[30]Robert Pollin, et al, Political Economy Research Institute, Economic Analysis of Medicare for All, at 2 (November 2018), https://bit.ly/2E6AhCw.
[31]*OECD.Stat – Health Expenditure and Financing*, Organization for Economic Co-Operation and Development, https://bit.ly/2sNaLux (viewed on January 27, 2019).
[32]Organization for Economic Co-operation and Development (OECD), Tackling Wasteful Spending on Health, at 232 (January 2017), https://bit.ly/2yVVrhT.
[33]Steffie Woolhandler, Terry Campbell and David U. Himmelstein, *Costs of Health Care Administration in the United States and Canada*, 349 New England Journal of Medicine 768-775, 772 (2003).
Alexis Pozen and David M. Cutler, *Medical Spending Differences in the United States and Canada: The Role of Prices, Procedures, and Administrative Expenses*, 47 Inquiry 124-134, (2010).
[34]Congressional Budget Office, Private Health Insurance Premiums and Federal Policy, at 27 (February 2016) https://bit.ly/1Qw9D0s.
[35]Nick Buffie, *Overhead Costs for Private Health Insurance Keep Rising, Even as Costs Fall for Other Types of Insurance*, Center for Economic and Policy Research (CEPR) Blog (February 6, 2017), https://bit.ly/2l6XVB0.
[36]David U. Himmelstein, et al., *A Comparison of Hospital Administrative Costs in Eight Nations: US Costs Exceed All Others by Far*, 33 Health Affairs 1586-1594, 1589 (2014).

3. <u>Medicare for All Would Reduce the Cost of Prescription Drugs and Medicare Services through Negotiation And Global Budgets</u>

The prices Americans pay for prescription drugs are outrageously high compared to similar countries. One recent study compared our health care spending with 10 other wealthy nations and found that the United States spent around $1,450 per capita on prescription drugs, the most of any wealthy country and more than double the roughly $750 per capita average spending of all 11 countries.[37] Further, an analysis by The *Wall Street Journal* compared U.S. prices across a number of drugs to prices in England, Norway, and Ontario, Canada. It found that U.S. drug prices were almost always higher, often significantly higher.[38]

Comprehensive negotiation on behalf of the entire U.S. population is therefore important benefit of a Medicare for All system. It would be a big improvement on the current Medicare program, which is prohibited from negotiating lower drug prices on behalf of the nation's seniors.[39] In contrast, the Veterans Health Administration (VHA) negotiates the price of drugs for the veterans it serves. As a result, veterans pay much lower drug prices than the general public. A 2015 study found that Medicare Part D would save around $16 billion a year if the agency were able to negotiate similar prices to those negotiated by the VHA on the same brand-name drugs.[40]

Given that Medicare for All would mean the government would have negotiating power on behalf of a much larger population—all Americans—drug prices would be even lower under Medicare for All than they are for the VHA. A recent estimate found that Medicare for All could save over $100 billion a year on drug costs.[41]

In addition to high drug prices, the cost of common medical procedures, such as appendectomies, hip replacements, and angioplasties, are often significantly higher in the United States than in other comparably wealthy countries.[42] In addition, basic health care prices for the same procedure vary wildly between health care providers, which reveals inefficiencies and overpriced services.[43] Providers and insurers generally negotiate prices behind closed doors and refuse to disclose their negotiated prices, citing trade secrets.

Allowing the federal government to use its full negotiating power would make health care pricing more rational and wring out a massive amount of waste from unnecessarily high prices. Under Medicare for

---

37 Irene Papanicolas, Liana R. Woskie and Ashish K. Jha, *Health Care Spending in the United States and Other High-Income Countries*, 319 JOURNAL OF THE AMERICAN MEDICAL ASSOCIATION 1024-1039, 1035 (2018).

38 Jeanne Whalen, *Why the U.S. Pays More Than Other Countries for Drugs*, THE WALL STREET JOURNAL (December 1, 2015), https://on.wsj.com/2pe6SiS.

39 JULIETTE CUBANSKI AND TRICIA NEUMAN, KAISER FAMILY FOUNDATION, SEARCHING FOR SAVINGS IN MEDICARE DRUG PRICE NEGOTIATIONS, at 1 (April 2018), https://bit.ly/2i1ffYI.

40 MARC-ANDRÉ GAGNON AND SIDNEY WOLFE, MIRROR, MIRROR ON THE WALL: MEDICARE PART D PAYS NEEDLESSLY HIGH BRAND-NAME DRUG PRICES COMPARED WITH OTHER OECD COUNTRIES AND WITH U.S. GOVERNMENT PROGRAMS, at 11 (July 2015), https://bit.ly/2p8FRIi.

41 Steffie Woolhandler and David U. Himmelstein, *Single-Payer Reform: The Only Way to Fulfill the President's Pledge of More Coverage, Better Benefits, and Lower Costs*, 166 ANNALS OF INTERNAL MEDICINE 587-588, 588 (2017).

42 INTERNATIONAL FEDERATION OF HEALTH PLANS, 2015 COMPARATIVE PRICE REPORT: VARIATION IN MEDICAL AND HOSPITAL PRICES BY COUNTRY, at 17, 22, & 24 (September 2016), https://bit.ly/2RS7R6K.

43 Elisabeth Rosenthal, *The $2.7 Trillion Medical Bill*, THE NEW YORK TIMES (June 1, 2013), https://nyti.ms/2yW7Gef.

All, the U.S. government would be able to negotiate reasonable prices for services and would prevent providers from charging vastly different prices for the same services.

Global budgets under Medicare for All would help ensure more rational prices for services. These comprehensive budgets – negotiated between the government and health care institutions (such as hospitals and nursing homes) – help control spending while ensuring Americans have access to medically necessary services.[44] Under global budgets, institutions have the incentive to control costs as they provide care. In contrast, our current system creates incentives for institutions to maximize revenue, for example by building expensive new hospital wings and then pressuring providers to refer patients for care, instead of furnishing the most sensible and medically necessary care.[45] Global budgets would have the potential to align providers' incentives with their missions to provide medically necessary care to those who need it.

Institutions are currently incentivized to maximize revenue by undertaking expensive renovations and on purchasing brand-new health care technology that can cost millions of dollars for a single machine. Under global budgeting, such purchases would be funded separately from an institution's operating expenses by creating a separate budget for capital expenditures. Capital purchases impose upfront costs on providers. As previously noted, once purchased, they create incentives to provide unnecessary care to recoup their investments.[46] By requiring separate budgets for the purchases of expensive medical equipment and building expansions, Medicare for All could ensure that such purchases are warranted by a community's needs and would thus reduce unnecessary spending, both on the capital expenses themselves as well as on spending for related services. Instead of having every hospital compete by purchasing complex new technology or building fancy new hospital wings, city and regional capacity would be considered to ensure access to needed care across the country.

IV. <u>CONCLUSION</u>

Once enacted, enrollment for Medicare for All would be similar to traditional Medicare but would happen at birth, establishment of residency, or other similar circumstances. Everyone in the United States would finally be covered and would remain covered throughout their lives. No one would experience loss of insurance when they change or lose a job or go back to school.

Under Medicare for All, our health care system would focus on health and wellbeing instead of generating profit and revenue for wealthy insurers. Hospitals, including many rural hospitals, would have the funds they need to serve their communities. Patients could get the long-term care they need in the setting of their choice. The U.S. would finally be able to ensure sufficient funding for public health, including future

---

[44]Stephen H. Long and M. Susan Marquis, RAND Corporation, Toward a Global Budget for the U.S. Health System: Implementation Issues and Information Needs, at 1 (July 1994), https://bit.ly/2O3v3YS.

[45]Robert A. Berenson, et al., Urban Institute, Global Budgets for Hospitals, at 2 (April 2016), https://urbn.is/2O2ExmU. Joshua M. Sharfstein, et al., The Commonwealth Fund, An Emerging Approach to Payment Reform: All-Payer Global Budgets for Large Safety-Net Hospital Systems, at 3 (August 2016), https://bit.ly/2Ra6awE.

[46]U.S. Government Accountability Office, Medicare: Higher Use of Advanced Imaging Services by Providers Who Self-Refer Costing Medicare Millions, at 16 (September 2012), https://bit.ly/2CDgusT. Dan Munro, *Why Physician Self-Referrals Have to Stop Now*, Forbes (January 26, 2015), https://bit.ly/2ArvYPd.

pandemics. And the nation could finally begin addressing massive health disparities in a comprehensive way.

As the pandemic has shown, everyone depends on the health care system throughout their lives. Whether we face a public health emergency like a global pandemic or simply need to meet routine medical needs, Medicare for All would ensure necessary treatments are available to everyone regardless of their ability to pay.

There would be no out-of-pocket costs or sudden loss of coverage, for example, due to unemployment, to get in the way of Americans receiving the care they need. Small businesses would not be further stressed by providing health care for their employees. In addition, under Medicare for All, Americans would have the freedom to choose a doctor or hospital to receive care wherever is most convenient during a crisis, instead of facing the additional burden of finding providers within narrow private insurance networks which may get overwhelmed during a pandemic.

While Public Citizen has been fighting for single-payer health since our founding over 50 years ago, we believe that the COVID-19 pandemic should serve as a crucial impetus for the U.S. to do to finally do what every other peer nation has already done, provide guaranteed universal health care.

Thank you again for the opportunity to provide comments for this historic hearing. **For questions, please contact me at ekemp@citizen.org.**

Americans for Tax Reform

May 12th, 2022

Dear Chairman Sanders, Ranking Member Graham, and Members of the Senate Budget Committee:

In light of your upcoming hearing entitled, "Medicare for All: Protecting Health, Saving Lives, Saving Money," we urge you to resist any new steps towards socialized healthcare. The Committee's hearing is another opportunity for the Left to promote a government takeover of the American healthcare system. The proposal, called "Medicare for All," replaces private insurance with government as the single payer.

An expansion of government healthcare would lead to extensive middle-class tax hikes and would reduce Americans' access to care.

Medicare for All Would Lead to Trillions in Middle-Class Tax Hikes

By Chairman Sanders' own admission, Americans making more than $29,000 per year would pay more in taxes under Medicare For All.

These tax hikes would hit American families at every income level and businesses large and small. The proposal increases taxes by $14.3 trillion over the next decade. This would pay for roughly half of the cost of single payer healthcare, which costs between $32 trillion and $36 trillion according to estimates.

The list of proposed tax hikes include:

- *A New, 4 Percent Employee Payroll Tax.* This would impose another 4 percent payroll tax on employees which he calls an "income-based premium paid by employees." This increases taxes on American families and individuals by $3.9 trillion.
- *A New, 7 Percent Employer Payroll Tax.* This would impose another 7 percent payroll tax on employees which he calls an "income-based premium paid by employers." This is a $3.5 trillion tax increase over ten years.
- *Eliminating Health Tax "Expenditures."* The proposal would ban employer-provided insurance and repeal the deduction for health care, increasing taxes on businesses by over $3 trillion over a decade.
- *This proposal would also repeal Health Savings Accounts,* which are utilized by an estimated 25 million American families. These tax advantaged savings accounts largely benefit the middle class – roughly half of all HSAs are owned by families earning between $60,000 and $200,000. The deduction for cafeteria plans and the medical expense deduction is also eliminated. In all, this will increase taxes on families and businesses by $4.2 trillion.
- *70 percent top tax bracket for ordinary income and capital gains income.* This would give America the highest income tax rate in the world. According to the Tax Foundation, a top 70 percent rate for ordinary income and capital gains income above $10 million will raise $51.4 billion over a decade. After accounting for macroeconomic effects, the proposal would actually cost the government $63.5 billion because the proposal suppresses investment and economic growth.
- *77 Percent Death Tax.* This would raise the death tax rate to 77 percent for inheritances. Under the proposal, the death tax would kick in at $3.5 million with a rate of 45 percent. This proposal will increase taxes by $315 billion over ten years.

- *Wealth Tax.* This would impose an annual wealth tax of 1 percent kicking in above $21 million in assets. This proposal will increase taxes by $1.3 trillion over ten years.
- *Bank Tax.* This would impose a tax on financial institutions totaling $800 billion over ten years.
- *Broaden the Self Employment Tax.* This would require business owners to report more of their business income as salary, increasing the amount of self-employment tax owed. This would increase taxes by $247 billion over ten years.

This plan would undoubtedly be footed by middle-income taxpayers, with estimates showing the program could raise taxes by $26,000 per household per year.

Medicare for All Would Reduce Americans' Access to Care

Medicare for All promises to eliminate the employer-based coverage which more than 180 million Americans rely on, even with about 81 percent of those people being satisfied with their coverage.

This proposal goes even further left than most foreign versions of socialized medicine. Canada, for example, has about 30% of its healthcare spending coming from the private insurance market; the proposal would have none.

Further, countries which have gone down a path of government control and socialized medicine haven't just seen higher costs; they've seen longer waits and dangerously poor care. In 2018, the UK's National Health System (NHS) cut or restricted access to 17 medical operations which they deemed 'unnecessary' in order to cut costs. In every country where it's been tried, a single-payer system eliminates choice and gives government the power to make healthcare decisions for regular people, often to their detriment.

In addition to poor care and long waits, socialized medicine would also reduce innovation, thus limiting future access to lifesaving, life-changing treatments. The U.S. is currently a world leader when it comes to medical innovation. According to research by the Galen Institute, 290 new medical substances were launched worldwide between 2011 and 2018. The U.S. had access to 90 percent of these cures, a rate far greater than comparable foreign countries. By comparison, the United Kingdom had access to 60 percent of medicines, Japan had 50 percent, and Canada had just 44 percent.

We urge you to resist any steps towards socialized medicine or Medicare for All. This system would lead to massive tax increases on middle-income Americans, would reduce access to quality care, and would decimate medical innovation.

Onward,
Grover G. Norquist
President, Americans for Tax Reform

AMERICANS FOR PROSPERITY

Hearing on Medicare for All

Submission for the Record

Senate Budget Committee

May 12, 2022

Chair Sanders, Ranking Member Graham, and distinguished members of the Committee:

Americans for Prosperity is pleased to submit this submission for the record on the important topic of health reform options, including Medicare for All. Our basic views in this area generally align with those of skeptics of Medicare for All, including today's panelists from the Mercatus Center and the Galen Institute.

About AFP

AFP is a national grassroots activist organization that works to empower every person to earn success, contribute to his or her community, and live a productive, meaningful life. AFP chapters in 35 states and Washington, together with thousands of activists across the country, advocate for a society of equal rights, openness, and mutual benefit based on the time-tested principles of human progress. We believe individual liberty, free enterprise, and bottom-up solutions offer the best way to meet people's needs.

Our health care vision

AFP works to create a health care system that continuously delivers better care at lower cost through markets rather than mandates. We believe markets work in health care when we let them. We hold that the best way to improve the welfare of patients is to let doctors, nurses, hospitals, manufacturers, and retailers compete freely in a robust, well-regulated marketplace, offering the best health care products and services at the best prices that meet patients' needs and respect patients' rights and preferences. We call this vision a "personal option," and in this submission for the record, we would like to outline some of the principles and reforms we believe are essential to making a personal option a reality.[i]

The current system

What problem does Medicare for All, or single-payer health care, seek to address? Surely it is not universal coverage since that goal has been effectively achieved in the United States.

Some 98 percent of Americans today are either covered by or eligible for some form of comprehensive, government-subsidized health insurance. While about 9 percent of Americans are officially uninsured, 7 percentage points of that group are eligible for public or private insurance but simply not enrolled. Just 2 percent of Americans are truly uninsured.[ii]

If we have achieved universal coverage, as a practical matter, why then would we put the government in charge of everyone's health care? Surely, not to improve quality. Eliminating private health insurance and granting the federal government a monopoly over providing standard health benefits to all residents of the United States would reduce competition. That would lead to lower overall quality, as we can see simply by looking at the experience of other nations that employ some form of government monopoly health care.

While certainly not perfect, the quality of care in American is generally very high. In many respects, Americans enjoy the best health care in the world. Our cancer survival rates, for example, are very good[iii] and continuously improving. We also tend to have shorter surgery wait-times.[iv]

What do Americans want?

When it comes to health care reform, Americans have historically been cautious, preferring incremental over radical change. That is still true today. Our polling finds 75 percent of Americans are generally satisfied with their current health care arrangements, and a similar percentage of Americans are not in the market for major changes or disruptions, preferring instead to fix what's broken in our system while preserving what works.[v]

That is not to suggest Americans are entirely satisfied. They are not. They think health care costs too much, they dislike being exposed to high and unpredictable out-of-pocket costs, they complain of the lack of price transparency, and the complexity and confusion of the system.

We believe these flaws arise because, in American health care today the patient is not the consumer, the patient is the product. Too many important decisions are made for patients instead of by them, by third parties, from insurance companies to hospital corporations to pharmacy benefit managers and other middle men that seem to operate without transparency or a true customer focus.

We believe this problem is not caused by the profit motive or market failures, bur rather by a number of well-meant but misguided government policies that shift power and responsibility from patients to third parties. This problem has its roots principally in the tax code, but also exists in the structure and incentives of numerous government programs, regulations, and subsidy schemes. The remedy is not to impose even more layers of government and bureaucracy, but rather to reform existing policies to give patients more choice and control. By making health care more like other markets, where the end-user controls the dollars and the essential decisions, we can increase choice and competition, and thus the quality and the abundance of medical goods and services, and thus the health, welfare, and happiness of patients and their families.

To put it more succinctly, we must do two things: empower patients to shop for value as true consumers, and remove the barriers standing between patients and the medical professional they trust.

Based on our polling and conversations with voters, it's clear that we Americans want:

- Good insurance at an affordable price
- Access to the latest life-saving drugs at a reasonable price
- To see the doctor of our choice, conveniently and affordably
- To know how much our care will cost, up front, before we pay for it

- The choice to try experimental treatments
- And strong government safety nets that protect the vulnerable

In a nutshell, Americans want we call a personal option. A personal option means giving you, the patient, the choice and control you want, with the quality you deserve, at prices you can afford, from the medical professionals you trust. Single-payer, government-run health care can never deliver those things.

False solution: Single-payer

Variations of a "public option" or "Medicare for All" have been tried many times, in many countries, and the results are not encouraging.

Peoples in countries with a single-payer system typically experience shortages and bureaucratic rationing. Access to a waiting list is not access to care. For example, in Canada, where private health insurance is effectively outlawed, health care is "free," yet patients pay for it in other ways.[vi]

- Canadians receive fewer cancer screenings than Americans do[vii] and have higher mortality rates for certain cancers.[viii]
- The median wait time in Canada for an MRI scan is more than two months — to be treated by a specialist, more than five months.[ix]
- And while Americans enjoy access to 89 percent of new drugs,[x] Canadians have access to only 44 percent — Greeks and Spaniards, a mere 14 percent — because their governments deem most new drugs "too expensive." [xi]

In these systems, people end up paying for their "free" care by being forced to endure needless suffering, lost income, and preventable death.

During the pandemic, we saw government failures that made it harder to get people the help they needed – things like providing testing kits that did not work, mask and ventilator shortages for frontline workers, and rigid state laws that kept hospitals from adding capacity and prevented doctors and nurses from going where they were needed.

By contrast, the bright spots of the pandemic – vaccines developed in record time, hospitals expanded overnight, nurses and doctors practicing across state lines, a telehealth revolution – all came about because policymakers wisely removed barriers between patients and the care they needed.

Realistically, a national single-payer program like Medicare for All would mean massive disruption and significantly higher taxes for American families, while potentially offering significantly less access to needed therapies. The Congressional Budget Office estimates that Senator Sanders's legislation would increase federal spending by more than $32 trillion over the first ten years.[xii] That cost must be paid, either in the form of higher taxes or lower reimbursement rates for doctors, nurses, and hospitals – or a combination of both.

True Solution: A personal option

So what should we do instead of Medicare for All? In the remainder of this submission, we will offer our suggestions for making a personal option a reality.

1. Help people, not insurance companies

Health care exists for patients. Government health insurance assistance should go directly to patients, rather than to insurance companies, similar to the way food stamps go directly to low-income families rather than to farmers or food producers. Congress should adopt more voucher-like approaches to existing health insurance subsidies, including Medicaid, Medicare, and the Affordable Care Act. It could, for example, start by adopting such an approach to fill in the so-called Medicaid coverage gap, the 2 million or so individuals who live in states that have not expanded Medicaid and who are not eligible for any form of government-subsidized health insurance. We could take some of the money we currently spend on Medicaid and deposit it directly into a tax-free Health Savings Account owned and controlled by the enrollee. Congress would require that this assistance be used to pay for health insurance premiums and legitimate out-of-pocket expenses but would not otherwise dictate how the recipient uses the funds. This approach would be more compassionate than current, top-down subsidy structures because it would be more efficient and dignified for the recipient.

2. Promote price transparency

In every market, consumers get to see the price up front – except in health care. We would never tolerate this at the gas station or grocery store. Unable to shop for value, patients grope in the dark and get hit with excessive charges and pay for needless middlemen and waste. Health care costs will not come down until we can see real prices. But how to get there? Some people favor top-down government mandates, forcing hospitals, insurers, and drugmakers to publish their list prices and their privately negotiated rates. The Trump Administration tried to do so through aggressive regulatory actions. While we strongly support price transparency, we do not believe a mandatory approach will actually help consumers in the long run. The only sure path to price transparency is to empower consumers to make the important purchasing decisions. When consumers are spending their own money, they shop for value, and prices become transparent naturally – just as they do at the gas station and the grocery store. A good place to start is to expand and strengthen special accounts that patients can use to save and pay for health care, tax-free. Such accounts help level the tax code playing field, effectively giving consumers the same kind of generous tax break for health care and coverage purchases that currently only employers receive.

3. Expand and strengthen tax-free HSAs

Tax-free Health Savings Accounts help 30 million American families pay their out-of-pocket medical expenses tax-free. Why not every family? An HSA is a tool that saves you anywhere between 10 to 40 percent off, each time you make a health care purchase. And it gives you greater control of your medical decisions. Studies show HSAs help reduce health care costs.[xiii] [xiv] [xv] Expanding this option is a prime way to put consumers in the driver's seat and bend the health care cost curve downward. Unfortunately, today only about 10 percent of Americans are able to have an HSA, because the law requires HSA owners to buy a narrowly defined, high-deductible health plan or HDHP. By removing this needless restriction, we can allow all Americans to save for health care, tax-free. It would also be desirable to significantly increase how much people can save in these accounts, as well as the array of items and coverage options they can buy with them, including, for example, direct primary care subscriptions and health insurance premiums. Examples of good bills that include these kinds of reforms include Senator Rubio's and Senator Tim Scott's

Health Savings Act (S.380, 2021), Senator Cruz's Personalized Care Act (S.153, 2021), and Senator Paul's Health Savings Accounts for All Act (S.4367, 2020).

4. Strengthen individual coverage HRAs

Current policy allows employers to set up, and employees to benefit from, special spending accounts known as individual coverage health reimbursement arrangements or ICHRAs. In addition to facilitating employees' out-of-pocket purchases using pre-tax dollars, these innovative accounts also enable employees to use tax-free money from their employer to buy health insurance that is personally owned and portable. This is a godsend, including for patients with costly pre-existing medical conditions. Thanks to ICHRAs, employees can now have the peace of mind that comes from knowing that they don't have to lose their health insurance coverage when they change jobs. Congress should reject efforts to eliminate or water down ICHRAs, and should facilitate educational efforts to increase employers' awareness and use of this exciting option.

5. Reduce mandates to make health insurance affordable

Insurance today is often a poor value for money. Thanks to well-meant but misguided mandates, federal and state, premiums in recent years have doubled, deductibles have tripled, and access to doctors and hospitals has dramatically narrowed. Happily, with some sensible insurance reforms we can reverse these harmful trends and actually bring down premiums while preserving protections for people with pre-existing conditions. Specifically, Congress should repeal costly, frivolous benefit mandates and ease or eliminate age-based community-rating price controls, so that more young, healthy people sign up voluntarily.

6. Reduce hospital market consolidation

Hospital services represent about 40 percent of all health expenditures in the United States. In recent years, hospital market consolidation has accelerated, reducing choice and quality, driving up prices, and tilting the playing field against physicians. Addressing and reversing this troubling trend requires legislative, judicial, and regulatory action, including modifications of antitrust laws, or at least modifications of their specific application. But there are other policy reforms that can help to reduce hospital market consolidation, and thus to improve the cost, quality, and abundance of hospital services.[xvi] Such reforms include the repeal of local certificate of need laws and reforms of Medicare to provide for site-neutral payments and an end to the moratorium on physician-owned hospitals. The latter two reforms are discussed more specifically, below.

6. Lift the federal moratorium on physician-owned hospitals

Section 6001 of the Affordable Care Act places an effective moratorium on participation in Medicare for new and expanded physician-owned hospitals (POH).[xvii] This prohibition is unjustified and should be repealed. Studies show that it unduly and needlessly limits competition and increases costs. For example, a recent literature review finds, among other things, that orthopedic and cardiac "focused factory" POHs offer consumers comparable or lower costs and higher quality care compared to other hospitals; patients with a wide range of serious conditions experience lower in-hospital and 30-day mortality rates in specialty POHs; patients with orthopedic conditions receive a greater number of conservative preoperative therapies prior to invasive procedures and experience shorter stays and lower risk-adjusted complication rates; general surgery POHs offer higher quality services compared to their competitors; and the cost and quality of general acute care POHs is not inferior to competitors. [xviii]

7. Move to site-neutral payment in Medicare

Medicare payment structures are built around the kind of facility in which care is delivered, rather than how efficiently and effectively it is delivered. Congress should move to site-neutrality, so that the Medicare payment for a medical service is the same whether it is delivered in a physician's office, a clinic, or a hospital setting. The Centers for Medicare and Medicaid Services issued a rule to accomplish site-neutrality on a limited basis.[xix] Congress should codify this site-neutrality policy and expand it to level the playing field among providers and remove the financial disabilities for medical professionals who would compete with hospital systems.

8. Modernize Medicare

Medicare is a popular but expensive and in critical ways outdated insurance product that fails to protect seniors from catastrophic costs and negatively distorts health care markets. We can do better by America's elderly and disabled citizens. Reform need not be partisan or polarized. There are incremental reforms that modernize and strengthen Medicare to give seniors more freedom and better access to doctors and therapies at lower cost. Because the private, competitive Medicare Advantage option often offers superior service with extra benefits at no or low out-of-pocket cost, more than 43 percent of Medicare enrollees have voluntarily opted into it. To increase competition within Medicare, we believe all new Medicare enrollees should be auto-enrolled into an affordable Medicare Advantage plan in their area, with a right to opt into original, fee-for-service Medicare if they wish. To increase competition within the over-65 market more generally, we believe seniors should be allowed to choose private coverage in lieu of Medicare without penalty, with reasonable policies to govern how and when they can opt back in, if they wish. Senator Braun's Fair Care Act (S.4796, 2020) includes a provision to do just that, as does Senator Cruz's Retirement Freedom Act (S.275, H.R.1166, 2021). We also endorse Representative Latta's Stop Penalizing Working Seniors Act (H.R.5563, 2021), which enable seniors enrolled only in Medicare Part A to save for and pay out-of-pocket health care costs, tax-free, through a personally owned and controlled Health Savings Account.

9. Make Medicaid reform a national priority

If there's something both sides of the aisle ought to be able to agree on, it's that we must eliminate waste in federal programs. Medicaid's improper payment rate has ballooned from 9 percent in 2018 to nearly 15 percent in 2019 and all the way to 21 percent in 2020 – possibly as high as 25 percent. Officially, Medicaid wastes on the order of $70 billion a year – enough to pay for health care for 12 million adults or 3.6 million disabled Americans for an entire year.[xx] Unofficially, the program probably wastes in excess of $100 billion a year. About 80 percent of these improper payments are due to payments to ineligible persons.[xxi] Meanwhile, the quality of care delivered by Medicaid has long been known to be inferior. Clearly, this broken program cries out for reform. Medicaid was never meant to be a middle-class entitlement that displaces private insurance options and busts the federal budget. It was meant to be a safety net. Congress should reform it to keep it focused on those who truly need help paying for health care. Congress should also help the working poor by using some of the money we currently spend on Medicaid as direct deposits into tax-free HSAs for low-income families.

10. Unleash the potential of telehealth

Telehealth technologies empower health professionals to remotely consult, diagnose, and treat patients without meeting in-person. Providers can safely and effectively deliver an array of health services through telehealth including primary care, mental health services, and emergency care. Patients can connect with health care workers through a variety of telehealth technologies including video conference apps, remote monitoring devices, instant messages, and audio phone calls. The pandemic has dramatically revealed how telemedicine can reduce costs and infections and ensure that people, especially in underserved rural and urban communities, can access health care in a timely manner.

A recent nonpartisan study by Americans Prosperity and the Progressive Policy Institute found that over the duration of the COVID-19 pandemic, the costs of telehealth care fell, suggesting that in a post-pandemic world telehealth could help increase access to medical care without increasing costs.[xxii] Expanding access to telehealth lowers health care spending by providing patients a low-cost alternative to expensive in-person care. The popular telehealth platform Teladoc reports the average telehealth consultation costs just $40. By comparison, the typical cost of an in-person primary care visit is $160. Virtual care also reduces costs by helping patients avoid expensive hospitalizations. Ascension Health, America's 2nd largest hospital system, found 60 percent of its telehealth patients would have visited an urgent care clinic or emergency room if they did not offer virtual care. This decreased costly outpatient services by 33 percent for Ascension's patients.[xxiii]

Prior to the COVID-19 pandemic, only 134,000 Medicare enrollees received virtual care every week. After the pandemic emergency reforms took effect, the number of enrollees receiving telehealth increased to 10.1 million, roughly one-third of all fee-for-service Medicare enrollees. Overall, Medicare enrollees purchased eight percent fewer primary care services between January and June 2020.[xxiv] From February to December 2020, the number of telehealth services delivered to privately insured patients increased over 1,500 percent. As a share of all health care services, virtual care increased from one percent to 21 percent during this period

Unfortunately, these important reforms are limited to the COVID-19 public health emergency. As soon as state and federal officials declare the pandemic over, these harmful telehealth barriers will resume and patients will lose access to essential virtual care. Our proposed solutions:

1. *Remove barriers on patient locations.* Under changes implemented by the CARES Act, CMS authorized health care providers to deliver care to patients located in any zip code and setting, including their home.[xxv] Prior to this reform, patients could only receive telehealth services from select health care facilities in rural areas.
2. *Remove barriers on provider locations.* Under the CARES Act, CMS announced that health care practitioners can deliver telehealth from an expanded array of facilities, including Federally Qualified Health Centers, Rural Health Centers, and their own homes.[xxvi]

3. *Expand the list of telehealth services.* Starting March 1, 2020, CMS announced that health professionals can deliver approximately 240 additional telehealth services to Medicare recipients, including mental health consultations, home health visits and emergency care.[xxvii]
4. *Expand the list of telehealth providers.* Prior to COVID-19, federal law authorized only nine types of health care providers to deliver telehealth services.[xxviii] Fortunately, the agency expanded the list of telehealth provider-types to include all practitioners who are currently authorized to deliver in-person care to Medicare recipients, including physical therapists, occupational therapists, and speech language pathologists.[xxix]
5. *End technology restrictions on telehealth.* Under the Cares Act, CMS authorized practitioners to deliver telehealth through audio-only phone calls.[xxx] In addition, the Office for Civil Rights (OCR) issued guidance allowing health care providers to deliver telehealth through any non-public facing telecommunication platform, including Zoom, Apple FaceTime, and Skype.[xxxi]
6. *Allow telehealth across state lines.* Prior to COVID-19, federal law prohibited health care practitioners from delivering telehealth to patients across state lines.[xxxii] Fortunately, CMS issued a waiver allowing health care providers to deliver telehealth in states that explicitly authorize out-of-state providers to provide virtual care without an additional license.[xxxiii]
7. *Empower insurers to offer comprehensive telehealth coverage.* Before COVID-19, federal law prohibited insurers from waiving deductibles for telehealth services for individuals with high-deductible health plans (HDHPs) associated with tax-free HSAs. Fortunately, the CARES Act allows insurers to offer telehealth services free of deductibles for individuals covered by these plans.[xxxiv] Examples of positive legislation in this area include Sen. Manchin's Protecting Rural Telehealth Access Act (S.1988, 2021), Senator Tim Scott's Telehealth Modernization Act (S.368, 2021), and Senator Schatz's CONNECT for Health Act of 2021 (S.1512, 2021).

11. Allow association health plans

Letting individuals and businesses band together to buy affordable coverage at group rates should be a no-brainer. Large businesses get such discounts, why not small businesses as well? Unfortunately, a federal court recently ruled that the U.S. Department of Labor does not have authority to clarify existing rules to permit AHPs federally. Therefore, congressional clarification is needed. Examples of good bills to do so include Senator Kennedy's Association Health Plans Act (S.896, 2021) and Senator Paul's American Healthshare Plans Act (S.3610, 2020).

12. Allow "truth in medicine"

The U.S. Food and Drug Administration imposes a speech restriction on drug manufacturers barring the sharing of scientific information with doctors about possible uses of drugs outside the current limits of the drugs' labeling – even when the information is truthful, non-misleading, and potentially life-saving. Congress should rescind this harmful gag rule.[xxxv]

13. Speed up FDA drug approvals

The pandemic and Operation Warp Speed have shown that a speedier FDA gets more life-saving drugs and medicines to people more quickly. It takes 10 to 15 years and $2.6 billion on average to bring a new drug to market.[xxxvi] Some drugs are approved in the United States only many years after they were approved overseas. Patients suffer and die needlessly. We can reduce this needless suffering and expense without harming patients by requiring FDA to recognize drugs and devices that have been approved by advanced countries we trust. Senator Cruz's RESULTs Act (S.154, 2021) would do just that. Another excellent proposal is Senator Braun's Promising Pathway Act (S.1644, 2021).

14. Improve Medicare drug coverage

There is bipartisan support for helping Medicare enrollee's deal with prescription drug costs by capping their total Part D out-of-pocket cost exposure and eliminating the infamous "donut hole" coverage gap. AFP supports these sensible reforms to help make prescription drugs more affordable.

15. Promote generic drug competition

Robust generic competition is critical to ensuring that costly medications and therapies become affordable, without harmful government price controls or infringing the just rights of inventors. It's time to end pay-for-delay schemes, patent evergreening, and abuse of FDA citizen petitions. Good places to start include Senator Crapo's Lower Costs More Cures Act (H.R.19, 2021)[xxxvii] and Senator Wyden's and Senator Grassley's Prescription Drug Price Reduction Act (S.2543, 2019, and S.4199, 2020).[xxxviii]

16. Legalize drug importation

Another way to put downward pressure on pharmaceutical costs is to legalize drug importation from abroad. The current restrictions on such importation unduly limit Americans' choices. While the pharmaceutical industry objects that such a reform would merely "import foreign price controls" into our country, it would actually put pressure on those countries to relax their price controls, which would be good for everyone. Importation should be allowed for individuals and importers, and not just governments.

17. Encourage pro-consumer state-level reforms

Not all reforms can be achieved solely at the federal level. Some require action by the states. The following state-level reforms are included in this discussion, not only for completeness, but because, in many cases, Congress can help support the states.

18. Liberate direct patient care

Direct patient care, also known as direct primary care, is a great new option that lets patients pay a flat fee for unlimited access to a primary care doctor and preventive services, with no insurance-company middle man. It's like a monthly Netflix subscription to your most trusted doctors. AFP supports legislation to legalize DPC at the state level, and encourages Congress to enact federal legislation to allow people to use their tax-free HSA and HRA funds to pay for DPC subscriptions out-of-pocket.

19. Strengthen access to short term renewable health plans

Short term renewable health insurance plans can be dramatically more affordable than traditional plans, up to 50 to 80 percent more affordable, because they are offer a streamlined, temporary option unburdened by excessive government mandates that drive up costs. While not a substitute for permanent coverage, these federally defined and state-regulated plans are an important option that everyone should have access to. About a dozen states have restricted them so severely, they are either unavailable or unaffordable. Five states have essentially outlawed them. Yet a recent study shows the only states where individual market premiums have increased since 2018 are the five that effectively prohibit these plans (California, Massachusetts, New Jersey, New York, and Rhode Island). Meanwhile, that states that allow short-term plans have lost fewer enrollees in the individual market, have had far more insurers offer coverage in the market, and have had larger premium reductions since 2018.[xxxix] Those hostile laws should be repealed, and we encourage states to conform their policies to current federal policy, which allows a plan duration of up to 12 months and renewable for a total of 36 months. Congress, meanwhile, should codify that existing policy while also allowing tax-free HSA and HRA funds to be used for short term plans.

20. Liberate hospitals to expand and compete

You shouldn't need a government permission slip or a political connection to provide a new medical service, purchase hospital equipment, or build a new facility. Local CON laws require government approval before private entities can do these things. Often, existing market participants have a veto over new entrants. Such protectionism harms patients and reduces the resilience we need to respond quickly to a crisis like COVID-19. A veritable mountain of studies and papers show that CON laws drive up costs and reduce quality, and that repealing them saves lives.[xl] While Congress wisely repealed the federal CON law back in the 1980s, and thus has no cause for federal legislation in this area, it can and should provide oversight on the issue, as well as moral support for state-level efforts to end this harmful protectionism.

21. Let nurses deliver the care they're trained for

The nearly 80 million Americans who do not have sufficient access to a health care provider would be served better if medical professionals like nurse practitioners were allowed to practice to the full extent of their education and training without having to pay a physician for the privilege. Senator Paul's Coronavirus Regulatory Repeal Act (S.969, 2021) would make this and similar pandemic reforms permanent, while giving Congress and federal regulators a chance to carefully review and block changes that would not be in patients' best interest.

22. Let doctors and nurses practice across state lines

The pandemic showed the vital importance of allowing doctors and nurses to care for out-of-state patients, including via telehealth. State and federal policies that effectively limit health care professionals to practicing within the borders of a single state reduce consumer choice, interstate competition, and the quality of care. States should amend their laws to automatically recognize out-of-state health professional licenses. And while federal programs including Medicare should respect state jurisdiction and policy choices, such programs should be reformed where possible to facilitate interstate care delivery. For example, Congress should make permanent Medicare policies adopted during the pandemic that allow state-licensed doctors and nurses to treat patients in and from other states.

Conclusion

Our system needs reforms. But overall, it is a good system. Americans enjoy superior quality and access, and, as a practical matter, universal coverage. Most are satisfied with their current coverage and are not looking for a radical overhaul. Instead, they want to fix what's broken and preserve what works. Instead of Medicare for All, or a public option, or further expanding existing government programs, Congress should enact a personal option that gives patients the choice and control they want, with the quality they deserve, at prices they can afford, from the medical professionals they trust. AFP stands ready to help you achieve this exciting vision.

---

[i] https://americansforprosperity.org/personal-option/
[ii] https://www.kff.org/uninsured/issue-brief/key-facts-about-the-uninsured-population/
[iii] https://www.healio.com/news/hematology-oncology/20180131/us-cancer-survival-rates-remain-among-highest-in-world
[iv] https://fee.org/articles/america-outperforms-canada-in-surgery-wait-times-and-its-not-even-close/
[v] https://americansforprosperity.org/voters-want-more-choice-control-health-care-survey/
[vi] https://www.encounterbooks.com/features/sally-c-pipes-on-the-false-promise-of-single-payer-healthcare/
[vii] https://www.thecentersquare.com/opinion/op-ed-health-care-a-personal-option-vs-the-public-option/article_c11a65e6-0a4f-11eb-b268-5f4c8d38b20f.html
[viii] https://www.cdc.gov/cancer/dcpc/research/index.htm
[ix] https://www.fraserinstitute.org/studies/waiting-your-turn-wait-times-for-health-care-in-canada-2019
[x] https://www.nationalreview.com/2020/08/canadian-single-payer-health-care-system-slow-inefficient/
[xi] https://galen.org/2019/examination-of-international-drug-pricing-policies-in-selected-countries-shows-prevalent-government-control-over-pricing-and-restrictions-on-access/
[xii] https://economics21.org/medicare-for-all-winners-and-losers
[xiii] https://www.nber.org/papers/w21031
[xiv] https://www.actuary.org/sites/default/files/pdf/health/cdhp_may09.pdf
[xv] file:///C:/Users/DClancy/OneDrive%20-%20Stand%20Together/dean%20files/policy/hc/hc%20-%20payment%20-%20decentralized%20-%20tax%20-%20hsa/hsa%20-%20studies%20etc/HSA%20effect%202019%20PA%20study.pdf
[xvi] https://www.heritage.org/health-care-reform/report/how-congress-can-help-reverse-hospital-market-consolidation
[xvii] https://www.healthaffairs.org/do/10.1377/hblog20210408.980640/full/
[xviii] https://www.mercatus.org/publications/healthcare/cost-and-quality-care-physician-owned-hospitals-systematic-review
[xix] https://www.govinfo.gov/content/pkg/FR-2019-11-12/pdf/2019-24138.pdf
[xx] https://thehill.com/blogs/congress-blog/healthcare/568825-medicaids-improper-payments-show-why-the-program-needs-reform
[xxi] https://nypost.com/2020/11/28/medicaid-hemorrhaging-100b-on-americans-ineligible-for-the-program/
[xxii] https://americansforprosperity.org/telehealth-expansion-improves-outcomes-and-lowers-costs-finds-new-bipartisan-report-from-ppi-and-afp/
[xxiii] https://connectwithcare.org/wp-content/uploads/2020/08/Ascension-Telehealth-Data.pdf
[xxiv] http://www.medpac.gov/docs/default-source/reports/mar21_medpac_report_ch14_sec.pdf?sfvrsn=0
[xxv] https://www.cms.gov/newsroom/fact-sheets/medicare-telemedicine-health-care-provider-fact-sheet
[xxvi] https://www.cms.gov/files/document/covid-rural-health-clinics.pdf
[xxvii] https://www.cms.gov/Medicare/Medicare-general-information/telehealth/telehealth-codes
[xxviii] https://www.law.cornell.edu/cfr/text/42/410.78
[xxix] https://www.cms.gov/files/document/summary-covid-19-emergency-declaration-waivers.pdf
[xxx] https://www.cms.gov/files/document/covid-19-emergency-declaration-waivers.pdf
[xxxi] https://www.hhs.gov/hipaa/for-professionals/special-topics/emergency-preparedness/notification-enforcement-discretion-telehealth/index.html
[xxxii] https://www.law.cornell.edu/cfr/text/42/410.78
[xxxiii] https://www.cms.gov/files/document/summary-covid-19-emergency-declaration-waivers.pdf
[xxxiv] https://www.congress.gov/116/plaws/publ136/PLAW-116publ136.pdf
[xxxv] https://goldwaterinstitute.org/free-speech-in-medicine/
[xxxvi] https://www.phrma.org/policy-issues/research-development
[xxxvii] https://republicans-energycommerce.house.gov/wp-content/uploads/2021/04/HR-19-Section-by-Section.pdf
[xxxviii] https://www.finance.senate.gov/imo/media/doc/PDPRA%20Committee%20Report%20092519%20FINAL.pdf
[xxxix] https://galen.org/2021/individual-health-insurance-markets-improving-in-states-that-fully-permit-short-term-plans-2/
[xl] https://www.mercatus.org/publications/corporate-welfare/certificate-need-laws

* * *

May 12, 2022
Senator Bernie Sanders
Chairman, Senate Committee on the Budget

Senator Lindsey Graham
Ranking Member, Senate Committee on the Budget
624 Senate Dirksen Office Building
Washington, D.C. 20510

Dear Chairman Sanders and Ranking Member Graham,

The title of the Senate Budget Committee hearing, "Medicare for All: Protecting Health, Savings Lives, Saving Money," scheduled for Thursday, May 12, could not be more misleading and inaccurate. Expanding a program that will be insolvent in four years will not save money or lives or protect anyone's health. On behalf of the more than one million members and supporters of the Council for Citizens Against Government Waste, rather than proposing to expand Medicare, I urge the committee to be focused on reforming Medicare.

Medicare Part A assists in paying for inpatient hospital services, hospice care, skilled nursing facilities, and home health services associated with hospital stays. The 2021 Medicare Trustees Report estimated that Part A will be depleted in 2026, the same date as the 2020 report. Congress must address this financial shortfall to minimize the negative impact on taxpayers and patients. Most proposals to "fix" Medicare include spending cuts, tax increases, and increasing the age of eligibility. None of these solutions are patient-centered and put individuals on Medicare at risk.

Government-run healthcare systems like Medicare for All lead to price controls, rationing, and long waiting lists to see a specialist or have surgery. There is a better way than adopting socialized medicine under which government bureaucrats and politicians decide what doctors patients can see and what treatments they can receive. Citizens Against Government Waste's 2021 report on government-run healthcare describes how this system would harm patients and eliminate consumer choice. Rather than Medicare for All, a free market approach to healthcare reform is essential to allow Americans retain control over their healthcare choices, with numerous options for coverage, and greater opportunities for more innovation. These ideas, among others, are included the Consensus Group's "Health Care Choices 2020: A Vision for the Future."

Medicare for All would expand Medicare to include all Americans, putting millions on government assistance and distorting the private insurance market. A Mercatus Center analysis estimated that Medicare for All would increase federal budget commitments by $32.6 trillion during its first 10 years of full implementation (2022–2031), assuming enactment in 2018. After analyzing a single-payer system, the Congressional Budget Office projected that federal subsidies would cost $1.5 trillion to $3 trillion higher in 2030 than under current law during the same year.

I urge you to reject Medicare for All and work instead to eliminate the waste, fraud, and mismanagement in the current program. Errors, false claims, and overprescribing or overcharging for Medicare services causes more than $60 billion in annual losses. Instead of addressing this mismanagement, supporters of Medicare for All wish to expand this failing government program and steer all Americans toward government health insurance.

Instituting a national one-size-fits-all health care system like Medicare for All will be a detriment to public health and the taxpayers. Congressional spending at current levels is unsustainable and expanding underfunded programs like Medicare is irresponsible and reckless. I strongly urge you not to support Medicare for All or any other government-run healthcare plan.

Sincerely,
Tom Schatz

FreedomWorks

May 12, 2022

Oppose Medicare for All

On behalf of FreedomWorks' activist community, I urge opposition to Medicare for All and any form of socialized medicine.

Medicare-for-all ultimately seeks to abolish private health insurance and would put us on a fast track toward placing all Americans on government-run health insurance. No longer would Americans be able to switch providers to get a better deal. There would be only one deal -- you, locked into whatever some bureaucrat decides is best for you.

At the same time, wait times at hospitals increase, and drug supplies become scarce under government-run health care. Premiums and deductibles would skyrocket at a faster rate than during Obamacare.

No longer are Democrats pretending to peddle the lie that President Obama told our country about Obamacare: "If you like your healthcare plan, you can keep it." Instead, they are embracing the idea of taking health decisions away from the American people and forcing them into a socialist scheme similar to many of those in Europe.

According to the Urban Institute, single-payer health insurance would cost $32 trillion over ten years. Such a plan would require massive tax hikes that hit the middle class. The Congressional Budget Office (CBO) warned that "patients might face increased wait times and reduced access to care" under a single-payer plan. In other countries, like England, that is a reality where wait times for surgeries recently reached a ten-year high.

For these reasons, I urge you to vigorously oppose any proposal that would move the United towards a single-payer system.

Sincerely,

Adam Brandon
President, FreedomWorks

Medicare For All would mean worse care for all

BY MICHAEL F. CANNON, OPINION CONTRIBUTOR - 05/04/22 5:00 PM ET

Senate Budget Committee Chairman Bernie Sanders (I-Vt.) has announced that as early as next week, his committee will hold a hearing "on the need to pass a Medicare for All single-payer program."

Sanders gets an "A" for passion, but an "F" in compassion.

The non-partisan Congressional Budget Office has cautioned that Sanders' Medicare for All bill would create "a shortage of providers, longer wait times, and changes in the quality of care."

Indeed, the non-partisan Medicare Payment Advisory Commission has warned since at least 2003 that Medicare's approach to health care quality "is largely neutral or negative." Enrolling 330 million people in the program would only make the problem worse.

Thankfully, there is a (potentially bipartisan) way to reverse Medicare's negative impact on quality: Apply "public option" principles not to the private health insurance market but to Medicare, where this traditionally Democratic idea would dramatically increase choice and competition.

Since 1965, Medicare has paid providers more for low-quality care than for high-quality care. For example, in 1995, Utah's Intermountain Health Care reduced mortality by improving how it treated pneumonia. Medicare rewarded those quality improvements by paying Intermountain *less*.

In 1999, Duke University developed a better way to treat congestive heart failure. Medication adherence increased. Hospitalizations fell. Resource use fell by half. Again, Medicare (and private insurers with similar payment rules) responded by reducing payments. Duke eventually had to shutter the program for lack of funds.

In 2002, Whatcom County, Washington improved glucose management for diabetics and stabilized congestive heart failure patients, saving $3,000 per patient. The county ended up shuttering the program for the same reason Duke did.

Need more evidence?

In 2009, Medicare *reduced* payments to Texas' Baylor Medical Center after the system cut heart-failure readmissions in half with no increase in mortality. Hospitals can nearly *double* net revenues if a Medicare patient develops post-operative complications. Medicare pays hospitals nearly $3,000 more per patient when low-quality care leads to more post-acute care and readmissions. Medicare paid a large urban hospital system more when it allowed urinary-tract or bloodstream infections than when it prevented them.

It doesn't have to be this way.

In the mid-1990s, Group Health Cooperative of Puget Sound improved diabetes care with an "average cost savings [] of $685-$950 per patient per year." Group Health's different payment rules—which markets developed a century before Congress enacted Medicare—allowed it to *profit* from those quality improvements.

What Sen. Sanders doesn't get is that medicine is so complex, no single payment system can promote all aspects of health care quality. Locking in *any* single set of payment rules—as a single-payer system by definition must—will always reward low-quality care and penalize progress.

Competition drives providers to improve all dimensions of quality—even those their own payment rules discourage. Improving care across the board requires letting all varieties of payment rules compete on a level playing field.

Public-option principles demand exactly that: a level playing field where consumers are the ultimate arbiters of quality and efficiency. Public-option supporters want a new government program to be one of the competitors.

But there's no need for a new program. Traditional Medicare is a government-run plan that already competes against private insurers. Economist Mark Pauly explains that Medicare "is essentially a risk-adjusted voucher program" that lets enrollees choose between a public option and private Medicare Advantage plans.

That playing field, however, is anything but level. Congress bars certain plans, encourages excessive coverage, and penalizes high-quality coverage. It further violates public-option principles by offering larger subsidies to healthy enrollees if they choose Medicare Advantage, and to sicker enrollees if they choose traditional Medicare.

Public-option principles demand eliminating all such distortions. Most important, they require that each enrollee's subsidy neither rise nor fall depending on which health plan, or how much coverage, he or she chooses. Only one type of subsidy can do that: cash.

Public-option principles *require* that Medicare mirror Social Security, which gives enrollees cash and trusts them to spend it. In 2022, Medicare will spend enough to give each enrollee an average cash subsidy of $12,100. Income- and risk-adjustment would give poorer and sicker enrollees thousands more to ensure they could afford coverage.

Enrollees would spend that money better than government bureaucrats do. Evidence shows that cost-conscious patients force providers to reduce prices and that when seniors control their health decisions, even those with cognitive limitations make good choices.

While Medicare for All would condemn generations to low-quality care, applying public-option principles to Medicare would improve health care through choice and competition. It's a Democratic idea even Republicans can love.

Michael F. Cannon is director of health policy studies at the Cato Institute and coauthor of "Would 'Medicare for All' Mean Quality For All?" (with Jacqueline Pohida, AGPCNP-BC, Quinnipiac Health Law Journal, 2022).

Democrats seize on cherry-picked claim that 'Medicare-for-all' would save $2 trillion

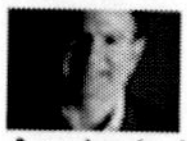

Analysis by Glenn Kessler
Staff writer
August 7, 2018
Share

"We know that Medicaid expansion and Medicare-for-all actually save this state and this nation $2 trillion if it were fully implemented."
— Andrew Gillum, Democratic candidate for Florida governor, in a primary debate, Aug. 2, 2018

This fact check has been updated
As our colleague David Weigel reported, Democrats have latched onto the catchy idea of "Medicare-for-all" (also known as M4A) as a way of expressing their support for universal health care.
On July 30, the Mercatus Center at George Mason University released a working paper on the 10-year fiscal impact of the Medicare-for-all plan sponsored by Sen. Bernie Sanders (I-Vt.), which would transition everyone in the United States from a mostly employer-provided health system to Medicare over four years. The report was written by Charles Blahous, a former economic adviser to George W. Bush and a public trustee for Social Security and Medicare from 2010 through 2015.
Gillum, the mayor of Tallahassee, was quoted in Weigel's article as having touted, during a debate, a $2 trillion cost-savings figure that is in the report. Sanders, too, has tweeted about this $2 trillion number, sarcastically thanking the conservative Koch brothers, whose foundation has contributed to Mercatus. "Let me thank the Koch brothers of all people for sponsoring a study that shows that Medicare for All would save the American people $2 trillion over a 10-year period," Sanders says in a video with the tweet.
But Blahous is crying foul, saying Medicare-for-all proponents are misrepresenting his findings. Let's take a look.

The Facts

We often warn readers that you can't get something for nothing. In the health-care realm, even relatively small shifts can lead to major dislocation and changes; President Barack Obama discovered that, to his chagrin. As former Lyndon Johnson White House aide Joseph A. Califano Jr. once noted, congressional dealmaking during the passage of Medicaid unexpectedly led to one-third of the Medicaid budget going to nursing homes — an industry that was literally built on Medicaid funding.
In doing his research, Blahous decided to follow the text of the Sanders plan and assume that providers — doctors, hospitals, and the like — would face an immediate cut of roughly 40 percent for the treatment of patients now covered by private insurance. (Note: an earlier version of this fact check incorrectly included a reference to drug

companies in the sentence above. The analysis found that drug costs would be $846 billion lower over ten years from an aggressive program to negotiate lower prescription drug prices but it would not be as much as a 40 percent decline.)

That in theory would reduce the country's overall level of health expenditures by $2 trillion from 2022 to 2031. But he makes clear that it's a pretty unrealistic assumption.

In the fourth sentence of the report's abstract, Blahous wrote, "It is likely that the actual cost of M4A would be substantially greater than these estimates, which assume significant administrative and drug cost savings under the plan, and also assume that healthcare providers operating under M4A will be reimbursed at rates more than 40 percent lower than those currently paid by private health insurance."

Under an alternative scenario, which assumes these cuts cannot be achieved, national health spending rises even faster than under current law because health-care demand would increase.

"To lend credibility to the $2 trillion savings number, one would have to argue that we can cut payments to providers by about 40 percent at the same time as increasing demand by about 11 percent," Blahous said.

The main point of his study is being ignored by Democrats — that even by generously accepting Sanders's assumptions that he could squeeze providers so much, the plan would still raise government expenditures by $32.6 trillion. This is in line with a 2016 estimate by the Urban Institute of an earlier version of the M4A plan — that it would cause federal expenditures to increase by $32 trillion. (Without the provider cuts, Blahous estimated the additional federal budget cost at nearly $40 trillion over 10 years.)

Sanders has said an earlier version of his plan would add $1.38 trillion a year in new spending between 2017 and 2026, paid for in part with new taxes on employers and an income-based premium — an estimate that one analysis in 2016 (disputed by Sanders) said was underfinanced by $1.1 trillion a year.

Blahous estimates total federal spending under M4A would be closer to $3.3 trillion a year. (Note: Some readers correctly noted these estimates are for different budget windows and spending pots and so are not directly comparable.)

"For perspective on these figures, consider that doubling all currently projected federal individual and corporate income tax collections would be insufficient to finance the added federal costs of the plan," Blahous wrote. (He's referring only to income tax collection, not existing Social Security and Medicare payroll taxes.)

Blahous told the Fact Checker: "Every table in the study (Tables 1-5) is very explicit that the additional costs arising from higher demand are substantially higher than the potential administrative efficiencies of going to a centralized national health insurance system. So whenever proponents argue that eliminating private sector insurance profits and overhead would enable us to cover more people for less money, that conflicts with the findings of the study."

Congress has passed cuts to health-care providers that do not come to fruition. Most famously, the 1997 balanced-budget agreement between President Bill Clinton and the GOP-led Congress included cuts that Congress deferred for 17 years with an annual provision known as the "doc fix." It was finally eliminated under a deal Obama reached with Congress in 2015, or else providers would have faced a cut of 21 percent. Other efforts to control spending in Medicare, however, have fared better, including as part of the enactment of the Affordable Care Act.

In 2012, Blahous wrote a study questioning the budget assumptions in the ACA, such as the political prospects for a tax on "Cadillac" health plans. He turned out to be right: The tax keeps getting pushed off and weakened. Health-care costs did decline after the passage of the ACA, but whether that pre-dated the law or not is a subject of continuing debate.

For the record, Blahous says the Kochs had nothing to do with his research. "It's academic research, it goes through a blind review process, and it represents my own work," he said. "I choose my own research subjects and follow the facts where they lead. You'd have to ask someone else about where funding comes from, I don't follow that and it doesn't affect me."

We shared Blahous's concerns with Gillum's campaign, which confirmed that he relied on the Mercatus study, and received this response: "The Mayor's a proud supporter of Medicare-for-All and this study shows the potential for significant savings," said communications director Geoff Burgan. "It would be a strong improvement over the Republicans' attempts to destroy our current system and rip health care away from people."

In response to this fact check, Sanders's office provided links to several articles, including in The Washington Post, that reported that Blahous concluded that the Sanders plan would reduce national health expenditures by $2 trillion. Blahous said these articles are good examples of the misinterpretation of his research: "It's precisely because people have been saying that, that the correction is warranted."

Note: Regular readers know we often provide links to thoughtful critiques of our fact checks. Economist Dean Baker, who has written carefully about the cost implications of shifting to Medicare-for-all, thought we were a little heavy-handed on the Pinocchios. He noted, however, that "I can sympathize with Kessler's complaint that the Democrats aren't giving the full story." Other attacks, however, were misinformed or highly ideological, apparently because Medicare-for-all advocates were upset that our analysis undermined an effective talking point. The Fact Checker does not take policy positions but merely outlines the facts. Our analysis was confirmed by fact checks by FactCheck.org, PolitiFact, the Associated Press and CNN. Blahous, the author, also wrote a question-and-answer article that explains how advocates have twisted his research for ideological purposes.

The Pinocchio Test

We don't intend to pick on Gillum, who appears to have picked up a talking point that is circulating among Democrats. But we do want to lay down a marker because this goes too far.

All too often, politicians mischaracterize conclusions that are contained in academic or think tank studies. At the Fact Checker, we rely heavily on how a study's author says the data should be presented. In this case, it's clear that Blahous bent over backward to accept Sanders's assumptions, only to find they did not add up. Democrats cannot seize on one cherry-picked fact without acknowledging the broader implications of Blahous's research.

Three Pinocchios

EXHIBIT 4

Health Care System Performance Compared to Spending

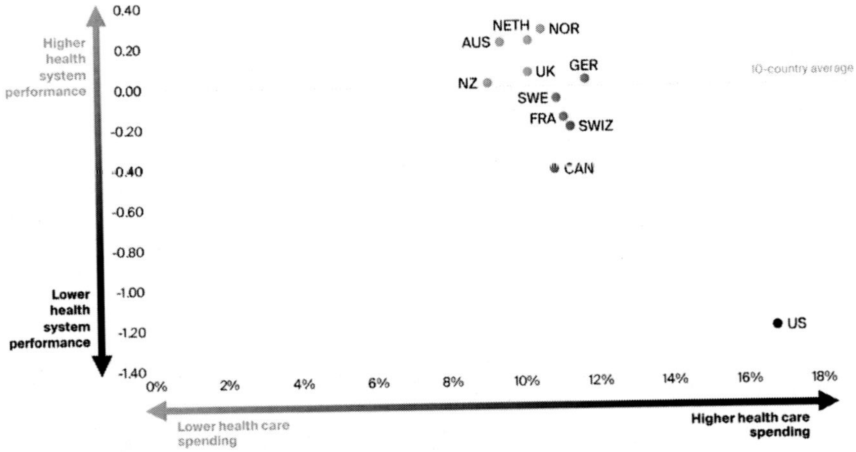

Note: Health care spending as a percent of GDP. Performance scores are based on standard deviation calculated from the 10-country average that excludes the US. See How We Conducted This Study for more detail.

Data: Spending data are from OECD for the year 2019 (updated in July 2021).

Source: Eric C. Schneider et al., *Mirror, Mirror 2021 – Reflecting Poorly: Health Care in the U.S. Compared to Other High-Income Countries* (Commonwealth Fund, Aug. 2021). https://doi.org/10.26099/01DV-H208

Chapter 2

Medicare Forever: Protecting Seniors by Making the Wealthy Pay Their Fair Share*

Committee on the Budget

Wednesday, September 27, 2023
Committee on the Budget,
U.S. Senate,
Washington, DC.

The hearing was convened, pursuant to notice, at 10:02 a.m., in the Dirksen Senate Office Building, Hon. Sheldon Whitehouse, Chairman of the Committee, presiding.

Present: Senators Whitehouse, Wyden, Kaine, Van Hollen, Padilla, Grassley, Johnson, Braun, and R. Scott.

Also present: Democratic staff: Dan Dudis, Majority Staff Director; Dan RuBoss, Senior Tax and Economic Advisor and Member Outreach Director; Sion Bell, Tax Policy Advisor; Anirudh Srirangam, Healthcare Policy Advisor.

Republican staff: Chris Conlin, Deputy Staff Director; Krisann Pearce, General Counsel; Nic Pottebaum, Professional Staff Member; Nick Wyatt, Professional Staff Member.

Witnesses:

The Honorable Marilyn Moon, Visiting Scholar Center for Medicare Advocacy, and Former Public Trustee of the Medicare and Social Security Trust Funds

---

* This is an edited, reformatted and augmented version of Hearing before the Committee on the Budget, United States Senate, One Hundred Eighteenth Congress, First Session, Publication No. S. HRG. 118–148, dated September 27, 2023.

In: A Healthier Tomorrow
Editor: Robert M. Deaton
ISBN: 979-8-89530-798-4

Ms. Chye-Ching Huang, Executive Director, Tax Law Center, New York University School of Law

Mr. James C. Capretta, Senior Fellow and Milton Friedman Chair, American Enterprise Institute

Opening Statement of Chairman Whitehouse[1]

Chairman WHITEHOUSE. Good morning. The hearing of the Budget Committee will come to order. I welcome our witnesses. I thank our ranking member. I welcome the members in attendance. Ranking Member Grassley and members of the committee, today's hearing is about guaranteeing Medicare's solvency, a good thing to do, by balancing the tax system so that it is less rigged and more fair. Another good thing to do.

So two good things. In July, the Budget Committee held a hearing on protecting social security by taking away tax tricks that let those at the top pay lower tax rates than teachers and firefighters. Today we turn to Medicare, our other pillar of American retirement security, whose insolvency is predicted to arrive sooner than social securities.

Right now, a government shutdown looms because house Republicans are once again trying to make the tax system even less fair to give more freebies to big business and billionaires. Republicans over there want to maintain the massive exemption for inheritances to wealthy heirs.

They want to keep tax breaks from multinational corporations that send their profits and jobs offshore, and they want to hamstring the Internal Revenue Service (IRS) from catching wealthy tax sheets. Nobody likes these policies, so they have to hold our government operations hostage.

It will cost billions and add to the deficit if they succeed at shutting the government down. At the end of the day their point is taking care of the billionaires in big corporations, the rest is smoke and mirrors. Any serious conversation about Federal spending and deficits must also include Medicare.

According to Congressional Budget Office (CBO), Medicare, along with Social Security, will make up more than half of spending growth over the next decade as America's population ages. And without new revenue, Medicare will cover less than 90% of scheduled benefits beginning as soon as 2031, only 8 years away.

---

[1] Prepared statement of Chairman Whitehouse appears on page 33.

Since its inception, Medicare has ensured that our nation's seniors do not become impoverished due to illness. As a result, older Americans live longer, live better quality lives, and get better care in the healthcare system. Today, nearly 80% of Americans either receive direct support from Medicare or have a family member or close friend enrolled in the program.

Almost every senior in this country will receive Medicare benefits which they have earned throughout their working lives and which let them retire in health and dignity. Rhode Island seniors understand the importance of Medicare on their quality of life. Joyce from Pawtucket said, "Medicare is a lifeline for me.

Reducing benefits would cause me to neglect medical problems, and I would actually end up in the hospital." Lisa from West Warwick said, "Without Medicare, I would exhaust my finances and go without care and medicines." And Anna from Providence said, "Medicare helps me in countless ways.

It helps pay for my wheelchair, shower chair, lift to get in and out of bed, doctor's visits and medicine among other things. All of these are essential and enable me to continue living my life." But for decades, some Republicans worked publicly to undermine Medicare. To have Medicare as former speaker of the House, Newt Gingrich put it; wither on the vine.

They proposed raising the Medicare eligibility age, turning Medicare to a private voucher program, and even sun setting Medicare altogether, then came the State of the Union address earlier this year when Republicans and Democrats together gave President Biden a standing ovation when he declared that cuts to social security and Medicare would be off the table.

That bipartisan consensus if it was real and not more smoke and mirrors leaves only one option, raise revenue. And we can raise revenue by unrigging our tax code. We can close loopholes that allow the super wealthy to avoid taxes. It would be good to level the playing field so the wealthiest in this country can't play by a special set of rules and avoid paying a fair share.

We can and must protect Medicare. We can and must do so without cutting benefits. And we can do that by making our tax code fairer. Win, win, win. According to the Centers for Medicare and Medicaid Services (CMS) chief actuary, the authority on Medicare solvency, my Medicare and Social Security Fair Share Act would ensure Medicare remains solvent effectively forever.

And we heard at our social security hearing that my legislation would also extend Social Security solvency indefinitely. As I told my Republican colleagues at our social security hearing, I'm more than happy to welcome serious proposals to protect Social security and Medicare without cutting benefits.

I've spent enough time in the Senate to know the difference between freewheeling chat and actual proposals. Actual proposals are what lead to actual agreements. So feel free to join in with an actual proposal. My proposal ensures Medicare solvency forever. It does so by unrigging a rigged tax system so those who can most afford to pay don't play by a different set of rules.

It is available for everyone to see and debate. We face simple arithmetic, raise revenue, or cut benefits. Those are the options if we are to preserve Medicare. If we abide by what seemed like a bipartisan commitment not to cut benefits, we must safeguard Medicare by raising revenue. It is literally life and death for millions of older Americans. Senator Grassley.

Opening Statement of Senator Grassley[2]

Senator GRASSLEY. Thank you for holding this very important hearing because we all recognize that Medicare as well as social security are very much a part of the social fabric of America. And they may be government programs, but they also interact with the private sector retirement and health benefits as well.

So it is not something that just government does, but private sector, retirement and healthcare programs plan on interacting with it. Republicans want to preserve and strengthen this program for future generations. For decades Medicare has provided seniors and those with disabilities access to routine and life-saving care at their local hospital, doctor's office, and pharmacy.

As then chairman of the Finance Committee, I'm proud to have led the effort in 2003 to modernize Medicare by establishing a prescription drug benefit. That effort required bipartisan cooperation from both chambers and presidential leadership.

In the first decade of Medicare Part D, the Federal government spent 36% less than CBO projected, while still improving access to prescription drugs for millions of seniors. That law also requires the Medicare trustees to review Medicare's finances annually.

For the past seven years, Medicare trustees have issued a funding warning because Medicare's outlays are expected to exceed its dedicated revenue by

---

[2] Prepared statement of Senator Grassley appears in the appendix on page 35.

45%. Medicare's hospital insurance trust fund is also in poor shape. Both CBO and the Medicare trustees expect it to be insolvent in about 10 years.

Upon insolvency and absent congressional action, Medicare Part A providers will see an 11% cut in reimbursements. We should be moving our healthcare system from volume to value, but we need to accurately account for what's working and not working.

As I stated at our Social Security hearing, the only way to make these critical programs sustainable is to follow the Ronald Reagan, Tip O'Neal model of 1983. And just as an aside, remembering some of the things you said in your opening statement, that would include more than just tax increases, that would include more than people putting proposals on the table as you're asking us to do, because I think they sat down at a table with nothing on it because they wanted everything to be negotiable.

And it ended up tax increases, it ended up changes in formula, it ended up changes in retirement age. And I suppose they thought they were going to save Social Security for 20 years, but as we see now, they saved it for 50 years.

And it is that bipartisanship that come between a Democrat speaker and a Republican president that we just can't let Social security fail, that led to their success. But everything being on the table, it wasn't a Republicans putting something out, Democrats putting something out because that gives people opportunity to shoot at things. So we've got to work in a bipartisan fashion and keep a range of options on the table. Unfortunately, anytime Republicans mention Medicare being in trouble, Democrats accuse us of trying to blow up the program. And blowing up the program is a pretty rich statement.

Considering Democrats have proposed and enacted major cuts to Medicare, often using the program as a piggy bank to pay for unrelated spending. Obamacare cut Medicare, including an annual 1% reduction in provider payments. I don't know whether we Republicans accuse you of cutting Medicare or not, but we could have, like we get accused of proposals we put forward.

Democrats have proposed cuts to Medicare advantage, which ignores the choice and competition these plans often offer consumers. On top of these Medicare cuts, the so-called Inflation Reduction Act passed only by Democrats and President Biden stole budget savings from Medicare to subsidize green energy tax credits.

Most of these democrat tax benefits will go to wealthier taxpayers. And let's not forget proposals like Medicare for all that would cost $30 to $40 trillion in the first 10 years, more than twice what Medicare costs today. Under this plan, hospitals would see a 16% reduction in revenue resulting in closures and reduced access to care.

Then there is President Biden's latest budget, which kicks the can down the road on Medicare, it for goes real solutions in favor of accounting gimmicks, massive tax hikes and price controls that will reduce access to lifesaving drugs and treatments.

The proposal currently touted by the Chairman would push the top marginal tax rates above 50%, impose a 37.4 percent top rate on capital gains. We don't talk much about the consequences of those policy decisions, but the CMS actuary concluded the proposal would address Medicare's long-term solvency, but with the caveat that he couldn't, "Independently assess the reasonability of the revenue estimates for the stated provisions." Based on an analysis of the proposal by Tax Foundation, which I ask unanimous consent to put in the record.[3]

Chairman WHITEHOUSE. Without objection.

Senator GRASSLEY. The chairmans proposed capital gains tax hike is a revenue loser. Moreover, the tax hikes as a whole will cost about 700,000 jobs. These tax hikes won't just hit high incomes Americans. While proponents claim only the top 2% will be affected, the proposed income thresholds not being indexed for inflation has a much broader effect than just the top 2%. As a result, the Social Security chief actuary estimates that up to 25% of the households will be captured by the end of the projection period. The truth is, taxes on the rich alone won't save Medicare for Children and grandchildren.

If Democrats believe otherwise, then request CBO and joint Committee on Taxation, analyze the proposals. So I think we'd like to have a more widespread investigation of these facts. Before you saw that, I was through with my remarks, but I wanted to just point out something that I gave a couple weeks ago on a speech on the floor of the Senate, and this won't take me maybe just a couple minutes. It is obvious that our healthcare system in the United States needs reform and accountability.

However, we shouldn't ruin it by turning it into a government run healthcare system. Whether you want to call it Medicare for all, single payer, or socialized medicine. I referred in my speech then to a Wall Street Journal article highlighting the failures of some government run programs. They wrote this about Great Britain.

---

[3] Statement submitted by Senator Grassley appears in the appendix on page 102.

"Now the state funded service is falling apart. People who suffer heart attacks or strokes wait more than one and a half hours on average for an ambulance. Hospitals are so full, they're turning patients away.

A record seven and one-tenth million people in England, more than one in 10, are stuck on waiting lists for non-emergency hospital treatment like hip treatment."

The article went on to say, "Delays in treating people are causing premature deaths of 300 to 500 people a week. And 1 in 5 British people were waiting for medical appointment or treatment at the National Health Service in December." If you could find—if you didn't find that alarming, I said, on the floor of the Senate, in May, British Columbia announced that they were sending cancer patients to Bellingham, Washington in the United States for treatment.

A Canadian news outlet wrote that health minister Adrian Dix announced, "That eligible breasts and prostate cancer patients will be sent to one of the two clinics in Bellingham for radiation treatment. The unprecedented move to send thousands of British Columbia patients to the United States (US) over the next 2 years is an attempt to address the backlog that the British Columbia has in one of the longest waits for radiation treatment in Canada."

Canada is taking this action because it's cancer patients face unacceptable waiting lines. When I read about Bellingham, it reminded me this, in the years that I've been fighting doctor owned hospitals, not having special treatment and not having, conflicts of interest and all that.

I used as one of my examples that there was a text in the hospital that said, if you have an emergency, call 911, that was posted in that hospital. So here we have British Columbia posting it in hospitals. If you need emergency action, go to Bellingham. And I think it is a crime that we would be thinking of things like that in America. Thank you for listening to me.

Chairman WHITEHOUSE. I'm always glad to listen to you. And I would simply say that I don't think we have to look as far as either British Columbia or across the Atlantic for models of how to do healthcare reform. I think the accountable care organizations from the Obamacare bill, I think the Center for Medicare and Medicaid Innovation (CMMI) work that is going on, we have really exemplary Accountable Care Organization (ACO) operating in Rhode Island.

I suspect you have some very good ones in Iowa as well. And I think they can lead a transition to patient-centered care and away from the fee for service treadmill that we have seen, improve the quality of care and lower the cost per patient. So I think there are good bipartisan ways to proceed and I look forward to working with my ranking member.

With that, our first witness is Dr. Marilyn Moon, a visiting scholar at the Center for Medicare Advocacy. She is an expert on healthcare financing and delivery with a particular emphasis on Medicare. She previously served as chair of the Maryland Healthcare Commission at the Congressional Budget Office and as a public trustee for the Social Security and Medicare Trust funds. She is a member of the National Academy of Medicine and is on the board of the Medicare right center. After she has made her statement, we will hear from Ms. Chye-Ching Huang, who is executive director of the Tax Law Center at the New York University School of Law.

Before starting the Tax Law Center, Ms. Huang was senior director of economic policy for the Center on Budget and Policy Priorities, where she worked on the analysis and design of a wide range of Federal tax, fiscal, and economic policy proposals in collaboration with tax, academics, practitioners, analysts and advocates.

We're also joined by Mr. James Capretta, a senior fellow and Milton Friedman chair at the American Enterprise Institute. He has also served as a senior advisor to the Bipartisan Policy Center and previously served as an associate director at the Office of Management Budget and senior analyst for the Senate Budget Committee and House Ways and Means Committee.

I welcome you all. Your full testimony will be made a matter of record. So if you could confine yourself to the five minutes for your opening statements, I'd be grateful. And then we'll have a chance for the members to ask questions. Ms. Moon, you may proceed.

Statement of the Honorable Marilyn Moon, Visiting Scholar Center for Medicare Advocacy, and Former Public Trustee of the Medicare and Social Security Trust Fund[4]

Dr. MOON. Thank you. Medicare represents one of our most successful Federal programs, helping seniors and persons with disabilities afford mainstream medical care. Sustaining it over time deserves careful attention to protect the valuable services it provides. Since Medicare's inception, life

[4] Prepared statement of Hon. Moon appears in the appendix on page 41.

expectancy at age 65 has risen by over 19 years as people have achieved access to life-saving care.

And Medicare has substantially held down the cost of what people would otherwise pay for this care. Medicare spending per capita was over $15,700 in 2022, an amount that totals 53% of the median income of persons 65 and older. Low and moderate income persons would never be able to afford the type of mainstream care that they enjoy today, if not for Medicare.

While the increase in cost of the program is often cited with alarm, in many ways, these costs signal Medicare's substantial success. Americans are living longer and receiving better care. Seeking ways to make the program function better and adopting new approaches to provide good care at lower cost certainly needs to be part of any discussion of Medicare's future. However, while substantial cost cutting over the last 30 years has meant that Medicare has grown at a slower pace than private health insurance, this cost cutting also means that Medicare has lagged behind coverage to many working Americans.

Medicare is not an overly generous program, and the substantial costs of healthcare not covered by Medicare remain daunting for many. Further limitations on coverage or reductions in provider payments could leave even more beneficiaries at risk. And policy debates should keep this in mind.

Indeed, there are strong arguments to be made for increasing benefits. Proposals to further cut benefits via increased premiums or cost sharing would exacerbate the inadequacy of the program. And premium support proposals and raising the age of eligibility are efforts at cost cutting that sometimes seem more benign, but can result in substantial increases in burdens on beneficiaries and increases in inequality and problems with access to care.

Thus, rather than focusing on further belt tightening as the means for keeping Medicare financially strong, it is important to consider additional sources of financing. Premiums and cost sharing, and the impact of taxes that finance Medicare mean that many older and disabled Americans are already paying substantial shares of their incomes for the cost of their care.

First, consider how much individuals pay out of pocket. A new study has found that it is over $6,500—substantially higher than what non-Medicare beneficiaries pay and a substantial share of the resources of moderate income beneficiaries.

In addition, the common view of Medicare is that younger taxpayers fund most of the program resulting in intergenerational burdens, but in fact, beneficiaries also contribute substantially to the taxes that fund the program. And these contributions have been growing over time.

After many years of Americans retiring early, more people now work past the age of 65 and contribute more to both income and payroll taxes. And the share of these taxes paid by persons over age 65 have increased. Seniors now pay about one-third of the income and tax revenues that go into financing Medicare.

And if premiums and copays are included, seniors are responsible for 41% of the costs of the Medicare program. To ensure stable future financing for Medicare, payroll taxes and personal income taxes likely need to be increased. For example, some approaches would include expanding personal income tax revenues to funding for part A.

Among these options, explicitly targeting those with higher incomes for revenue increases would better protect modest Medicare beneficiaries. For example, the Biden administration has proposed raising the rate that higher income persons now must pay under current law to 5% on those with incomes above $400,000.

Expanded contributions from those with higher incomes can be justified on a number of grounds, although the cap on wages subject to tax was eliminated a number of years ago, burdens on higher income individuals are still substantially smaller than on middle income taxpayers because higher income people receive a much greater share of their incomes from sources other than wages and salaries.

A commitment to maintaining Medicare over time deserves nothing less than taking a serious look at financing issues. Thank you.

Chairman WHITEHOUSE. Thank you very much, Dr. Moon. Ms. Huang, please proceed.

Statement of Chye-Ching Huang, Executive Director, Tax Law Center, New York University School of Law[5]

Ms. HUANG. Chairman Whitehouse, Ranking Member Grassley, and distinguished members of the committee, I'm honored to join you today. The tax base is the foundation for the Federal budget and it supports the nation's priorities like social security, defense, education, and healthcare, including Medicare.

---

[5] Prepared statement of Ms. Huang appears in the appendix on page 50.

But our Federal tax base isn't broad enough to ensure the most solid financial footing for Medicare and other national priorities for generations to come. Some income from vast fortunes is completely carved out of the Federal income tax base and goes untaxed over decades, lifetimes, or generations.

Large multinationals can still report profits offshore so that they're subject to little or no US tax. And a raft of other loopholes and preferences shrink the tax base and attract tax avoidance and evasion instead of productive investment innovation and work.

An example that directly hurts Medicare and the other trust funds is that gaps in the Medicare taxes mean that some high income business owners don't have to pay into the system in the same way that workers and other business owners do, but they can instead avoid hundreds of billions in taxes.

The tax base is also weakened by a stark Federal tax gap. More than half a trillion dollars of taxes owed under the law just aren't paid each year. So don't contribute to important national programs. And some $100 billion of that amount should have been paid directly into the Medicare social security and Unemployment Insurance (UI) trust funds, but wasn't.

So while I just mentioned that some business owners take advantages of loopholes in the law to avoid owing any Medicare taxes, other filers are just not paying the taxes that the law says that they do owe.

Sometimes that can be because filers try to undertake aggressive but lawful tax avoidance and in doing so, step over the boundary into unlawful tax evasion. So for example, the IRS has been taking a really close look at certain hedge fund owners and private equity managers and other wealthy business owners that they say have been unlawfully underpaying hundreds of millions of dollars in self-employment contributions each.

So where do we start to broaden the Federal tax base and shrink the tax gap? Here are three ways. The first is by rejecting proposals that are on the table right now, but would increase tax cheating and shrink the tax base. That means maintaining IRS discretionary and mandatory funding. Cutting the IRS budget even more deeply than agreed to in the debt ceiling deal would hurt deficits, hurt honest filers, and benefit tax cheats. It also means rejecting proposals to weaken new information reporting tools that help the IRS find and focus on tax evasion. And it means building on rather than reversing the corporate base broadening that was enacted in 2017.

For example, the stronger limit on interest deductions claimed by large businesses should be retained. It helps reduce the tax systems tilt towards debt financing. But if law makers do choose to weaken some of the 2017 laws based broadens, the cost should be offset with tax increases on corporations. Second, lawmakers can address the three big areas of the tax base that need attention.

Income from large fortunes that never gets taxed, tax subsidies on multinationals foreign profits, and the complex and patchy taxation of pass through entities. A really good example of a priority in that pass through entity area is closing those loopholes in the Medicare taxes and sending the revenues directly to the trust funds. Third, lawmakers can choose from a broad menu of other options, large and small to broaden the tax base.

One would be further strengthening the Bipartisan Corporate Transparency Act that I know many members on this committee helped to lead and secure. Stopping cryptocurrency traders from gaming the timing of their tax losses, and reducing tax compliance—tax non-compliance in the market for expensive art.

The Tax Law Center has proposed or analyzed several dozen options to broaden the tax base. And they are linked too in my testimony. Law makers of both parties, including members of this committee, have often looked to base broadening as an economically sound way to raise revenues and improve the fairness and integrity of the tax system. And there continue to be really good options in this space. Lawmakers can choose the revenues to use the revenues to protect Medicare and other Federal priorities from cuts that would cause families hardship, to reduce long-term deficits and to make new investments that would raise health and living standards and help build an economy that is dynamic, inclusive, and resilient. I would be so happy to take your questions.

Chairman WHITEHOUSE. Thank you very much Ms. Huang. And now Mr. Capretta the floor is yours.

Statement of James C. Capretta, Senior Fellow and Milton Friedman Chair, American Enterprise Institute[6]

Mr. CAPRETTA. Thank you, Mr. Chairman. Thank you Ranking Member Grassley and other members of the Committee. I'm very pleased to be here to have this conversation with you today. The headline focus of today's session is the impending depletion in the Medicare Hospital Insurance Trust Fund. Given the potential harm that exhaustion might cause, that is of course, a very important matter for Congress to take up as soon as possible.

---

6 Prepared statement of Mr. Capretta appears in the appendix on page 67.

But the imbalance between Hospital Insurance (HI) spending and outgo is actually a manifestation of a larger problem, which is the widening gap between Medicare's total costs for both HI and supplementary medical insurance to pay for both trust funds expenses.

As I show in my testimony in Figure 1, data for all of Medicare's costs and receipts from the 2023 trustees reports shown as a percentage of gross domestic product show that there is a rapid growth in spending across the years. In 1990, total program spending equaled 1.9% of Gross Domestic Product (GDP), three decades later it had reached 4% of GDP.

And the Medicare trustees expect it will reach 4.9% of GDP in 2030 and 6% in 2050. Related to this is the very large increase in general fund transfers to Medicare over time. These are the amounts that come out of the general fund of the Treasury uncapped, and really unregulated in any way that go into the SMI trust fund to cover any expenses not covered by premiums.

This is not a well-known part of the program, but it is very important. Over the next 10 years alone, $6.6 trillion will come from the General Fund of the Treasury into Medicare. By 2050. The annual transfer will equal 2.8% of GDP up from 0.5% in 1990. So that shows you how much growth there has been in this part.

For Medicare, the trend is what is most alarming. Going forward as population ages the unfunded liabilities of Medicare measured— in this context measured as any spending above and beyond the taxes and premiums collected. The Treasury Department does a calculation of this every year. It's now at about $52 trillion over the infinite horizon.

Okay. It is a big number. But I think the thing to focus on is it is gone up a lot even in the last 7 years. It is when—2016 it was $20 trillion less. So this number of sort of trying to assess where we're going with Medicare keeps worsening and worsening and worsening over time. And it is related to, obviously a lot of it has to do with population aging.

So there is a big challenge ahead. Just real one last point on the big picture here. This is all wrapped up in a fiscal challenge that continues to worsen very rapidly and really does deserve the attention of the Congress in the near term. Right now the deficit is scheduled to be close to $2 trillion this year.

By 2050, just to put this in context, in 1980, let me go back in time. Spending on Social Security and Medicare were 5.5% of GDP in total. In 2050 they're scheduled to be 13.1% of GDP. So there is just been a fundamental transformation of our fiscal situation associated largely with this. And of course, CBO projects that by 2050 mostly related to this question, Federal debt is on track to go to 170% of GDP.

So, you know, there is some big things ahead if some corrections aren't put in place. Now—what—what I recommend, I have seven, I'm going to go through them real quick in my last minute. First, I would very much recommend that this be both a revenue and a spending side of the equation discussion.

And that it be bipartisan that that will bring more stability to the program over the long term if there is wide agreement about how to finance the program and try to make it as efficient as possible. Second, I would try to move toward a single insurance benefit instead of the fragmented benefit we have today. Today we have A, B, and D.

It'd be better if you designed a single insurance benefit going forward, much like people experience in the non-Medicare market. I'd improve this choice structure for the beneficiary. So it is much clearer what they're picking when they sign up for their various coverage options. Today, it is a very confused and fragmented choice structure that is been set up for them. They often have to rely on brokers. I promote premium competition between the private side of Medicare and Managed Medical Assistance (MMA) plans and the traditional program, and also competition amongst the providers in terms of the prices they're charging.

Last two quickly, Mr. Chairman, I would reform the trust funds so that they are reflective of the combined program. Instead of having an A and B side that can add to confusion about the financing. And finally, I'd build in some automatic adjustments so that once you make a deal that deal sticks over time through other adjustments that might be necessary to keep it always permanently stable. Thank you.

Chairman WHITEHOUSE. Thanks Mr. Capretta. Ms. Huang, you mentioned in your testimony that for instance, private equity managers can avoid paying into Medicare by structuring their income. How do they do that? What is the trick?

Ms. HUANG. Yeah. So I mean, I think it is really important that the vast majority of Americans do in fact contribute to Medicare by taxes, either on in—on income from their work or from their businesses. And the problem is that some of these wealthy filers can avoid those taxes just by using a loophole that exempts income made from various types of pass through entities used to own businesses.

And those are entities of the sort that certain hedge fund and private equity managers use that invites hundreds of billions of dollars of wasteful tax avoidance. And as I mentioned, some of that tax avoidance gets so aggressive that it arguably becomes tax evasion, because people are just not paying what they're lawfully supposed to.

Chairman WHITEHOUSE. It is a fairly expensive proposition to set up all those pass through entities to enable that. So presumably we're talking about very high income people who embark on this strategy?

Ms. HUANG. Indeed. And—and I—I think the estimates are that closing this loophole would raise more than $300 billion and some 85% of that would come from people with incomes above a million dollars a year.

Chairman WHITEHOUSE. Mr. Capretta, you mentioned, the need to revisit the taxes used to pay for Medicare and the need for new revenue. On the revenue side, what would you recommend? Your mic.

Mr. CAPRETTA. I have a little bit of a historical perspective on this, which is that when Medicare was created, it was in a sense an addendum to social security with a payroll tax. And the—the idea was that this was going to be, in a sense, contributions from workers at least partially paying for Medicare through their payroll tax contributions. I think breaking from that entirely and having a very different revenue stream into Medicare is possible. I'm not ruling it out.

Chairman WHITEHOUSE. What—what would you recommend, though? My time is short, so I'm trying to get——

Mr. CAPRETTA. I'd recommend———

Chairman WHITEHOUSE [continuing]. If you've got a recommendation.

Mr. CAPRETTA. I'd recommend a straight increase in the payroll tax, which would generate a fair—a fair amount of revenue.

Chairman WHITEHOUSE. And how about the people who are dodging the payroll tax through mechanisms like Ms. Huang just described. Should we reach out to them?

Mr. CAPRETTA. I'm not against—I'm not against closing——

Chairman WHITEHOUSE. You're not here to defend that behavior?

Mr. CAPRETTA [continuing]. Loopholes. I'm not against changing.

I think some of that to address income inequality might be best addressed outside of Medicare, but I'm not against any reasonable way to look at making sure the tax base is fair.

Chairman WHITEHOUSE. So you also have nice things to say about ACOs, accountable care organizations. Indeed, you recommend them as a new coverage option. I'm a big fan of ACOs because I've seen them succeed spectacularly in Rhode Island, reducing costs, sending millions of dollars back to Medicare and causing somewhere between relief and joy through the patient population because of the new services that are enabled when doctors are freed from the fee for service treadmill. But what are your reasons?

Mr. CAPRETTA. Very similar to yours. I would say that Medicare would benefit greatly from a provider run managed care plan option.

Chairman WHITEHOUSE. Yeah.

Mr. CAPRETTA. That there is sort of a distrust sometimes with insurance led managed care and a provider led managed care option that was robust and people could opt into and not just be placed in, I think would be a benefit to the program.

Chairman WHITEHOUSE. Yeah. And our experience for what it is worth in Rhode Island has been that what's really worked has been when a primary care provider group does this on its own. The more different influences you add, the more it slows down and bogs down. But some of our best primary care providers chose early on to go this route, and they really have made—made us very proud.

Let me put it that way. Dr. Moon, let's just say we don't get this squared away. We don't do something bipartisan. We don't do something that lowers costs and raises revenues, and we hit the 11% hit to the system from the predicted cash crunch. What does that look like to a senior?

Dr. MOON. I think it looks like pretty much like disaster to a senior. A large number of moderate income seniors whose incomes are between, say, 200% and 400% of poverty simply would do without a lot of care because they could not afford additional costs that they would have to incur.

The other problem is who would be providing the services if there were big cuts in payments to providers? More people might opt out of the system who are providers of care. One of the benefits of Medicare over time has been that almost all doctors and hospitals participate in the program making it assured that people will get mainstream care when they need it. And that is something I think we do not want to even contemplate putting at risk.

Chairman WHITEHOUSE. Thanks very much. Senator Grassley.

Senator GRASSLEY. Thank you.

Chairman WHITEHOUSE. And then just for everybody's awareness, the order after Senator Grassley is Senator Padilla, Senator Johnson, Chairman Wyden, and Senator Scott.

Senator GRASSLEY. Mr. Capretta I mentioned in my opening comments, and I think the Chairman agrees that this has to be done in a bipartisan fashion. And with a whole range of options on the table. Too often Democrats claim that Republicans want to cut Medicare every time we mention the troubles facing the program.

So Mr. Capretta Democrats have a record of proposing and enacting Medicare cuts. I've already mentioned some in my statement. I'd like to have you elaborate if you agree with my statement.

Mr. CAPRETTA. Well, both parties, I would say, have sometimes put Medicare changes on the table. They have reduced spending. You can call them cuts of course. And, you know, in the Affordable Care Act (ACA) there—there was a very substantial change in particularly for inpatient hospital services, something called a productivity adjustment factor.

Which is still in place and permanent and has a very large cumulative effect on spending. So I think many people view it as a good thing because it is brought down hospital spending quite a bit. The question is, is it sustainable over the long run?

We're relying very heavily on it to keep the numbers down, but it may—the actuaries are always warning that it might be overdone.

Senator GRASSLEY. Under Medicare for all Mr. Capretta, what happens to provider reimbursement rates and how would that affect care, particularly in rural America?

Mr. CAPRETTA. Well, Medicare for all, I think needs to be viewed for through a political economy lens. How does it get managed over time? You know, and it is very easy to, when you're facing a budget crunch, just to pay people less. And of course, when you pay providers less, eventually there is supply changes.

That means fewer providers actually provide the services at the lower rates. That is how you end up with queuing problems. So I do think that our multi-payer system, much as we dislike many aspects of it, keeps open revenue streams that makes it so that providers are not dependent on any one player to make sure they can serve patients. And so I think we—we shouldn't move away from that.

Senator GRASSLEY. We always hear this business about raising taxes on the rich. During President Obama's tenure, rich was arbitrarily defined at $200,000. So as part of Obamacare, Democrats enacted three and eight-tenths percent net investment tax on—at these thresholds, but didn't index them. Knowing it would eventually hit middle income taxpayers.

Since its enactment, the number of taxpayers hit by this money grab have more than doubled from 3 million to 7 million. Now they're proposing to quadruple the tax and claim it'll only apply to 2% of the taxpayers. So you can understand why I'm skeptical about that statement. Mr. Capretta, much like three and eight-tens percent tax enacted on Obamacare, wouldn't the number of taxpayers affected by this supercharged tax increase over time capturing more than 2% of the taxpayers?

Mr. CAPRETTA. If you don't index the income threshold upon which a tax is applied of co—over time, the nominal value—the real value of those thresholds, of course erode due to inflation. So we've had bracket creep the—in the past in our tax system, and it is sometimes it is sustainable and sometimes not, depending on what is going on. There usually is eventually some pushback on it.

Senator GRASSLEY. Yeah. President Biden's Medicare proposal and President Obama's Affordable Care Act both double counted Medicare revenue. So Mr. Capretta, these are obviously underhanded gimmicks in the budget. How does this impact Federal deficits and debt?

Mr. CAPRETTA. Well, I—I do think this is an under-reported phenomenon, which is when you include on the Pay As You Go (PAYGO) scorecard, Medicare savings and HI in particular, you can end up double counting it. It can make the solvency of Medicare improve, which allows higher payments for Medicare down the road.

And it also could be used to finance another bill, you know, through the PAYGO scorecard. So I think there—what we should try to avoid when we're working on Medicare solvency is taking credit for it on both sides of the budget. Especially, you know, a lot of times it is not big enough to make a real big difference, but Medicare's big. And so when you put a lot more money into Medicare and then also claim you can spend it under PAYGO for something else, that is when you end up with a problem.

Senator GRASSLEY. Thank you, Mr. Chairman.

Chairman WHITEHOUSE. Thank you. Senator Grassley. Senator Padilla, followed by Senator Johnson.

Statement of Senator Padilla

Senator PADILLA. Thank you, Mr. Chair. Just want to remind us that during last week's hearing, several of our colleagues discussed the impact of the American Rescue Plans expanded child tax credit. It was nothing short of striking that the national child poverty rate hit a record low of 5.2% in 2021.

And that included a decline in the rate of Hispanic children from 14.7% in 2020 to 8.4% in 2021. That is something I think we're all proud of, both sides of the aisle. Recent census data shows however, that many of these families stood back into poverty upon the expiration of the expanded child tax credit.

Now I can't help but notice that a lot of the Republican proposals for spending suggest delaying or reducing benefits that have been earned and are meant to be retirement security for older Americans. The poverty rate amongst US seniors 65 and older is already nearly doubled that of the Organisation for Economic Co-operation and Development (OECD) average in just three countries have worse income inequality among this age group.

Question for Dr. Moon. What are the expected impacts of these proposals to cut Medicare on senior poverty rates and inequality?

Dr. MOON. Thank you. I think that the important thing to keep in mind here is that older and disabled Americans are like all the rest of the population. That is, there are some who have very modest incomes and some who have much more substantial incomes.

But the number of seniors who rely upon Medicare and Social Security to a massive degree, is much higher than many people appreciate. And for those with moderate incomes not very far above the poverty level, because our low income protections for seniors are not that generous, this is a real potential burden.

They're already paying a substantial amount, often more than a quarter of their incomes for their healthcare costs, for example. And further cuts in the Medicare program or further requirements for them to pay more would have a substantial impact.

It doesn't always show up in terms of the formal poverty rates because we base that on—on income and not on Medicare. But people who look at the in-kind contributions that are made in alternative measures would often note with alarm what would happen, if you were to, for example reduce spending on Medicare.

Senator PADILLA. Thank you. Now, unsurprisingly, a lot of our Republican colleagues are focusing on cuts, cuts, cuts across the board. And the budget in Medicare is no different. Focusing on cuts to benefits, cut—cuts to coverage and cuts to access. When I believe what we should be discussing is ways to preserve and build on Medicare's many successes.

Now, efforts to strengthen Medicare and save on costs don't have to be mutually exclusive. For example, the Collaborative Care models is an evidence based and cost-effective strategy for treating common behavioral health problems in primary care that remains underutilized. About 1 in 4 Medicare beneficiaries live with mental illness.

I mean, that is the population at large. But only 40% to 50% receive treatment. It is also more pervasive in beneficiaries from American Indian, Alaska, Native, and Hispanic communities. Now, the President's fiscal year 24 budget laid out a plan to extend the life of the Medicare Trust Fund, while also lowering costs for mental health services.

And specifically, it eliminated cost sharing for some mental and behavioral health visits and required parody between physical health and mental health coverage under Medicare. We knew mental health was a crisis before the pandemic.

It is only been exacerbated and spotlighted by the pandemic. And since Dr. Moon, how have these cost cutting debates influenced the scope of Medicare coverage, including for mental health services?

Dr. MOON. I think that mental health is a good example, like a number of other benefits that have often been underappreciated. Home health was one of them for a long time. Hospice care is another example. And often in a zeal to cut costs, the notion is if we expand the services that are offered there will suddenly be abuse and costs will go up.

Rather than thinking about what the appropriate way to provide care is. I think that reforms that are aimed at improving the quality of care by making it the right care at the right time always makes sense and should always be an effort.

And I think mental health would be one of those things. What you want to be very careful about is not doing—assuming that there are cost cutting that is less careful in terms of protecting the things that need to be protected.

Senator PADILLA. Yeah. Thank you. And if I heard you let me sort of rephrase for the folks back home, just as with physical health treating mental health in emergency room settings is not the most cost effective approach.

Dr. MOON. I totally agree with that.

Senator PADILLA. Thank you, Mr. Chair.

Chairman WHITEHOUSE. Thank you Senator Padilla. Senator Johnson.

Statement of Senator Johnson

Senator JOHNSON. Hey, Mr. Chairman. Had I not read my schedule, I would've thought maybe this hearing would've been titled Our Broken Tax System. Which by the way, anytime we have the Chairman of the Finance

Committee, anytime you two want to sit down and work to simplify and rationalize our horribly complex and broken tax system, I'm—I'm all in.

But this is hearing on Medicare and unfortunately, you know, I think Mr.—the—the Chairman and so many Democrats are pretty much one trick ponies. Whether the social security, whether it is Medicare, the only solution is increasing taxes. Which again, I don't think we ever generate the revenue by increasing taxes because it harms economic growth.

From my standpoint, if you're looking at how to fix Medicare, you've got to look at the root cause of problem. And I would argue the root cause of problem is the cost of healthcare. You know, why is it so grossly expensive? You know, and out of whack with other nations?

There are many reasons, but I would argue we have largely removed the benefit of free market competition out of healthcare across the board. And again, I come from the private sector. I—I didn't like competition. I would love to have been a monopolist because—but because I had to compete, my prices were a lot lower, my quality was a lot higher, as well as my level of customer service was a lot higher.

That is what a functioning free market system does. Unfortunately, in healthcare, only about 10 cents of every dollar is paid by the patient and 90 cents is paid by somebody else. And so we have no idea what anything costs. There is—there is really no consumerism involved. There is not cons—consumers making wise choices and, you know, calculating what—what something costs versus what the benefit is.

So, Mr. Capretta, you did in your testimony mention three forms of competition. You said choice, you talked about premium competition, you talked about provider competition. I mean, would you basically agree with my—my assessment there that the root cause of this is we need to interject the benefits of a competitive marketplace into healthcare. And that is what we ought to be talking about here.

Mr. CAPRETTA. The answer is yes. But it is complicated as you know, which is why it hasn't been done. The—in healthcare, I think it is important to understand there has to be some structure. There are some market failures in healthcare.

I wrote a book recently maybe I'll make a plug for it. US Health Policy in Market Reforms and Introduction. Kind of covers the, you know, as an introductory matter, sort of different things that need to be done to bring more discipline from the marketplace into the health system. It can't be done though just by deregulation on its own.

It has to be structured so that the person who is making a choice can see very clearly a price difference based on the same insurance plan or the same medical service. So that means in the, you know, in the insurance context, standardization of the benefits so that the premium difference is very clear.

Senator JOHNSON. Let me quickly interject. I think also you need to separate healthcare costs in terms of the catastrophic costs that need insurance and the non-catastrophic that people could pay for out of their pocket. I think, you know, if we could separate that in some way, shape, or form as opposed to paying for everything. I have limited time.

I also want to talk about figure 1. You talked about the fiscal challenge. I would call it a fiscal crisis. You know, it is a slow moving train running right at us and it is, you know, Washington DC is not addressing it. We're, as you said, about a $2 trillion deficit this year.

We're spending $1.9 trillion more this year than we did just four years ago. And your figure 1 is pretty stark showing that about half of Medicare costs are going—going to be provided by the general revenue fund. That we're going to have the same problem with Social security. The trust fund runs out.

If we're going to plus up those benefits, we're going to need revenue out of the general fund. And I—the question I have is will we have the financial wherewithal to plus up those benefits. To, you know, meet the requirements of what Medicare is going to need in terms of financing? And that start—starts to speak to prioritization of spending.

We used this committee for climate change and the budget. You know, talking about—by the way, in testimony over $5 trillion has been spent globally combating climate change. I would argue it— it obviously, hasn't made a dent because we still have climate change alarmists. $5 trillion!

In the Inflation Reduction Act, another $1.2 trillion according to Goldman Sachs study, is what is going to be spent because of that piece of legislation. You know, we need to start prioritizing what limited resources we have to the priorities of government. And again, I would say Social Security, Medicare, those promises we made to seniors would be top priorities.

And maybe these green energy boondoggles that are not going to fix climate change would probably be a lower priority for spending. Would you like to comment on that?

Mr. CAPRETTA. No, I don't think so. I don't—I'm not an expert on the climate——

Senator JOHNSON. Okay. Set aside climate change. Just in terms of we need to get our arms around these massive deficits, this massive debt, or we're not going to have the financial wherewith. We'll have a debt crisis and then—then this all comes crashing down; correct?

Mr. CAPRETTA. I do think we are headed towards some major dislocation if we don't get fiscal discipline into our budget process. So I would very much recommend on a bipartisan basis that both sides get together and start working through some of the challenges of getting the debt down, deficits down.

So we don't pile up as much as we're projected to in the coming decade. And certainly over the coming 30 years. It is really a very big problem, and it is going to require both taxes and spending.

Senator JOHNSON. But also prioritization of spending. Okay. Thank you Mr. Capretta. Thank you Mr. Chairman.

Chairman WHITEHOUSE. Thank you, Senator Johnson. Now we turn to the distinguished Chairman of the Finance Committee who has spent more time fighting for seniors, and I think hardly, almost anybody in Congress going back to his early Gray Panther days in Oregon.

Statement of Senator Wyden

Senator WYDEN. When I had a full head of hair and rugged good looks. Thank you Mr. Chairman, and good to be working with my colleagues. See a number of members from the finance committee. Colleagues, the fact is the ultra-wealthy can fire off a text to their accountant and say, make sure I don't pay income or payroll taxes this year.

And they go on and say, what kind of tax workarounds can you get me so I don't have to pay those taxes? And the fact that these schemes are legal, underline, legal, highlights the fact that if the ultra-wealthy paid their fair share of taxes, there wouldn't be such a serious Medicare shortfall.

And you contrast what I just described, which can happen every day, be illegal to older Americans who worked hard all their lives, paid their fair share of taxes year in and year out, didn't have accountants who get them this special deal, and those older Americans are now staring down the barrel of a serious Medicare shortfall uncertainty.

And I'm all in colleagues on transformational Medicare reform. Before he retired, Chairman Orrin Hatch of our committee and I joined in a landmark kind of reform that I'm going to ask you about in a minute, Ms. Moon. But I want to start with a question on the revenue side. A proposed colleagues as chairman of the finance committee, a menu of ideas for colleagues to choose from.

A menu. Not I'm going to require you do this and this. The menu includes; wealthy partnerships paying their fair share. Back when I was coming up, partnership were a couple people who ran a sporting goods operation. That is not these big partnerships now.

The billionaires paying their fair—close—fair share, closing the self-employment, you know, loophole and more. This seems fair to me and it sure will strike the millions of working Americans who pay taxes day in and day out. Those taxes are collected on them and they don't have all these breaks.

Ms. Huang, what do you think? What are your thoughts with respect to something that is fair? And by the way, gives everybody in America the chance to be successful. We want people to be successful, we just want everybody to do it. Your thoughts?

Ms. HUANG. Completely agree that there is a—a wide menu of really economically sound ways to broaden the tax base. And,—and we have our own, you—you have yours. There is a lot to choose from there.

But let's start with the one where if I were to get the text message from my multi-billionaire client about how I can, you know, spend all I want this year without paying any taxes, well the first thing I would do is look at that billionaire's $100 billion worth of stock and say, well, why don't you just take out a credit line against that stock?

You can—you can borrow $10 billion, put that stock up as collateral, spend it on whatever you want, and you won't be facing any capital gains tax or income tax on that. So that is income that doesn't ever see the tax system or the tax returns in the year that it is made or in the year that it is spent. And that is one of the biggest holes in one of the first places I would be looking to make the tax system fairer.

Senator WYDEN. Okay. A—as you know, our theory is give everybody in America a chance to get ahead. And that is what the menu's all about. Now, let's go to transformational change Ms. Moon, and thanks for all your good work. Before he retired, the late Orrin Hatch and I said, Medicare today is not the Medicare we had when we were coming up.

It is mostly about chronic illness, cancer, diabetes, heart disease, strokes, and not just acute care. And a very large percentage of seniors has two or more of these conditions. So Chairman Hatch and I wrote what I think is a transformational update of the Medicare guarantee. It is not a voucher, it is a guarantee, that we'll use reforms like telemedicine.

We'll use simple preventive steps. Colleagues, you want to help seniors, let's get grab bars in showers, costs a few dollars, seniors save untold injuries and costs. Those are the kinds of reforms that make sense, that update the Medicare guarantee.

So we've talked about revenue, Ms. Moon, you've been one of our leading authorities. Chronic illness is what Medicare today is all about, wasn't—it was acute care when I was coming up. Your thoughts?

Dr. MOON. I think you're absolutely right.

The Medicare program has not changed with the times in that way. It is changed in a number of ways that have improved. But I think part of the problem has been that when new ideas come along, the fear is you're just going to add that on and it is going to be another add-on to the cost.

And so there is a reluctance to do it. On the other hand, one way that people often talk about is, well then let's turn it over to the private sector and just give them an amount of money and let them decide. That solution hasn't worked very well either because we have not had the kinds of oversight and controls.

There are very good Medicare Advantage plans out there, for example, that serve the needs of the people that they function for. But there are others that are in it just for making money as in— as good insurers. And I can tell them exactly how to do it and they know how to do it very well and they—they're very successful at it. But it hasn't necessarily improved our healthcare system.

Senator WYDEN. I'm—I'm—I'm glad you made that—that point because not all Medicare advantage plans are created equal. And I think, you know, the Senate Finance Committee, and we've had a number of colleagues here, has been leading the fight to crack down on those abuses. I know my time is expired, but thank you for the kind words about the new focus on chronic illness because I think dollar for dollar was some very small investments in prevention. We can get big savings. Thank you. Thank you, Mr. Chairman.

Chairman WHITEHOUSE. Thank you. Next is Senator Scott, but before his clock starts, I just wanted to add 30 seconds of chairman time to point out that things like grab bars in showers are the very kind of things that doctors in ACOs are able to arrange for their patients because it makes sense and creates savings when they install those kind of things.

We have had our doctors in Rhode Island who do this. Do things as simple as make sure rugs are non-slip in people's houses in order to save money for the system, keep people healthier, and do their work better. So with that observation, let me turn it over to Senator Scott.

Statement of Senator Scott

Senator SCOTT. Thank you, Chairman. You know, when the—it is interesting that Senator Wyden brought up the idea that there is rich that take advantage of the system. Joe Biden and his wife actually did that.

They—they took money from income that should—that they should have paid Medicare tax on, they put into a S Corporation so they could take money that they—from paid speeches and books put in there so they didn't pay the 3.8% Medicare tax under the Affordable Care Act.

And that is something that it clearly ought to be fixed. Because that is—it is—it is clearly unfair that—that people are doing that. I have a—I think it is very important to every state, but clearly my state that we don't see a reduction in benefits for Social security and Medicare.

So I have a bill that would stop that. Unfortunately, I haven't had the opportunity to get Chuck Schumer to—Senator Schumer to put on the floor, but it would be—it—I think none of us should be supporting it. And there is lots of ways to reduce the cost of delivery of healthcare. But one thing we shouldn't be doing is ever talking about doing anything to reduce the benefits of Medicare and Social Security.

And I know Senator Johnson brought this up, if we don't get this budget under control, how is interest expense going to come down? So, Mr. Capretta what do you think? Do you think if we continue to run $2 trillion a year deficits the interest—interest costs for not just us—not just for the Federal debt, but for buying a house.

Mortgages are now up to a eight—almost 8% for a 30 year mortgage. Car interest rates are up to a 23 year high. I think credit card might be the highest ever. So if we don't get the budget in control, is our interest expenses going to come down?

Mr. CAPRETTA. No. According to CBOs, current projections, by 2050, the net interest payment on the accumulated debt would be 9.4% of GDP, which essentially means, you know—you know, every dollar that comes in, you know, half of what we're raising in revenue would basically be going toward net interest payments under current projections.

So that is too much, obviously. And so well before 2050, we're— we're going to need some action by Congress, I think to kind of do both the revenue side and the spending side.

Senator SCOTT. And is—is Medicare dependent—Medicare—paying for Medicare depending on what, you know, how much money we have in revenues? So if we're going to spend it on interest expense or we're going to have less money to—to put it into Medicare?

Mr. CAPRETTA. Well, actually it doesn't quite work that way. I mean, the way the Medicare Trust fund, HI trust fund works is, at least in theory, if it ran through its reserves, the spending is going to be cut across the board probably.

So that is one reason why this is such a big issue. And exhaustion of the trust fund is a concern. Now a lot of people think, well, that would never happen. Congress would step in and say, well, we're going to pay the benefits anyway and borrow the money. So in some sense, what CBO is projecting is we're just going to end up paying the Medicare benefits one way or another and have to borrow it from somewhere.

And I think that is the cycle that we're in that needs to be thought through about how to get out of it.

Senator SCOTT. So there is been a lot of proposals by Democrats to raise taxes to pay for Social security and—and Medicare. Medicare in particular. So right now, under part—parts B and D, do the rich get subsidies? Are there—are there—are their payments subsidized? So like—like right now, if you make say, $500,000 a year, do you pay the full cost for part—part B and Part D?

Mr. CAPRETTA. Not yet. They do pay—they are starting to pay income related premiums, but they don't cover the full cost of the program yet. So no, they still get some subsidy. And that is in part because they, the—the people who wrote—wrote that provision wanted to make sure there is still large participation, even amongst—it is supposed to be a universal program, at least in theory.

That everybody participates in, higher income and lower income. And so that is the theory behind giving at least some subsidy for B and D to the high income.

Senator SCOTT. But—but just put it in perspective, they are subsidized?

Mr. CAPRETTA. Yes.

Senator SCOTT. Okay. Do you know how many taxpayers make more than $500,000 a year? Like if we—if you're going to—if you're going to tax the wealthy, I assume that'd be over $500,000 a year. I don't know. Maybe it is $200,000. How many taxpayers are there?

Mr. CAPRETTA. Well, you might want to direct that to our tax expert here. I'm not sure I have that number at the top of my head, but it is going to be a small number relative to the——

Senator SCOTT. How many—how many taxpayers make more than half a million dollars a year?

Ms. HUANG. Well, less than 2%.

Senator SCOTT. Say—say again.

Ms. HUANG. Sorry. Did you—well, less than 2%.

Senator SCOTT. So what is the number? So that make—how many—how many make less? Be less than 2 million, right?

Ms. HUANG. Somebody's got a calculator on them?

Senator SCOTT. Yeah. It is less—it is less—less than 2 million. How——

Ms. HUANG. 300 million—2.5 people per household.

Senator SCOTT. Okay.

Ms. HUANG. 2% of that.

Senator SCOTT. Okay. It is—it is less than 2 million. How much should their taxes go up? And what are they—what are they paying now? If they make—if—what's the average person that makes $500,000 a year or more pays? What are they paying now in taxes and what—what should it go up to—to make sure that, you know, there is never a cut in any program?

Ms. HUANG. Yeah, so I mean, like, if you want to look at an even smaller slice. The top 1% say, they—they—they hold—they get about 21% of all of the income in the nation, and they pay about 24% of all the taxes. That is Federal, state, and local, and all types of Federal taxes. The one thing that is a little bit somewhat misleading about that—that statistic is that included in their income is not all of the gains on the—the very large growth of their assets. So when you take into account that kind of income, and if you look at an even smaller slice of people, they only pay about 8% of their incomes in tax.

Senator SCOTT. But when they sell it, they pay taxes.

Ms. HUANG. Yes. But the—the problem is that they don't have to sell it and they can hold it over their lifetimes or even generations.

Senator SCOTT. What would you take it up to? What rate would you take it up to?

Ms. HUANG. I think that there is a long way to go from something like 8% to either the—the marginal or even the average rates that, you know, most ordinary filers face. So if you look at the middle of the income distribution, they pay about——

Senator SCOTT. What would it take—what would it take to make sure we don't have a deficit?

Ms. HUANG. To make sure——

Chairman WHITEHOUSE. We're getting well into Senator Van Hollen's time. If you could wrap it up.

Senator SCOTT. I just want to ask her what what number would have to go—go up to?

Ms. HUANG. Well, if we would assess, just say, reverse the— the—the total deficit impact of the Trump and Bush tax cuts, that would be——

Senator SCOTT. And that would be—we'd have a have a balanced budget?

Ms. HUANG. About 3% of GDP, that would be enough to completely wipe out the increase in the debt to GDP ratio over the long term.

Senator SCOTT. We—we would have a balance——

Chairman WHITEHOUSE. Senator Van Hollen.

Statement of Senator Van Hollen

Senator VAN HOLLEN. Thank you Mr. Chairman, thank all of you for your testimony. Mr. Capretta, I think in your testimony you acknowledged that in order to address the Medicare shortfall, there needs to be a revenue component.

And I heard you say that you would support closing some of the tax loopholes. Would that include closing what is known as the Gingrich Edwards loophole?

Mr. CAPRETTA. I don't know what that is, so I'm—I can't comment.

Senator VAN HOLLEN. That is—that is the loophole where people manipulate the amount of their income that comes in wages versus in business income.

Mr. CAPRETTA. Yeah.

Senator VAN HOLLEN. To lower their—their Medicare tax.

Mr. CAPRETTA. Yes. I'm not against that in theory. I think that might be best handled and put into our income tax side. Medicare, going back to the history of it, we added a new me payroll tax for Medicare in 1965 in a sense being a contribution from working wages that paid for their hospital coverage in retirement. I'm not adverse to changing that kind of original deal.

Senator VAN HOLLEN. Yeah.

Mr. CAPRETTA. But I think we should be cognizant that we are going to change it if we start introducing very different tax bases.

Senator VAN HOLLEN. If I—if I may, because—just because my time is short. We're—we're talking about closing a loophole that allows people to manipulate what part of their income is wage income and—and therefore the Medicare tax applies. But no—no, I do appreciate the fact that you recognize and support that we need a revenue component that we need to close loopholes.

I wish that was a bipartisan conclusion right here in the Senate. I would welcome any of my Senate Republican colleagues joining me today to introduce a bill to begin to close these loopholes to help address the Medicare Trust Fund issue. And I do want to applaud the Chairman of this committee Senator Whitehouse for the bill that he introduced.

I'm proud to co-sponsor that bill. But at least it puts a plan on the table. You know, our colleagues can agree or disagree with it. They disagree with it, apparently, but I've just been looking at what the House Budget Committee passed this last week with respect to Medicare. And here's what they said.

We're going to get $400 billion in savings over the next 10 years through, "bipartisan solutions." In other words, they just totally kicked the can down the road. They refuse to put a plan on the table as Senator Whitehouse, myself, and others have put a plan on the table.

And so there is a big difference between you know, complaining about the democratic plan and actually putting a Republican plan to deal with the Medicare solvency issue on the table. Now, I—I do applaud the Republican Study Group for at least putting a plan on the table. Dr. Moon that plan is going back to the idea of voucherizing Medicare.

You know, I recall when Paul Ryan was the Chairman of the Budget Committee, he put forward a plan. I disagreed with it, but I credit him and his colleagues with at least putting forward an idea. There's no idea right now apparently on, in terms of the Republican Budget Committee, and I haven't seen a plan from my colleague. Could you talk about what voucherizing Medicare would mean to seniors?

Dr. MOON. I think if you're using it as a means for holding down spending, it is pretty clear that what you're doing is kicking the can down to the providers or insurers who are going to get those funds and have to make them stretch to provide the Medicare benefits.

That is a difficult thing because we have not seen incredible creativity on the part of such individuals, particularly insurance companies, of finding ways to hold down costs, aside from doing things like denying care and raising premiums.

There are ways in which you can improve efficiencies and you can be creative, but those are much harder to do and much less likely to be put in place by somebody who simply wants a quick buck from the payment that they're going to get. That is what has tended to happen in some of the poorly operating Medicare Advantage plans.

I think that is an indication for what would happen under the voucherizing of the program. I think ultimately Medicare has to be a responsibility between providers of services and the government to try to figure out how to find ways to be more creative and efficient in the healthcare system. Just giving it over to someone and saying, it is your problem now. I don't think we'll solve the problem.

Senator VAN HOLLEN. I appreciate it. And Ms. Huang, if I could just get a very short answer to you on a—a question, because I— I think you've mentioned this, but I just want to make sure I understand. Many of us are trying to make sure the IRS has the resources it needs to crack down on very wealthy taxpayers who are not paying current taxes that are due and owing.

And I think you've indicated that about $100 billion each year that would go into the Medicare Trust fund as well as to Social security and an unemployment trust fund, $100 billion a year in what's due is not being collected because the IRS does not have the expertise at this point in time to do that.

Ms. HUANG. That is exactly—that is exactly right. And you know, if you have a service that has lost 40% of its expert auditors and it can't get staplers and—and pens for some of its sites, that—that is going to happen. And that is why cutting IRS appropriations and mandatory funding will hurt deficits, will hurt the funds, and will also hurt filers that want the IRS to pick up the phone.

Senator VAN HOLLEN. Right. So, Mr. Chairman, just in closing, I would point out that while the—the—the House Republican budget doesn't put forward any plan on Medicare, the fact that they want to turn back the resources for the IRS would actually make the situation worse. Thank you.

Chairman WHITEHOUSE. Senator Braun.

Statement of Senator Braun

Senator BRAUN. Thank you, Mr. Chairman. I'd like to point out, because the comment was made earlier about the Trump tax cuts, whether you calculate that at $2 trillion or $1.5 trillion, that is either $150 billion over each year for 10 years. I, when I point that out, or $200 billion.

And I'd also like to point out that our deficit is now $2 trillion a year. So complaining about that is such a small part of the total deficit that we're living with that is now amounting to a trillion dollars every six months. Medicare social security are the drivers of it. So we need to do something if we're going to save them.

We never talk about on social security, that is fairly easy. You get three or four variables. Do we have the political will to do it if we want to save the system for those that are going to be retiring down the road. I don't think anybody's worried about the fact that we'll borrow enough money to backfill to get folks nearing retirement or in it.

Never hear about the underlying cause of healthcare costs because of the industry itself. In my own business, I created consumer involvement and transparency for them to work with, and we were able to put a big dent in it. Of course, that is skin in the game. Nobody wants skin in the game anymore.

They either want the employer to pay for their healthcare costs or the government. And that was not that big a deal 30, 40 years ago when it was under 10% of our GDP. Now it is approaching 20% of our GDP. I'd like each one of you to comment on anything we do with taxation. That is a political endeavor that no one wants to take on. Even when the other side of the aisle, I've had the argument with Senator Van Hollen, we've never been able to generate much more than 18% of our GDP in tax revenue. Raise the rates, you get a little more into the treasury, your economic growth goes down.

So it is doable if we take on the healthcare industry to make them transparent, competitive, that is big hospitals insurance, try to get it to where it does what most other industries do. Is that even something that anybody thinks about? You could get probably 10 Republicans interested with maybe all Democrats. If it was based on competition and transparency. It would make the cost for government as the payer to come down.

And I know it works because it is worked on things like Laserassisted in situ keratomileusis (LASIK) surgery, it is worked on enterprising private health insurance plans that keep their employees safe from catastrophic risk through injury or illness. Did it in my own company 15 years ago. We haven't had a premium increase in 15 years.

Just using the user or demand side of the equation. Like each of you with a minute, minute and-a-half, just tell me, is that doable? Do you ever think about it? And why wouldn't that be part of the solution that would help all healthcare, whether it is Medicare, Medicaid, or through private insurance? Start here.

Mr. CAPRETTA. I'll be very quick. The answer is yes. I think a lot can be done in this area. As I said to Senator Johnson earlier, we need to put some structure around the choices, some standardization, and make it absolutely clear to the consumer when they can save some money and when they would benefit.

So you got to standardize what their pricing in the medical services market, not insurance. And you got to standardize insurance too, so they can see clearly the premium difference. Right now, it is very obscured and complex. And you got to take a lot of the risk out for the patient. It is all got to be win-win for them, pick a less expensive option, they save money.

Senator BRAUN. Sounds like an excellent plan. The remaining two witnesses, the other side of the aisle generally looks for more revenue. I have not found an easy way in my nearly five years here to get any new revenue that is going to meet the—the agreement of 60 senators. Or you'd have to do it through reconciliation. What about reforming the industry? Is that something you'd be interested in?

Ms. HUANG. Well, I—I think I'm a little I'm still an optimist and I actually saw a little bit of cross partisan agreement around closing a big loophole that affects the Medicare taxes today. And that would save around $300 billion over 10 years. And I—I also——

Senator BRAUN. Think that is only 30 million a year.

Ms. HUANG. And I think that there is a——

Senator BRAUN. And that is a band aid. Your big issue is your 20% of the GDP currently. So, go ahead.

Ms. HUANG. Well, I think that base broadening is one of the areas where members of both parties have looked to over time, in part because a lot of that you can think of as spending that goes through the tax code. And some of it is very inefficient and in effective at what it does. And there are very many responsible ways of raising revenues through that approach.

Dr. MOON. I think that we should always be looking for ways to make the program more efficient, to work better to meet the needs of patients. And I think some of what Dr. Capretta had to say makes a lot of sense. But I would add the caveat and caution that people, when they're faced with very high medical expenses, which is where most of the costs of healthcare come from, aren't good at making choices.

They're in a crisis. They're trying to figure out what they're going to get. And we have a very complicated healthcare system that does not work well to provide either information to people or to help them make choices.

Senator BRAUN. I think you've just made my case right there. So we're running out of time. I like what you're saying because that is true. I would offer that if we're going to do anything in the near term, it—it is going to be difficult to raise revenues.

We've already done some stuff in our help committee to where taking on reforming the healthcare industry. Remember the providers are going to still be there. The government either pays for it or employers do. You make them more competitive, you get rid of the barriers to entry, you harness entrepreneurialism.

That is the only way you take it from being 20% of our GDP down closer to what most other countries get it at, which is 12% to 13%. There's room, I think for bipartisan maneuvering there.

Chairman WHITEHOUSE. And I think Senator Braun, you have a track record of accomplishing just that. So I do look forward to working with you. Senator Kaine is walking in as his time comes. Would you like a moment to get yourself——

Senator KAINE. Mr. Chair, if anyone else hasn't asked questions, I rather if they go before me or—or has anyone else?

Chairman WHITEHOUSE. Well, Senator Johnson has already had his round.

Senator KAINE. Okay.

Chairman WHITEHOUSE. But he's been waiting patiently for a second round, so I'd be more than happy to give him five minutes and then turn to you.

Senator KAINE. That would be great. Let's do that.

Senator JOHNSON. Well really just to——

Chairman WHITEHOUSE. Your next around, Senator Johnson.

Senator JOHNSON. I appreciate that. So just to make the point.

Senator Braun was talking about year revenue percentages and— and spending percentages. Year 2000 spending—total spending was 17.7% of GDP according to Mr. Capretta's table 2. Revenue was 20%.

So we had a surplus. This year, 2022 revenue was 19.6%. Those are pretty historic highs. The Senator Braun, you know, generally we're somewhere between 17–18%. So we're, you know, historically high. By the way, in that

17%, 18% is regardless of what the maximum tax rate is. And we, we've had tax rates in excess to 70% and you're still raising about 17, 18%. Because again, we have such a broken and complex tax system, all kinds of loopholes. The government can only collect X percent. And kind of 20% is sort of the top level right there. But the difference this year is spending is 25.1%.

So again, when we had a surplus, seven—spending was 17.7%. Now that we have massive deficits spending's up to 25.1%, which brought me to the conclusion that we better start prioritizing spending. We—we just can't continue to spend a quarter of our GDP through the Federal government because we'll never be able to raise the revenue.

No matter what you do, you just can't get 25%. You can't squeeze that out of the—the American taxpayer. So we better recognize that reality. And again, I would point out that the solutions, what Senator Braun was talking about is, how do you reform the healthcare system?

And as I was talking about, to reintroduce consumerism. And— and I'll say, separate out the two different types of spending. And I wouldn't mind Mr. Capretta talking a little bit more about that, you know, medical services.

I mean the—the routine care that we all go in that, for example, Medicare, you know, we got a waiver during—during COVID for telehealth that then expires. And you know, all the medical providers in Wisconsin are saying, can you extend that exemption? Because telehealth worked really well.

Why would they even need an exemption? Because it's government run, it is bureaucratic and makes no sense. So when you have government regulation, government bureaucracy, it just prevents providers from—from, you know, being imaginative. You know, showing some real progress in terms of how to deliver things more efficiently.

Again, what this free market does. Best possible price, best quality, best level customer service. Again, that is what the free market does. Why don't we introduce more of that? Ms. Capretta, just real quick, would you like to respond to that?

Mr. CAPRETTA. Yeah. I think we're—we're—we're on the cusp of maybe doing some of that with the price transparency requirements that have been put in place. Some of it might be statutory if—if the Congress moves ahead. But there needs to be more standardization of packaged benefits.

And by the way, I would agree with the comment that not all of healthcare is going to be subject to consumer discretion. There are a lot of studies of this, and it is going to be probably about 40%. So there is some big ticket items where you can't shop.

Senator JOHNSON. Okay. So real quick.

Mr. CAPRETTA. But there are some things where you can——

Senator JOHNSON. You're saying about 40% would be kind of what you earlier referred to as medical services?

Mr. CAPRETTA. Yes.

Senator JOHNSON. And then the—then 60% would be, again, the catastrophic care, the things you need insurance for?

Mr. CAPRETTA. Yes.

Senator JOHNSON. Correct?

Mr. CAPRETTA. Correct. It'd be big things where you're—it—it is not really a packaged discernible item. It is going to be some ongoing event with unknown outcomes. And so you're going to spend a lot of money and you can't really shop for it.

Senator JOHNSON. Well, you—you mentioned transparency. I know there is a lot of talk about that. Again, you introduce free market competition, you automatically get transparency because consumers are asking, what does it cost?

My concern about government regulated transparency, it'll be fudged. I mean, it is just—it is just not going to work as efficiently as a free market system that just demands price transparency. And that is—nobody knows what anything costs in healthcare.

Mr. CAPRETTA. Yeah.

Senator JOHNSON. I mean, nobody knows.

Mr. CAPRETTA. The only point I would make there, senator on the other side is that when a consumer wants to buy a—a surgery, for instance, they need to have the surgeon in, the anesthesiologist, the radiologist, the diagnostics.

Senator JOHNSON. Yeah. But that—that is——

Mr. CAPRETTA. They need a package benefit that they can figure out and price.

Senator JOHNSON. That is—that is the insurance market.

Mr. CAPRETTA. That is going to require regulation.

Senator JOHNSON. That is the insurance side. You know, the example I use is eye care. You know, people do pay for that out of pocket. So, you know, LASIK surgery has dramatically come down in price because consumers know what it costs. They understand the benefit.

If we get more of healthcare in that model and then look at the insurance model, and again, pre-package it, have it very standardized. When I was in—in business, it drove me nuts buying insurance because you always had to look at, well, what does this plan exempt? It made no sense.

I mean, they're just exempted certain conditions to save money. So there wasn't transparency in that insurance. And that is where I would definitely go toward specific models. This, you know, coverage A covers all these things. Coverage B covers this and have that standardized. That you would require government regulation.

Mr. CAPRETTA. I—I'm very much for that. Yes.

Senator JOHNSON. Okay, good. Well, yeah——

Chairman WHITEHOUSE. With that we turn——

Senator JOHNSON [continuing]. We got some solutions here, Mr. Chairman.

Chairman WHITEHOUSE. With that, we turn to the patient Senator Kaine.

Statement of Senator Kaine

Senator KAINE. Not patient. I needed to adjust my brain into the right committee. So thank you, Senator Johnson and Mr. Chair. A recent New York Times article caught my attention. The article was entitled, A huge threat to the US Budget has receded and no one is sure why. I'd like to introduce that New York Times article for the record, Mr. Chair.[7]

Chairman WHITEHOUSE. Without objection.

Senator KAINE. The article outlines that since 2010 Medicare spending has been significantly lower than expected. According to the CBO, between 2010 and 2020, that cost was about 9% lower than what they had expected. And the most interesting part is that nobody's a hundred percent sure why.

Is it a combination of legislative changes, new laws, economic changes, technical changes? Which CBO estimated led to some passed overestimation of spending per beneficiary. And the majority of the decrease has come in this category, less spending per beneficiary. I'd like to understand a little bit more about this.

I wonder whether the passage of the Affordable Care Act and the extension of health insurance to working Americans in the millions who had never had insurance before, might have led them to live healthier and thus need less healthcare immediately upon obtaining Medicare eligibility age.

---

[7] Statement submitted by Senator Kaine appears in the appendix on page 103.

But Dr. Moon, might you speak to that trend and offer any thoughts that you have about why Medicare spending over the last decade was lower than expected?

Dr. MOON. I agree that we don't know exactly and it is very hard to parse it out. But we do know, for example, from studies that have been done of people who come onto the Medicare program when they did not have insurance before they came on, they spent much more in the first few years, and it lasted for a number of years than other beneficiaries who had insurance.

So undoubtedly the Affordable Care Act will have had a very large impact. I think there'll be eventually studies that show that.

The other thing that people don't focus on so much is that this is a period of time when the baby boom generation was first becoming eligible for Medicare. And 65 year olds are much cheaper to provide care for than 85 year olds. And when we baby boomers get a little older, we'll be adding to the cost. So some of that may not stick.

I think we're also finding some ways in which people are a little more skeptical and concerned about their care and asking better questions. Some of that comes from competition, some of that may help. But I'm also skeptic that we have a system that is very receptive to people making good choices. This is really important stuff to people. They don't want to mess around.

They're not going to go out and shop 14 different Magnetic Resonance Imaging (MRIs) before they choose which one they're going to get, et cetera. We're going to have a real difficulty wrestling this to the ground. And I think this is going to have to make a concerted effort to provide more consumer information, better investment in providing that information to people so they can make good choices, but also better government controls and insight into how we manage this very cumbersome but important system.

Senator KAINE. Well, there is—there is an overlap in—in your comment and what Senator Johnson was saying, a market where people don't know what the costs are or shopping for the price of 14 different MRIs to decide which one to take is not the way people will approach their healthcare choices.

We've got to figure out a way more information, more transparency, I think all can agree on that. Ms. Huang, I want to ask you a question. Your testimony describes how wealth—the wealthy can often structure their affairs to choose their tax rates and when even if ever their income is taxed.

I'm a co-sponsor of a bill by Senator Baldwin, it is called the Carried Interest Fairness Act. And that would address this issue, at least with respect to closing the carried interest loophole. Could you—could you describe how reforms in this space could help address the two-tier tax system that you described?

Ms. HUANG. Thank you, Senator. It is a really great example of how preferences in the tax system sort of attract avoidance and— and sometimes even evasion and in complex ways. So the carried interest loophole, as you know, is—is how some hedge fund managers can choose capital gains treatment on compensation that should really be taxed as salaries.

In other words, they can just elect to have a lot of their income tax at a lower rate. So closing this loophole would just mean that the labor of fund managers would be taxed similarly to workers who are employed and, you know, at the same companies that these hedge fund managers are investing in.

And, you know, the 2017 tax law did take a small step towards addressing this issue, but bills like yours and others would more comprehensively close the loophole.

Senator KAINE. I—I'm very much a believer that we ought to move to a system where income is income. I—I would want it to be progressive with rates that would be higher as income goes up, but a system that would not advantage structuring your income as, you know, capital gains rather than salary, or carried interest rather than salary, or interest rather than dividends.

You know, we—we just give people who have the ability to hire sharp accountants and lawyers the ability to, you know, essentially choose their own tax rate. Most people don't get that deal. And we should move to a system and that would be more fair.

And it would be one way we could also address some issues like the solvency and—and funding solvency of programs like Medicare. Really important. As I yield back, I am really intrigued with this Medicare cost issue. As you said, Dr. Moon, even though this particular question about ACA expansion and connection of Medicare costs, there may not be enough data yet.

There has been significant studies about the Medicare spending per beneficiary of people at health insurance before they reach Medicare age and those who didn't. And just the healthier you can keep yourself during in life, the healthier you're going to be when you reach Medicare age.

And if you don't have access to good healthcare or health insurance, you're going to have a lot of deferred maintenance on the body when you get to Medicare. And that will drive costs up. And so I think the—if the—if the past studies hold, I think we would likely see that the expansion of affordable health insurance, both through Medicaid expansion, but also just providing subsidies so that people can buy insurance on the exchange at a lower cost rate. That expansion is going to be a significant factor in the reducing—the reduction over what we might've expected Medicare per beneficiary costs. So I look forward to more discussion on that. And with that, Mr. Chair, I yield back.

Chairman WHITEHOUSE. Thanks, Senator Kaine. Let me thank the witnesses for appearing before the committee today and for the many colleagues who participated. Let me also thank the advocates and the District of Columbia seniors who joined us here in the hearing today. Appreciate very much your presence.

I would say that perhaps some faint outlines of progress began to emerge in this hearing. I think we had folks on both sides talk about the need to raise revenues. I would favor doing that by unrigging loopholes that benefit very wealthy people. But certainly the prospect and the need for additional revenue seems to have emerged on both sides of the hearing.

The opportunity to save costs in Medicare seems to be also a mutually agreed prospect. I would recommend using the Accountable Care Organization payment reform escape from fee for service treadmill strategies. But I do think that there are cost savings that we—proven cost savings that we can pursue.

I would think that we could take advantage of the bipartisan standing ovation at President Biden's State of the Union to lock in an iron clad guarantee as we reform this, that there will not be benefit cuts. And that no benefit cuts becomes a core guiding principle of our conversations.

And then finally, that the purpose of the exercise should be to extend Medicare solvency. And I would recommend that we plan to extend Medicare solvency essentially forever the way my piece of legislation does. Without objection, I'll submit letters for the record from AARP, the American Federation of State County Municipal Employees, the National Committee to Preserve Social Security and Medicare, the Alliance for Retired Americans, the Medicare right center, the Rhode Island Alliance for Retired Americans, the Senior Agenda Coalition of Rhode Island, and the Rhode Island Geriatric Education Center at the University of Rhode Island.

Questions for the record are due by 12 noon tomorrow, and we will ask witnesses to respond to any questions that we may forward to you within seven days of receipt. With no further business before the committee, the hearing is adjourned. Thank you all.

(Whereupon, at 11:42 a.m., Wednesday, September 27, 2023 the hearing was adjourned.)

Opening Statement for "Medicare Forever: Protecting Seniors by Making the Wealthy Pay Their Fair Share"

Ranking Member Grassley and members of the Committee, today's hearing is about guaranteeing Medicare solvency by balancing the tax system so it's less rigged and more fair — two good goals.

In July, the Budget Committee held a hearing on protecting Social Security for all by taking away tax tricks that let those at the top pay lower tax rates than teachers and firefighters. Today, we turn to Medicare, our other pillar of retirement security, whose insolvency is predicted to arrive even sooner than Social Security's.

Right now, a government shutdown looms because House Republicans are—once again—trying to make the tax system even less fair, to give more freebies to big businesses and billionaires.

Republicans want to maintain the massive exemption for inheritances to wealthy heirs. They want to keep tax breaks for multinational corporations that send profits and jobs offshore. And they want to hamstring the IRS from catching wealthy tax cheats.

Nobody likes this, so they hold our government operations hostage. It will cost billions and add to the deficit, if they succeed at shutting the government down. At the end of the day, the point is taking care of the billionaires and big corporations. The rest is smoke and mirrors.

Any serious conversation about federal spending and deficits must also include Medicare. According to CBO, Medicare, along with Social Security, will make up more than half of spending growth over the next decade. And without new revenue, Medicare will cover less than 90 percent of scheduled benefits beginning in 2031. That is only eight years away.

Since its inception, Medicare has ensured that our nation's seniors do not become impoverished due to illness. As a result, older Americans live longer, live better-quality lives, and suffer less discrimination in the health care system.

Today, nearly 80 percent of Americans either receive direct support from Medicare or have a family member or close friend enrolled in the program. Almost every senior in this country will receive Medicare benefits, which they have *earned* throughout their working lives, and which let them retire in health and dignity.

Rhode Island seniors unerstand the importance of Medicare on their quality of life.

Joyce from Pawtucket said, "Medicare is a lifeline for me. [Reduction in benefits] would cause me to neglect medical problems and I would actually end up in the hospital."

Lisa from West Warwick said, "Without Medicare I would exhaust my finances and go without care and medicines."

And Ana from Providence said, "Medicare helps me in countless ways. It helps pay for my wheelchair, shower chair, lift to get in and out of bed, doctor's visits, and medicine, among other things. All of these are essential and enable me to continue living my life."

But for decades, some Republicans worked publicly to undermine Medicare, to have Medicare, as former Speaker of the House Newt Gingrich put it, "wither on the vine." They have proposed raising the Medicare eligibility age, turning Medicare into a private voucher program, and even sunsetting the program altogether.

Then came the State of the Union address earlier this year, when Republicans and Democrats gave President Biden a standing ovation when he declared that cuts to Social Security and Medicare were off the table.

That bipartisan consensus, if it was real and not more smoke and mirrors, leaves only one option: raise revenue.

And we can raise revenue by unrigging our tax code. We can close loopholes that allow the super-wealthy to avoid taxes. It would be good to level the playing field so the wealthiest in this country can't play by a special set of rules and avoid paying a fair share.

We can and must protect Medicare. We can and must do so without cutting benefits. And we can do that by making our tax code fairer.

According to the CMS Chief Actuary—the authority on Medicare solvency—my Medicare and Social Security Fair Share Act would ensure Medicare remains solvent effectively *forever*. And we heard at our Social Security hearing that my legislation would also extend Social Security solvency indefinitely.

As I told my Republican colleagues at our Social Security hearing, I welcome serious proposals to protect Social Security and Medicare without cutting benefits. I've spent enough time in the Senate to know the difference between free-wheeling chat and actual proposals. Actual proposals are what lead to actual agreements, so join in.

My proposal ensures Medicare solvency forever. It does so by unrigging a rigged tax system, so those who can most afford to pay don't play by a different set of rules. It's available for everyone to see and debate.

It's simple arithmetic: raise revenue or cut benefits. Those are the options if we are to preserve Medicare. If we abide by what seemed like a bipartisan commitment not to cut benefits, we must safeguard Medicare by raising revenue. It's life and death for millions of older Americans.

Prepared Opening Statement by Senator Chuck Grassley of Iowa, Ranking Member, Senate Budget Committee, Hearing on Medicare Solvency, Wednesday, September 27, 2023

Thank you, Mr. Chairman, for holding this very important hearing, because we can all recognize Medicare and Social Security are very much a part of the social fabric. They may be government programs, but they also interact with the private sector, retirement and health benefits as well. It's not something that just government does; but private sector, retirement and health care programs plan on interacting with it.

Republicans want to preserve and strengthen this program for future generations.

For decades, Medicare has provided seniors and those with disabilities access to routine and life-saving care at their local hospital, doctor's office and pharmacy.

As then Chairman of the Finance Committee, I'm proud to have led the effort in 2003 to modernize Medicare by establishing a prescription drug benefit.

That effort required bipartisan cooperation from both chambers and presidential leadership.

In the first decade of the Medicare Part D, the federal government spent 36 percent less than CBO projected, while still improving access to prescription drugs for millions of seniors.

That law also requires the Medicare Trustees to review Medicare finances annually.

For the past seven years, the Medicare Trustees have issued a Funding Warning, because Medicare's outlays are expected to exceed its dedicated revenue by 45 percent.

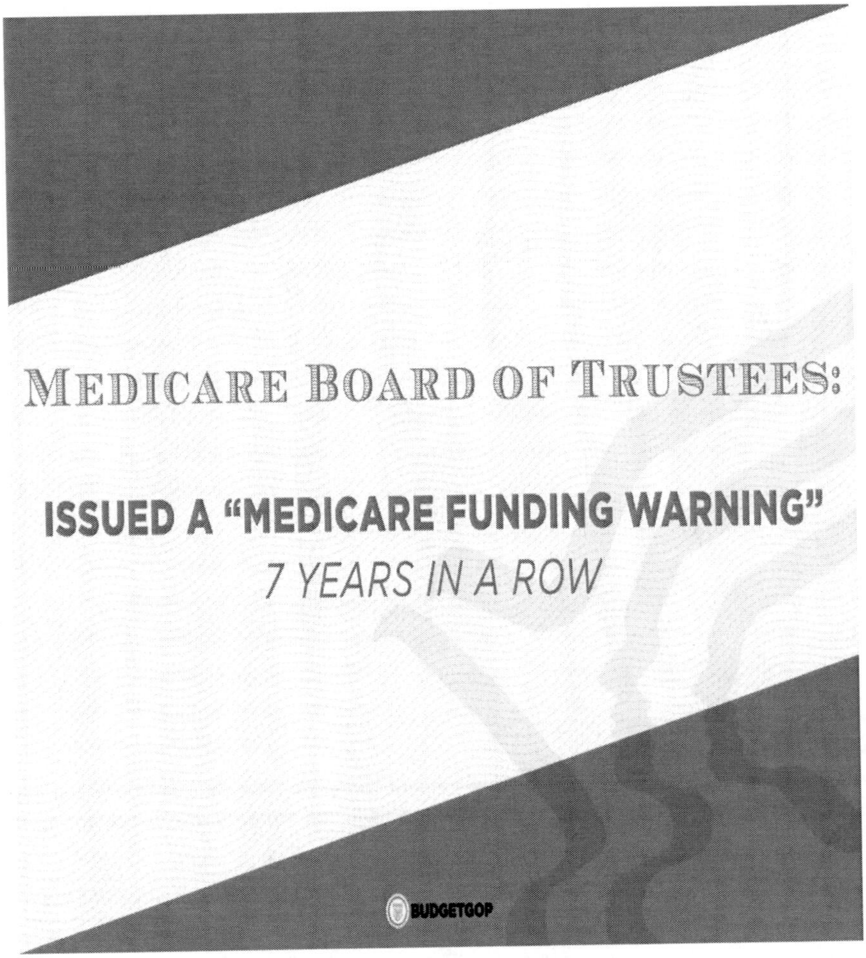

Medicare's Hospital Insurance Trust Fund is also in poor shape. Both CBO and the Medicare Trustees expect it to be insolvent in about ten years.

Upon insolvency and absent congressional action, Medicare Part A providers will see an 11 percent cut in reimbursements. We should be moving our health care system from volume to value, but we need to accurately account for what's working and not working.

As I stated at our Social Security hearing, the only way to make these critical programs sustainable is to follow the Ronald Reagan-Tip O'Neill model of 1983. And just as an aside, remembering some of the things you said in your opening statement, that would include more than just tax increasers; that would mean more than people putting proposals on the table as you're asking us to do. Because I think they sat down at a table with nothing on it because they wanted everything to be negotiable, and it ended up tax increases, it ended up changes in formula, it ended up changes in retirement age.

I suppose they thought they were going to save Social Security for 20 years, but as we see now, they saved it for 50 years. It's that bipartisanship that [came from] a Democrat speaker and a Republican president that we just can't let Social Security fail, that led to their success. But everything being on the table, it was the Republicans putting something out, Democrats putting something out, because that gives people opportunity to shoot at things.

So, we've got to work in a bipartisan fashion and keep a range of options on the table.

Unfortunately, any time Republicans mention Medicare being in trouble, Democrats accuse us of trying to blow up the program. Blowing up the program is a pretty rich statement, considering Democrats have proposed and enacted major cuts to Medicare, often using the program as a piggybank to pay for unrelated spending.

Obamacare cut Medicare, including an annual one percent reduction of provider payments. Democrats have proposed cuts to Medicare Advantage, which ignores the choice and competition these plans offer consumers.

On top of these Medicare cuts, the so-called "Inflation Reduction Act" passed only by Democrats, and President Biden stole budget savings from Medicare to subsidize green energy tax credits. Most of these Democrat tax benefits will go to wealthier taxpayers.

And let's not forget proposals like Medicare-for-All that would cost 30 to 40 trillion dollars in the first 10 years – more than twice what Medicare costs today.

Under this Democrat plan, hospitals would see a 16 percent reduction in revenue, resulting in closures and reduced access to care.

Then there's President Biden's latest budget, which kicks the can down the road on Medicare. It forgoes real solutions in favor of accounting gimmicks, massive tax hikes and price controls that will reduce access to life-saving drugs and treatments.

The proposal currently touted by the Chairman would push the top marginal tax rate above 50 percent and impose a 37.4 percent top tax rate on capital gains.

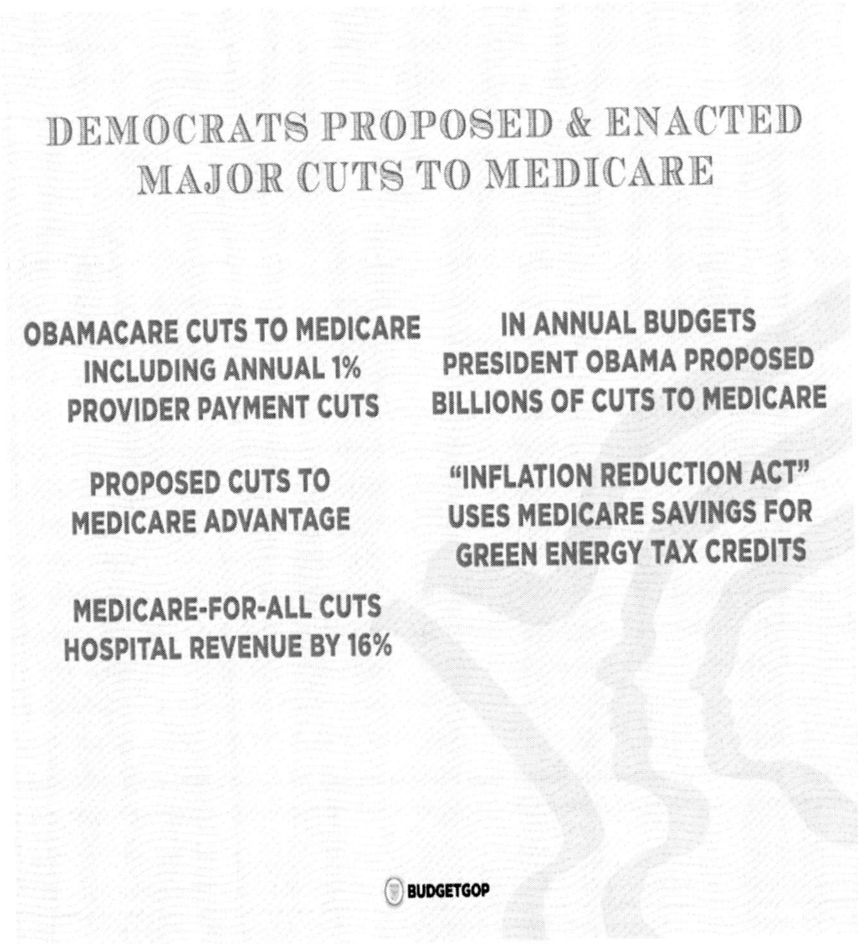

We don't talk much about the consequences of those policies, but the CMS actuary concludes the proposal would address Medicare's long-term solvency – but with the caveat that he couldn't "independently assess the reasonability of the revenue estimates for the stated provisions."

Based on an analysis of the proposal by the Tax Foundation – which I ask unanimous consent to put in the record – the Chairman's proposed capital gains tax hike is a revenue loser. Moreover, the tax hikes as a whole will cost about 700,000 jobs.

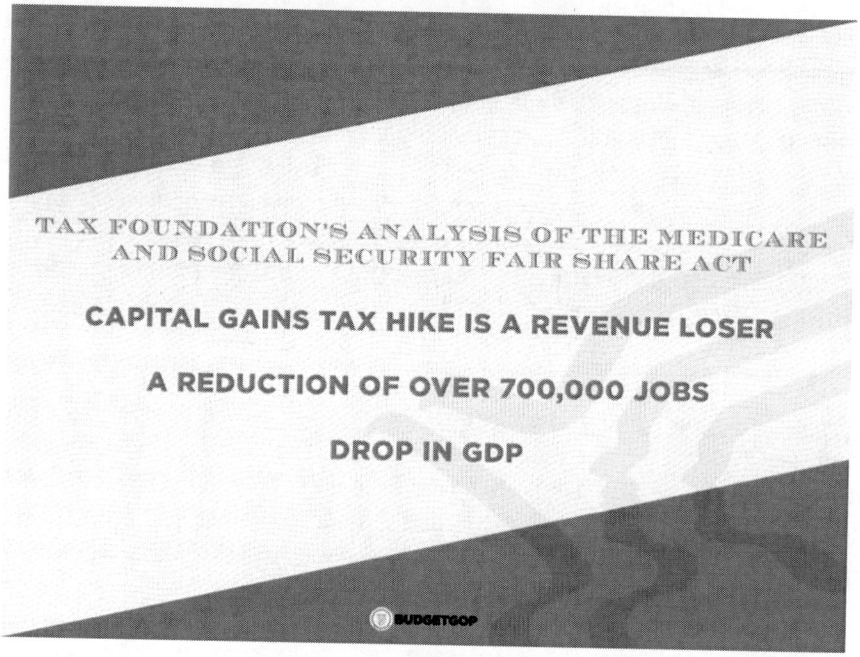

These tax hikes won't just hit high-income Americans. While proponents claim only the top two percent [of households] will be affected, the proposal's income-thresholds not being indexed for inflation has a much broader effect than just the top two percent. As a result, the Social Security's Chief Actuary estimates that up to 25 percent of households will be captured by the end of the projection period.

The truth is, taxes on the rich alone won't save Medicare for our children and grandchildren. If Democrats believe otherwise, then request the CBO and the Joint Committee on Taxation analyze the proposal. So I'd think we'd like to have a more widespread investigation of these facts.

You thought I was through with my remarks, but I wanted to just point out something that I gave a couple of weeks ago in a speech on the floor of the [Senate], and this won't take me maybe just a couple minutes.

It's obvious that our health care system in the United States needs reform and accountability. However, we shouldn't ruin it by turning it into a government run health care system, whether you want to call it Medicare for all, single payer or socialized medicine.

I referred in my speech then to a *Wall Street Journal* article highlighting the failures of some government run programs. They wrote this about Great Britain: "Now, the state funded service is falling apart. People who suffer heart attacks or strokes wait more than one and a half hours on average for ambulance. Hospitals are so full, they are turning patients away. A record 7.1 million people in England, more than one in 10, are stuck on waiting lists for non-emergency hospital treatment like hip treatment,"

The article went on to say "delays in treating people are causing premature deaths of 300 to 500 people a week, and one in five British people were waiting for medical appointment or treatment at the name health service in December." If you didn't find that alarming, I said on the floor of the [Senate], in May, British Columbia announced that they were sending cancer patients to Bellingham, Washington in the United States for treatment.

A Canadian news outlet wrote that health minister Adrian Dix announced "that eligible breast and prostate cancer patients will be sent to one of the two clinics in Bellingham for radiation treatment." The unprecedented move to send thousands of British Columbia patients to the U.S. over the next two years is an attempt to address the backlog that British Columbia has in one of the longest waits for radiation treatment in Canada. Canada is taking this action because its cancer patients face unacceptable waiting lines.

When I read about Bellingham, it reminded me of this: in the years that I've been fighting doctor-owned hospitals not having special treatment and not being conflicts of interests and all that, I used as one of my examples that that there was a Texas hospital that said if you have an emergency call 911 – that was posted in that hospital. So here we have British Columbia posting in hospitals, if you need emergency action, go to Bellingham. And I think it's a crime that we would be thinking of things like that in America.

Testimony Submitted to the Senate Budget Committee, September 27, 2023, Considering the Impacts on Beneficiaries in Medicare Financing, Marilyn Moon

Medicare has grown rapidly since its inception in 1966, rising from 0.71 percent of GDP in 1970 to 3.72 percent in 2022, making it a frequent target in discussions about reducing federal government spending.[8] Medicare's total spending growth reflects both expansion in the number of beneficiaries (from

---

[8] Unless otherwise noted, most of the statistics reported here come from Board of Trustees, *2023 Annual Report of the Boards of Trustees of the Federal Hospital Insurance and Federal Supplementary Medicare Insurance Trust Funds*, 2023, Washington, D.C.: U.S. Government Printing Office.

20.4 million in 1970 to 64.9 million in 2022), and increases in the per capita costs of health care. The increase in costs of the program is often cited with alarm, but in many ways, higher costs for Medicare over time signal substantial success: Americans are living longer and receiving better care. It is to be expected that costs would rise.

The solvency of the Part A Trust Fund also garners substantial attention and over the years has periodically faced the prediction of impending insolvency. The most recent projection is that the fund will be depleted by 2031. That provides additional urgency for dealing with Medicare's issues, but it should not be viewed as a judgement about Medicare's success or the need to cut back on the program. The Part A Trust Fund and its projections were essentially put into place to offer an early warning sign for the need for funds to assure that Medicare would continue to function without interruption. It is not a signal of the need for cutting back on services. Social Security and Medicare provide vital support for the most vulnerable of our citizens and should not be dealt with as short term budget issues.

Challenges from the aging of the Baby Boom generation and expanded life expectancies were both anticipated when Medicare passed in 1965, and discussions about the need for increasing tax rates over time were part of the legislative debate and early planning for Medicare's needs.[9] It was well known at that time that payroll tax revenue would not increase at the same rate as the costs of Medicare and hence rates would need to be raised periodically.

Indeed, in the early years of the program, both current and future scheduled rates changed several times. In more recent years, much of the improvement in the solvency outlook of Medicare has come from cost cutting efforts and changes in the way that care is delivered rather than from continuing to increase payroll tax rates.

Substantial cost cutting over the last 30 years has meant that Medicare has not grown faster than other costs of health care. In many years, it has grown at a slower pace than private health insurance. Moreover, as a share of GDP, Medicare has been stable for the last four years despite the challenges of the pandemic. However, this cost cutting also means that Medicare has often lagged behind coverage available to many working Americans. Consequently,

---

[9] Robert Myers, *Medicare*, Irwin Press, 1970.

Medicare is not an overly generous program,[10] and studies have documented the unmet needs of these most vulnerable of our citizens.[11]

Seeking ways to make the program function better or adopting new approaches to provide good care at lower cost certainly needs to be part of any discussion of Medicare's future. And there are some areas (such as payments to Medicare Advantage plans) where reforms could yield important savings. Part D changes made in the Inflation Reduction Act will also help to hold down costs in the future (and help beneficiaries better afford the costs of drugs). But, further limitations on coverage or reductions in provider payments could leave even more beneficiaries at risk for getting good care, and policy debates should keep this in mind. Indeed, there are strong arguments to be made for increasing benefits—improvements in post hospital and long term care and better protections for those with modest incomes are just two examples. But concerns about financing Medicare have often precluded serious considerations for improving the program. Thus, rather than focusing on further belt tightening as the sole means for keeping Medicare financially strong, it is important to consider additional sources of financing.

The Contributions That Medicare Has Made to Its Beneficiaries

When Medicare began, many seniors could not afford mainstream medical care. The program changed that and proved to be remarkably successful from its very start. Suddenly access to mainstream care was available as nearly all hospitals and doctors participated in the program (despite initial skepticism that they would do so), making care available to nearly all persons 65 and over. Further, Medicare is often lauded as having accelerated the integration of hospitals in the U.S., ensuring that minority patients as well as white Medicare beneficiaries would be served. Medicare's initial success continues today as the program remains popular and continues to give seniors (and since 1972 persons with disability) access to lifesaving care.

---

[10] Kaiser Family Foundation, "How Does the Benefit Value of Medicare Compare to the Benefit Value of Typical Large Employer Plans? A 2012 Update," by Frank McArdle, Ian Stark, Zachary Levinson, and Tricia Neuman, April 2012. https://www.kff.org/health-reform/issue-brief/how-does-the-benefit-value-of-medicare/.

[11] Kaiser Family Foundation, "How Much is Enough: Out of Pocket Spending Among Medicare Beneficiaries: A Chartbook,", July 2014; "Problems Getting Care Due to Cost or Paying Medical Bills Among Medicare Beneficiaries," by Juliet Cubanski, Tricia Neuman and Anthony Damico, April 2, 2020. www.kff.org/coronavirus-covid19/issue-brief/problems-getting-care-due-to-Cost-or-paying-medical-bills-among-medicare-beneficiaries.

In 1965, less than 58 percent of Americans age 65 and over had insurance for hospital costs; once Medicare was fully phased in that share jumped to over 97 percent.[12] And while many factors contribute to reductions in life expectancy, growth in life expectancy between 1950 and 1960 was just 0.4 years as compared to an increase of 0.9 years between 1960 and 1970.

And by 1975, that number rose by another 0.9 years. Access to lifesaving care certainly contributed to these life expectancy increases, which have continued to rise over the years. By 2016, life expectancy was 19.4 years for those reaching age 65 as compared to 14.3 years in 1960.[13]

Medicare spending per capita was $15,727 in 2022—an amount that totals 53 percent of median per capita income for persons 65 and older. Thus, for most older Americans, without Medicare, the costs of health care would be well beyond their means—and it is unlikely that subsidized retiree insurance would defray those costs for many.[14] It is not hard to understand how much Medicare has contributed to the living standards of older and disabled Americans, undoubtedly reducing poverty substantially.[15]

Despite the important role that Medicare has played in assuring retirement security for nearly 60 million current Americans—and in providing assurances to younger persons planning for retirement—the substantial costs of healthcare that are not covered by Medicare remain daunting for many. Requirements to pay premiums and cost sharing–and to contribute through taxes to Medicare's financing mean that many older and disabled Americans are already paying substantial shares of their incomes for the costs of their care.

Contributions to Medicare from Beneficiaries

Before exploring options for new sources of financing, it is important to examine the status of Medicare beneficiaries since explicitly or implicitly

---

[12] Marilyn Moon, "What Medicare has Meant to Older Americans," *Health Care Financing Review*, Medicare Advancing Towards the 21st Century 1966-1996, Vol. 18, Winter 1966, pp.49 59.

[13] Centers for Disease Control and Prevention, *Health, United States*, National Center for Health Statistics; www.cdc.gov/nchs/hus.

[14] Even though employer retirement health subsidies only cover what Medicare does not, still only a minority of employers offer such coverage and that number has been declining over time.

[15] Measures of poverty that include the value of Medicare routinely reduce the share of seniors in poverty substantially although these estimates are to some extent still considered "experimental."

many proposals for reducing the costs of Medicare would adversely affect them. As I have already noted, Medicare is not currently a very generous program, placing considerable burdens on those the program serves. And proposals to further cut benefits, for example, indirectly through premium support proposals (limiting the government's contribution to Medicare) or raising the eligibility age, or directly via increased premiums or cost sharing would exacerbate the inadequacy of the program. That is particularly important when considering how much individuals now pay out of pocket.

A new study by KFF found that the out of pocket burden of Medicare continues to rise over time—now standing at $6,557 in 2021—substantially higher than what non-Medicare beneficiaries pay.[16] In 2010, the amount was $4,734 and in 2000, $3,293. Moreover, the burdens are heaviest on those with incomes in the $20,000 to $40,000 range. Those beneficiaries do not have low income protections (because of the strict eligibility requirements for such benefits) and often lack the supplemental insurance that higher income people often receive at subsidized rates from former employers. Further, these costs are rising faster than the median incomes of Medicare beneficiaries—and particularly for those with incomes below 300% of the federal poverty level. For example, for those with incomes between 100 and 200% of poverty, the share of income going to out of pocket spending has risen to 26 percent in 2021 compared to 23 percent in 2000. While the expansions in insurance protections for younger families have improved since Obamacare was passed in 2010, Medicare beneficiaries' situation has not.[17]

In addition, the common view of Medicare is that younger taxpayers fund all but the beneficiary premiums and copayments, resulting in intergenerational burdens. But in fact, beneficiaries also contribute substantially to the taxes that fund Medicare—and these contributions have been growing over time. After many years of Americans retiring early, more people now work past the age of 65 and hence contribute more to both income and payroll taxes. In fact, the shares of these taxes paid by persons over age 65 have increased over time. Seniors now pay about one-third of the income

---

[16] Kaiser Family Foundation, "Medicare Households Spend More on Health Care than Other Households," July 2023, by Nancy Ochieng and Juliette Cubanski.

[17] These numbers are reflective of out of pocket spending for those in traditional Medicare. The Medicare Advantage program is often touted as helping to lower these costs but data are not reliably reported and in some cases, out of pocket spending would not be lower. These protections also come at other costs such as lack of access to certain provider and more restrictions on care. Much more analysis needs to be undertaken before concluding that expanding Medicare Advantage would readily be a "solution" to the costs of care for older and disabled Americans. See, for example, Marilyn Moon.

and tax revenues that go into financing Medicare. And if premiums and co-pays are included, young taxpayers were responsible for just 59 percent of the costs of Medicare services while beneficiaries, their families or former employers were responsible for 41 percent in 2016.[18] And the share that beneficiaries pay is continuing upward. Thus, policies directed at explicitly increasing burdens on beneficiaries do not represent a good strategy for the future.

Financing Options

Since the last payroll rate increase in 1986, Medicare's share of the population and total spending per capita have nearly doubled. Some of the need for increased revenue has been filled by general revenues (mainly the personal income tax), largely because of changes in the health care system. The shifting of medical care away from inpatient hospital to outpatient settings has meant that Part B—financed by premiums and general revenues--represents a greater share of spending as compared to Part A. The share that payroll taxes cover for all Medicare has fallen from 61.8 percent in 1970 to 36.4 percent in 2019.

To ensure stable future financing for Medicare, payroll taxes and/or personal income taxes will need to be increased. Payroll taxes have always been popular because they are simple, administered by employers with no filing requirements by workers, and dedicated to Social Security and Medicare. Traditionally, economists have criticized the payroll tax because it is assessed only against wages and hence falls disproportionately on lower income persons.

Progressivity (the extent to which a tax burden falls more on higher income persons) for Medicare's portion of the payroll tax improved when the taxable wage cap was eliminated and when additional requirements for higher income taxpayers and beneficiaries to pay more were added. But wages have also declined as a share of incomes for Americans over the years, with income from interest and dividends rising particularly for those with higher incomes, making the payroll tax *less* progressive. There is still substantially more room to improve the progressivity of funding for Part A.

A modest increase (for example, a 0.5 percentage point increase each on employers and employees) could raise substantial new revenues for

[18] Marilyn Moon and Jing Guo, "Who Pays for Medicare?" Center on Aging at Americn Institutes for Research, Issue Brief Series.

Medicare's Part A Trust Fund, extending its life substantially and keeping the dedicated nature of the tax that funds most of Part A. It would need to be phased in over time and to be paired with other changes to enhance progressivity.

And since general revenues by law will naturally increase over time to fund Parts B and D, this approach would mean that both types of taxes will expand to fund Medicare.

Additional approaches would include expanding personal income tax revenues to the funding for Part A. This would mean that there would be no extra burden on individuals whose incomes come mainly from wages, since the burden would be more evenly spread across all income sources, or options could focus on those with higher incomes in general. A variation of this approach could target certain types of income to be devoted to the Part A Trust Fund rather than a general rate increase. Closing various tax loopholes (for both personal and corporate income taxes) and increasing IRS enforcement capabilities are often popular proposals and have been advocated for a variety of purposes.[19] Further, an increase in the tax on capital gains could be used to explicitly supplement the existing payroll tax and hence enhance the progressivity of Medicare taxation.

To further protect modest income Medicare beneficiaries, another approach would explicitly target those with higher incomes to achieve increases in revenues. We have already moved in that direction with the requirement that individuals with incomes above $200,000 (and couples with incomes over $250,000) to pay an income tax surcharge of 3.8 percent. This amount could be increased for those with even higher incomes. For example, the Biden administration has proposed raising the rate to 5 percent on those with incomes above $400,000. (And, revenues from the existing high income tax and any expansion should be directly credited to the Part A trust fund.) Estimates from the Medicare Actuaries indicate that this option for improving revenues would extend the solvency of the Part A Trust Fund indefinitely.

Expanded contributions from those with higher incomes can be justified on a number of grounds. Although the cap on wages subject to tax was eliminated a number of years ago, improving the progressivity of the payroll tax, burdens on higher income individuals are still substantially smaller than on middle-income taxpayers because higher income people receive a much greater share of their incomes from sources other than wages and salaries. This

---

19 See for example, Paul Van de Water, "President Biden's 2024 Budget Would Strengthen, Improve Medicare," May 3, 2023, Center on Budget and Policy Priorities.

trend has been going on for some time and will likely continue. It is one of the reasons why payroll taxes are declining as a share of GDP (and why the share of income going to the wealthiest Americans is increasing). Bolstering the Part A Trust Fund in this way would help to offset the decline in revenues coming into the fund because of the shift away from wages and towards greater inequality in Americans' incomes.

Conclusion

Whatever choices are made for financing Medicare for the future, protecting Medicare's viability in ensuring the health and security of those it protects should be the guiding principle in considering how to proceed. Beneficiaries are already making strong contributions toward the costs of Medicare and the program's benefits remain modest, so they should not be expected to bear unusual burdens for protecting its future. Rather, it is appropriate to consider broader financial contributions from all Americans in the form of additional revenues. Medicare remains one of the most popular and successful programs of the federal government and a commitment to maintaining it over time deserves nothing less.

Strengthening the Tax Base, Written Testimony for Hearing, "Medicare Forever: Protecting Seniors by Making the Wealthy Pay Their Fair Share," Chye-Ching Huang, Executive Director of the Tax Law Center at NYU Law, the United States, Senate Committee on the Budget, September 27, 2023

Chairman Whitehouse, Ranking Member Grassley, and distinguished members of the Committee, thank you for the opportunity to testify.[20] I am the Executive Director of the Tax Law Center at NYU Law, a public interest initiative that seeks to improve the integrity of the tax system. The Center is

---

[20] This testimony draws heavily on my prior work including: *Building Back Better: Raising Revenue to Invest in Shared Prosperity,* Testimony Before the U.S. Joint Economic Committee (October 6, 2021); *How U.S. International Tax Policy Impacts American Workers, Jobs, and Investment,* Testimony Before the Senate Committee on Finance (March 25, 2021); *Depletion of IRS Enforcement Is Undermining the Tax Code,* Testimony Before the House Ways and Means Committee (February 11, 2020).

staffed by tax lawyers with expertise in tax administration, private practice, and the tax legislative process, and our work draws on extensive networks of public interest minded tax practitioners and experts.

Summary

The federal tax base should be broadened and strengthened to more securely support the nation's priorities.

A building needs a strong foundation. It should be wide enough to support what's resting on it. It should also be solid, without gaps and cracks.

The federal tax base is the foundation for the federal budget, which invests in national priorities including, social security, defense, economic security programs, benefits for veterans and federal retirees, education, transportation and healthcare – including Medicare.[21] But currently:

- The federal tax base is not broad enough. Too much income—especially of the largest corporations and highest-income individuals—is excluded. For example, certain pass-through business income is excluded from the net investment income tax (NIIT) and Self-Employed Contributions Act (SECA) taxes, allowing business owners to avoid paying their fair share of taxes, lowering both general and trust funds revenues. Exclusions from the tax base can attract wasteful and aggressive tax avoidance.
- The federal tax base is unacceptably leaky. Before lawmakers acted to restore the IRS's ability to address tax compliance, it was estimated that more than $500 billion per year would leak out of the "tax gap,"[22] with some $100 billion each year lost to the Medicare, Social Security, and UI trust funds on account of taxes owed but not paid.[23]

---

[21] CBPP (CBPP), *Policy Basics: Where Do Our Federal Tax Dollars Go?* (July 28, 2022).

[22] *See* Internal Revenue Service (IRS), Federal Tax Compliance Research: Tax Gap Estimates for Tax Years 2014-2016, Publication 1415, 27 (August 2022) ("Tax Gap Estimates for 2014-2016").

[23] For 2014 to 2016, parts of the tax gap that affected these trust funds included the $7 billion annual self-employment tax non-filing gap; the $82 billion annual employment tax underreporting tax gap; the $5 billion annual employment tax underpayment gap; and the $6 billion annual underreporting of taxable Social Security benefits. *Id*, at 11, 20. Portions of unpaid SECA and FICA taxes, as well as the tax on taxable Social Security benefits, are directed to the Medicare Trust Fund if paid. Centers for Medicare and Medicaid Services, How is Medicare Funded? (last visited September 24, 2023); *see also* I.R.C. §§ 1401, 3101, 3111.

Some of this loss comes from tax avoidance overstepping the boundaries of the law into illegal tax evasion.

Broadening the federal tax base and shrinking the federal tax gap is a sound way to raise revenues and will put the federal budget and the critical priorities it funds on a more solid and lasting foundation:

- *Enhanced revenue can protect critical federal priorities from cuts, address long-term deficits, and finance new investments* to meet national challenges, including lifting the health and living standards of low-and moderate-income families; and supporting an aging population.
- *Well-designed measures to strengthen the tax base can support economic growth* by ensuring more resources flow to productive activity and preventing wasteful tax avoidance and evasion. Would-be tax avoiders and evaders should not gain an advantage over businesses that pay what they owe and choose to focus on their products, customers, and innovation rather than play tax games.
- *Strengthening the tax base complements proposals to raise tax rates:* each percentage point of tax would cause less economic and revenue waste from tax avoidance and evasion.
- *A stronger tax base can help both general revenues and dedicated revenue streams including the Medicare trust fund* (that has relied on general revenues from time to time).

Three ways lawmakers can secure a broader tax base and shrink the federal tax gap are:

1) Reject proposals currently on the table that would increase tax cheating and non-compliance and weaken the tax base. That means:
   a) *Maintain IRS base discretionary funding and do not subject IRS mandatory funding to more damaging cuts below levels agreed to in the debt ceiling deal.*
   b) *Do not undermine new tax compliance provisions* that will help honest filers comply with their tax obligations, help the IRS to detect tax cheating, and reduce random audits of taxpayers who have filed accurately.

c) *Build on, rather than reverse, the limited base broadening in the 2017 law.* Corporate base broadeners used to offset part of the cost of permanent corporate tax cuts should take effect and continue—or if weakened, the cost should be offset with other corporate tax base broadening or rate increases. Costly provisions that narrowed the tax base in ways that encourage tax avoidance—such as the 199A pass-through deduction and the doubled estate tax exemption—should expire on schedule. Base-protecting mechanisms such as the GILTI minimum tax should be strengthened.

1) *Address the "big three": the non-taxation of income from extraordinarily large fortunes; the non-taxation of certain foreign profits; and pass-through taxation.* Each of these areas combines a too-narrow tax base with major non-compliance issues. For example, ensuring that all pass-through business income of high-income taxpayers is subject to either the NIIT or SECA tax and ensuring that all the revenues flow to the relevant trust funds would directly help Medicare's finances.
2) *Choose from a large menu of big and small options to strengthen the tax base.* The Tax Law Center at NYU Law (Tax Law Center) has compiled a broader menu of options to strengthen the tax base, "Broadening the US Federal Tax Base," that the Tax Law Center has designed or analyzed in the course of our work (such as submitting on the Priority Guidance Plan and Green Book) and that we intend to update. These include closing the capital gains loophole for exchange-traded funds, strengthening the bipartisan Corporate Transparency Act's (CTA's) reporting requirements to ensure it more effectively addresses the most complex types of tax evasion and corruption, and extending broker reporting to high-value art transactions.

Part I: Federal Revenue and the State of the Tax Base

Federal tax revenue should rise. This is necessary to meet the fiscal challenges associated with an aging population, and to protect and enable investments that the nation needs to make to raise health and living standards for low-and moderate-income families; secure an innovative, dynamic, and inclusive economy; and address global challenges.

The long-run projected growth in federal spending stems primarily from the retirement of the baby boomers and the related rise in health care and retirement security costs.[24]

Federal revenues are currently about 18.4 percent of GDP, but CBO projects this to fall through 2025, and to rise only modestly afterwards. However, a large part of the projected rise is due to the scheduled expiration of large parts of the 2017 tax law, which some lawmakers are proposing to halt in full.[25] Revenues would be about 3 percent higher, as a percentage of GDP, without the two rounds of tax cuts first enacted under President Bush and then under President Trump: those tax cuts alone are enough to explain the entire projected increase in the debt-to-GDP ratio over the coming decade, as testimony explained to this Committee earlier this year.[26]

Revenues must rise to meet our national fiscal challenges and other priorities. Relative to the size of the economy, U.S. tax revenue is substantially lower than that of most other Organisation for Economic Co-operation and Development (OECD) countries.[27] Revenue measures can be paired with responsible policies to contain cost growth across the federal budget, like the provisions of the Inflation Reduction Act that allow Medicare to negotiate lower prices for certain drugs, which are estimated to deliver about $25 billion in savings through 2031.[28] A balanced combination of revenue increases and cost control—inside the Medicare trust fund and across the budget—can protect against spending cuts that would both increase hardship and undermine the nation's ability to secure an inclusive, sustainable, and dynamic economy.[29]

To increase federal revenues, addressing tax rates will need to be one part of the picture, which can include reversing some of the 2017 tax law's deep tax rate cuts for corporations, allowing rate cuts for high-income filers to

---

[24] Congressional Budget Office (CBO), The 2023 Long-Term Budget Outlook 6 (June 2023).

[25] *Id.* at 20.

[26] Brian Deese & David Kamin, *Principles for the 2025 Tax Debate*, Tax Notes (forthcoming) (manuscript at 5) (on file with author); Bobby Kogan, *The Rich Get Richer, Deficits Get Bigger: How Tax Cuts for the Wealthy and Corporations Drive National Debt,* Testimony Before the Senate Budget Committee n.xxvi (May 17, 2023).

[27] *See* Tax Policy Center (TPC), *Fiscal Facts: Total Tax Revenue for OECD Countries* (June 19, 2023); TPC, *Briefing Book (Federal Budget): How Do U.S. Taxes Compare Internationally?* (May 2020).

[28] CBO, How CBO Estimated the Budgetary Impact of Key Prescription Drug Provisions in the 2022 Reconciliation Act 11 (Feb. 17, 2023). CBO estimates that the negotiation program will lower Part D spending by $14 billion, Part B spending by $9 billion, and other federal spending by $1 billion. *Id.*

[29] *See* Paul Van de Water, Medicare Is Not "Bankrupt," CBPP (February 13, 2023).

expire, and considering proposals to increase tax rates on revenue sources dedicated to the Medicare trust fund and other specific parts of the budget.[30]

But the tax base should be strengthened in tandem, and this is the focus of my testimony. The tax base is not broad enough and too much tax that is owed goes unpaid.

It is convenient to look at base broadening and the tax gap as separate problems, but they are deeply linked, and the line between them is not always clear-cut. Carve-outs from the tax base attract aggressive tax avoidance seeking to push even more income into the special preferences and out of the tax base. In doing so, filers can blur or even step over the boundary of the law into outright tax evasion. Meanwhile, Treasury and IRS interpretations of the tax law that are overly generous to taxpayers but that are not the best application of the law can unnecessarily widen tax breaks, shrink the tax base, and hurt public finances in doing so.

1. The Tax Base Is Not Broad Enough

The tax base is *what* gets taxed at the relevant tax rate schedule. The bulk of federal revenues comes from taxes on incomes (both individual and corporate) and payrolls.

Various deductions, exclusions, and other preferential treatments carve income out of the federal tax base.[31] These targeted tax breaks for specific types of income or filers are sometimes called "tax expenditures,"[32] or "spending through the tax code" because their economic and budgetary impact is like a spending program designed to subsidize a particular activity.[33]

Tax expenditures shrink the tax base by reducing the amount of income taxed at normal tax rates. Individual and corporate tax expenditures are

---

30 *See* Department of the Treasury (Treasury), General Explanations of the Administration's Fiscal Year 2024 Revenue Proposals, 72-74 (March 9, 2023); U.S. Senate Committee on the Budget, Sen. Whitehouse: We Can Protect Social Security for All Without Cutting Benefits (August 12, 2023).

31 *See* Treasury, Tax Expenditures (last visited September 24, 2023).

32 TPC, *Briefing Book (Tax Expenditures): What Are Tax Expenditures and How Are They Structured?* (May 2020).

33 The Congressional Budget Act of 1974 requires that a list of "tax expenditures" be included in the budget and defines them for these purposes as "revenue losses attributable to provisions of the Federal tax laws which allow a special exclusion, exemption, or deduction from gross income or which provide a special credit, a preferential rate of tax, or a deferral of tax liability." *See* Congressional Budget and Impoundment Control Act of 1974, Pub. L. No. 93-344 §3(a)(3), 88 Stat. 297, 299 (1974).

estimated to cost about $1.5 trillion (about 6 percent of GDP) in FY2022,[34] more than the cost of Medicare and Medicaid combined, or either defense or non-defense discretionary spending.[35]

Tax expenditures, just like other types of federal spending, are not inherently sound or unsound policy.[36] But many carve-outs from the tax base are costly, fail to achieve their aims, and create new problems. Overall, the value of individual tax expenditures flows towards high-income filers that need little help or incentive to undertake the activities—such as building wealth through homeownership, education, or saving—that the subsidies are meant to support.[37] This makes them ineffective at achieving their purported goals while increasing income, wealth, and racial inequality.[38] On the business side, many business tax breaks are portrayed as benefiting "small businesses" and innovation but are in fact tilted towards large corporations that can use them for tax avoidance, giving them another unfair tax advantage over smaller and startup firms.[39]

Exclusions from the tax base can also attract tax avoidance, sheltering, and gaming that pulls investment away from more productive activities.[40]

---

[34] *See* Treasury, *supra* note 12; Bureau of Economic Analysis, Gross Domestic Product, Fourth Quarter and Year 2022 (Third Estimate), GDP by Industry, and Corporate Profits (March 30, 2023). Totals do not account for interactions.

[35] FY2022 outlays for Medicare, net of offsetting receipts, and Medicaid totaled $1.3 trillion. *See* CBO, The Budget and Economic Outlook: 2023 to 2033 14-15 (February 15, 2023). Defense discretionary spending was $746 billion, while nondefense discretionary spending was $910 billion. *Id.* at 17.

[36] For example, the Child Tax Credit is a tax expenditure that is a powerful tool for lifting families out of poverty. *See* CBPP, *Policy Basics: The Child Tax Credit* (December 7, 2022).

[37] The CBO estimates that in 2019 18% of the value of major individual income tax expenditures flowed to the highest-income 1 percent of filers. *See* CBO, The Distribution of Household Income, 2019 (November 2022). TPC estimates of individual income tax expenditures for 2022 are not aggregated. *See* TPC, *Individual Income Tax Expenditures (December 2022)* (December 2022). We are not aware of recently updated aggregate estimates that include effects of the Inflation Reduction Act.

[38] *See* CBPP, *Policy Basics: Federal Tax Expenditures* (December 8, 2020). For analysis of racial disparities in tax expenditures, *see* Assistant Secretary for Tax Policy Lily Batchelder & Deputy Assistant Secretary for Tax Analysis Greg Leiserson, Disparities in the Benefits of Tax Expenditures by Race and Ethnicity, Treasury (January 20, 2023).

[39] *See How to (Not) Support Small Businesses Through the Tax System*, The Tax Law Center at NYU Law (Tax Law Center) (June 9, 2023).

[40] This effect can be described as a reduction in "allocative efficiency." For a review of the empirical literature suggesting that allocative efficiency effects can be more substantial than supply-side impacts in the context of individual income tax reform, *see* William Gale & Andrew A. Samwick, *Effects of Income Tax Changes on Economic Growth*, Brookings Institution (February 1, 2016).

Prominent exclusions from the federal tax base that shrink it in unproductive ways are:

- *The ability to wipe out accumulated tax on the capital gains of assets held until death.* This means large incomes of the wealthiest filers never face income tax at any rate, either during their lifetime or their heirs' lifetimes.[41] Even capital gains and dividends that do face income tax get a lower tax rate than income from salaries, and combined with the complete exclusion of some capital gains from the tax base, these preferences for income from wealth are carve-outs from the individual income tax base.[42]
- *Large amounts of foreign income of large multinationals are entirely or partially exempt from the US tax base.* The 2017 tax law set up an international tax framework that affords complete exemptions[43] and zero or low rates to certain foreign income of US multinationals, meaning that it faces rates far below the 21 percent top domestic corporate tax rate.[44] Even with the requirement that some of those profits face a minimum level of tax under the new global intangible low-taxed income (GILTI) regime, these exclusions and reduced rates amount to a tax break on multinationals' foreign profits worth some $45 billion annually.[45] This is the largest corporate tax expenditure.[46] The US tax base also excludes specific types of foreign income including from foreign oil and gas extraction.[47]
- *Holes in payroll taxes and the "Medicare tax" on unearned income.* The Affordable Care Act enacted the "unearned income Medicare contribution" or NIIT to ensure that high-income filers—who earn most of their income from wealth rather than from wages and

---

[41] *See* Huang, *Building Back Better, supra* note 1 at 10 (October 6, 2021).

[42] *See, e.g.*, Congressional Research Service (CRS), Tax Expenditures: Compendium of Background Material on Individual Provisions 5, U.S. Senate Committee on the Budget (December 2022). Note that these numbers consider only permanent tax expenditures reported in FY2020.

[43] *See* Kimberly Clausing, *Profit Shifting Before and After the Tax Cuts and Jobs Act*, 73 National Tax Journal 4, 11 (2020).

[44] Huang, *How U.S. International Tax Policy Impacts American Workers, Jobs, and Investment, supra* note 1 at 2.

[45] *See* Joint Committee on Taxation (JCT), Estimates of Federal Tax Expenditures for Fiscal Years 2022-2026 32 (December 22, 2022).

[46] *See id.*

[47] *See* I.R.C. § 907; *see also* Huang, *How U.S. International Tax Policy Impacts American Workers, Jobs, and Investment, supra* note 1 at 3.

salaries—faced tax rates on their income comparable to the Medicare payroll tax rates faced by wages and salary earners. The 3.8 percent NIIT rate is the same as the 2.9 percent combined employee and employer Medicare payroll tax faced by all earners plus the 0.9 percent high-earner Medicare rate on wage and salary income. The NIIT means that most high-income taxpayers pay a 3.8 percent tax on income above $200,000 for a single filer or $250,000 for a married couple, either through employment taxes (FICA or SECA) or through the NIIT. FICA and SECA revenues flow to the Medicare trust fund, but NIIT revenues currently do not.

The NIIT somewhat reduces incentives for high-income filers to try to convert their salary and wages into other types of income in order to avoid FICA and SECA. The NIIT was originally intended to apply to all forms of income not covered by those employment and self-employment taxes,[48] but lawmakers left large gaps in this tax base that allow high-income filers to avoid facing any payroll tax or NIIT when their income flows through certain pass-through businesses.[49] Specifically, high-income filers who own limited partnerships or S corporations and are actively involved in the business can avoid both the NIIT *and* the additional 0.9 percent high-earner Medicare tax.[50]

There are many other large and small ways that the tax base has been shrunk. Many appear explicitly in tables and analyses of tax expenditures or revenue raising options prepared by congressional and administration estimators, such as the 1200-page compendium that the Congressional Research Service prepared for this Committee in December 2022.[51] Others are not as visible, because they flow from questionable regulatory decisions,[52] are

---

[48] *See* Jason Furman (@jasonfurman), X (formerly known as Twitter) (October 28, 2021, 12:13 PM), https://twitter.com/jasonfurman/status/1453756934985850889.

[49] *See* Karen C. Burke, *Exploiting the Medicare Tax Loophole*, 21 Fla. Tax Rev. 2 570, 606 (September 22, 2017).

[50] For full analysis of gaps in the bases of these taxes, *see* CRS, The 3.8% Net Investment Income Tax: Overview, Data, and Policy Options (June 30, 2023); Treasury Office of Tax Analysis, Gaps Between the Net Investment Income Tax Base and the Employment Tax Base (April 14, 2016).

[51] CRS, *supra* note 23.

[52] Regulatory decisions can show up in the estimate of a broader tax expenditure, but not be separately listed.

smaller or hard to estimate, raise difficult methodological questions, or are newly emerging.[53] Part II.2 returns to this broader set of options.

2. The Tax Base Is too Leaky

Before the enactment of the Inflation Reduction Act (IRA), the "tax gap" of federal taxes owed under law but not paid amounted to $496 billion annually from 2014 to 2016,[54] an estimated $540 billion annually between 2017 and 2019,[55] and approximately $7 trillion over the coming decade.[56] About 28 percent of the individual income tax underreporting gap is attributable to the highest-income one percent of filers.[57]

---

53 For example, tax expenditure estimates do not regularly attempt to estimate payroll tax expenditures, or focus on the payroll tax implications of provisions that are also individual income tax expenditures. Difficulties involved include considering and estimating the tax expenditure on benefit eligibility (especially in Social Security). *See* JCT, JCX-22-22, Estimates Of Federal Tax Expenditures For Fiscal Years 2022-2026 4 n.8 (2022); CBO, The Distribution of Major Tax Expenditures in 2019, 33-34 (October, 2021). This has the somewhat counterintuitive effect that provisions like the NIIT, which policymakers consider primarily as a measure to address the payroll tax base issues, are counted as "negative" tax expenditures for the income tax. It also means that measures used to plug holes in the base via an alternative default tax base (such as the Corporate Alternative Minimum Tax (CAMT)) can be treated as "negative" tax expenditures, but carve-outs from the alternative tax base (such as the exclusion of depreciation from the CAMT base) are not. Finally, some effects that are arguably tax expenditures can appear when new business and technology developments do not fit neatly into the default tax rules. For example, the current exclusion of digital assets from the "wash sale" rules, *see* Taylor Cranor & Mike Kaercher, *Congress Should Extend Wash Sales Rules to Digital Assets*, Tax Law Center (April 17, 2023), is arguably a departure from the normal tax base but one that has only become evident as the market for digital assets has developed.

54 IRS, *supra* note 3, at 11. This is the "gross" tax gap for the most recent years available. The net tax gap, subtracts the amount of the tax gap the IRS anticipates will be recovered and was $428 billion annually between 2014 and 2016. *Id.* IRS estimates may understate the true amount of tax non-compliance because they cannot account for certain types of sophisticated avoidance and evasion. *See* IRS Updates Tax Gap Estimates; New Data Points the Way Toward Enhancing Taxpayer Service, Compliance Efforts, IRS-2022-192 (October 28, 2022) ("IRS Updates Tax Gap Estimates").

55 IRS, *supra* note 3, at 27. The net tax gap over the same period is estimated at $470 billion annually. *Id.*

56 Treasury, The American Families Plan Tax Compliance Agenda, at 3 (May 2021).

57 Andrew Johns & Joel Slemrod, *The Distribution of Income Tax Noncompliance*, 63 Nat'l Tax J. 397, 406 (2010); Jason DeBacker et al., *Tax Noncompliance and Measures of Income Inequality*, Tax Notes Federal 7-8 (February 16, 2020). Estimates of the total tax gap and the share attributable to the highest income filers vary and are difficult to make given limited sightlines of the IRS into some major categories of non-compliance (including offshore income, digital assets, and income held through complex layers of entities). *See* Daniel Reck et al., Washington Center for Equitable Growth, *Tax Evasion at the Top of the U.S. Income Distribution and How to Fight It* (March 22, 2021); IRS Updates Tax Gap Estimates, *supra* note 35.

These leaks directly deplete the Medicare trust fund. Taxes owed, but not paid, to the Medicare, Social Security, and Unemployment Insurance trust funds total some $100 billion each year (IRS estimates do not currently divide this impact between the funds).[58]

A striking example of potential tax non-compliance leading to losses from the trust funds is currently before the courts. The IRS announced a campaign in 2018 to examine arrangements where individual partners have "inappropriately claimed to qualify as 'limited partners' not subject to SECA tax."[59] This illustrates how a tax base that is not broad enough can invite wasteful tax avoidance as filers try to push their income out of the base—and how aggressive tax avoidance can then also blur or overstep the line into unlawful tax evasion. Currently, Point 72 Asset Management, a hedge fund founded and owned by billionaire Steve Cohen, is challenging a tax assessment on $344 million of earnings for failing to pay SECA.[60] The case is one of several objections to assessments arising from the IRS campaign.[61]

A decade of damaging cuts to IRS enforcement funding beginning in 2010 left the IRS unable to adequately fulfill its basic function of upholding the tax law and ensuring that filers pay what they owe. Before the recent IRA, the IRS lost about 40% of its auditors, including those experienced enough to review the most complex returns of large businesses and high net worth individuals.[62] At some sites, the IRS even lacked basic supplies, such as pens and staplers.[63] Under resourcing also hampered the IRS's ability to do the research needed to understand the root causes of the tax gap and new emerging areas of non-compliance, including offshore tax evasion and tax evasion involving digital assets.[64]

---

[58] *See supra* text accompanying note 4.

[59] *Large Businesses and International Active Campaigns*, IRS (September 15, 2023). The IRS has paused the campaign while these cases are being concluded. *See* Kristen A. Parillo, *IRS Pauses New Audits Under SECA Campaigns*, Tax Notes (September 26, 2023).

[60] Miles Weiss, *Steve Cohen Fights a $10 Million Tax Bill to Derail an IRS Plan*, Bloomberg News (August 18, 2023).

[61] *See* Respondent's Motion for Partial Summary Judgment, *Soroban Capital Partners LP v. Comm.*, No. 16218-22 (T.C. March 1, 2023); Petition for Readjustment of Partnership Items Under Code Section 6226, *Denham Capital Management LP v. Comm.*, No. 9973-23 (T.C. June 21, 2023).

[62] *See* Chuck Marr et al., *Rebuilding the IRS Would Reduce the Tax Gap, Help Replenish Depleted Revenue Base* (December 16, 2022).

[63] Alan Rappeport, *Decades of Neglect Leave I.R.S. in Tax Season 'Chaos'*, New York Times (March 4, 2022); *see also* Michael Kaercher & Chye-Ching Huang, *Cracks in the System: The Consequences of Underfunding the IRS*, Tax Law Center (April 15, 2022).

[64] *See* Treasury Inspector General for Tax Administration, *Actions are Needed to Improve the Completeness, Development, and Review of IRS Tax Gap Estimates* 6 (March 23, 2023).

To rebuild and transform taxpayer service and ensure that high-income filers and large corporations pay more of the taxes they already owe, the IRA provided the IRS an additional $80 billion to be spent through the end of 2031. CBO estimated that this funding would raise a *net* $180.4 billion between 2022 and 2031 by simply collecting more tax revenue that is already owed under the law. This is a rare example of spending that pays for itself many times over.

The debt limit deal undermined this effort. If implemented, it will result in $21.39 billion in cuts to IRA funding and *add* to deficits by a net of some $20 billion over the next ten years in increased tax non-compliance.[65]

It would be a mistake to think that because the IRS has some ability to change the timing of its spending of IRA money so that cuts are accounted for on the "back end" that the damage to its ability to improve tax compliance and service will not be felt far earlier.

The reason that lawmakers provided the IRA money as a mandatory stream over a decade was to enable transformational projects—IT upgrades and systems modernization, hiring and training expert staff, and dramatic improvements to taxpayer services[66]—that need multiple years of funding to plan and execute well, and some confidence of continued funding. By cutting some 27% of the IRA funding, the deal moves forward a cliff in IRS funding to FY2030 or sooner.[67]

A nearer cliff may cause the IRS to commit to less ambitious transformation. As it approaches, it will be impossible for the IRS to responsibly hire or plan for multi-year projects as though the funds will continue, and the IRS will be forced to slow or reduce compliance and service improvements. The IRS cannot move faster to compensate: its workforce and systems are depleted, limiting how quickly it can hire and train new staff without taking existing staff off frontline activities and harming service and compliance. House proposals to cut IRS funding even below the levels agreed to in the debt ceiling deal would worsen the damage.[68]

---

65 Thalia Spinrad & Chye-Ching Huang, *Impact of House and Senate IRS Funding Proposals,* Tax Law Center (July 18, 2023).

66 Chuck Marr, Samantha Jacoby & Jabari Cook, *Success of the IRS Rebuilding and Tax Gap Reduction Effort Depends on Sufficient Funding Through Annual Appropriations*, CBPP (December 7, 2022).

67 Thalia Spinrad & Chye-Ching Huang, *supra* note 46; Chye-Ching Huang, Thalia Spinrad, & Kathleen Bryant, *Debt Ceiling Deal's Cuts to IRS Funding Bring the IRS Funding Cliff Closer: Appropriators Should Not Compound Harm*, Tax Law Center (June 28, 2023). Moreover, House bills have proposed to rescind all of the remaining IRA funds and thus would, if enacted, move the funding cliff up to FY2024. *Id.*

68 Thalia Spinrad & Chye-Ching Huang, *supra* note 46.

Some lawmakers are also proposing to undo or undermine the statutory tools the IRS will need to focus on the most egregious non-compliance rather than random audits of honest and accurate filers.[69] New bipartisan "third party" information reporting requirements on digital asset brokers will allow those who invest in digital assets to track their income and comply with their tax filing obligations. And new information reporting applying to the corporations that run online peer-to-peer payment platforms will increase voluntary compliance by helping gig workers and others who use these platforms to track and report income. These measures can help discourage the use of payment platforms or digital assets to hide income and evade taxes.[70] They can also help the IRS to steer its audit and other compliance activity away from audits of accurate filers and towards those who try to deliberately evade taxes on income generated through online payment platforms or digital assets.[71] These measures should be implemented, not weakened.

Part II: Forging a Strong Tax Base

Lawmakers can strengthen the tax base in four key ways.

1. First, do no harm by rejecting proposals that will increase tax non-compliance and shrink the tax base. That means:

a) *Maintain IRS base discretionary funding and do not subject IRS mandatory funding to more damaging cuts below levels agreed to in the debt ceiling deal.* The US Senate Committee on Appropriations has passed a proposal setting IRS base funding for FY2024 at a nominal freeze.[72] This is $1.8 billion below the level requested by the President's Budget and does not keep pace with inflation. This will require more repurposing of IRA funds just to fill the hole in the base levels of operations that further IRS transformation would then build

[69] Grace Henley et al., *Undermining Information Reporting Requirements for "Gig" Companies and Other Online Platforms Would Hurt Honest Filers, Cost Revenue, and Reward Tax Evaders,* Tax Law Center (June 12, 2023); Michael Kaercher & Taylor Cranor, *Taxing Digital Assets: What's at Stake?*, Tax Law Center (August 4, 2022).

[70] Grace Henley et al., *supra* note 50; Chye-Ching Huang, *U.S. Will Likely Lose Billions Due to Unacceptably Long Delay for Digital Asset Reporting Requirements,* Tax Law Center (August 24, 2023).

[71] Grace Henley et al., *supra* note 50; Kaercher & Cranor *supra* note 50.

[72] Chuck Marr & Samantha Jacoby, *Bipartisan Senate Action Passes Minimal Test for IRS Funding While Multiple House Republican Bills Fail,* CBPP (July 20, 2023).

on.[73] This is far less damaging, however, than the House proposals that would effectively result in the rollback of all IRA funding.[74]

b) *Do not undermine new tax compliance provisions that will help honest filers comply with their tax obligations and will help the IRS detect tax cheating while reducing random audits of compliance taxpayers.* This means rejecting proposals to repeal or weaken 1099-K information reporting for third-party settlement organizations (requiring online marketplaces and "gig" platforms to provide information reporting to document business transactions over $600) and section 6045 cryptocurrency broker reporting.[75]

c) *Build on, rather than reverse, the limited base broadening included in the 2017 law.* The 2017 tax law included some base broadening measures, such as the elimination of business expense deductions for entertainment, and limitations to individual tax expenditures including itemized deductions.[76] Its phase-ins and sunsets mean decisions must be made about what parts of the law to retain, fix, and let expire.[77] In general, lawmakers should retain and build on sound measures that broadened the federal tax base—but let expire or scale back costly, inefficient and regressive provisions that shrank the tax base.[78] For example:

- *Corporate base broadening measures in the 2017 tax law should be allowed to take effect and strengthened.* For example, the 2017 tax law introduced a stronger limitation on deducting interest expenses to 30 percent of adjusted taxable income for businesses with gross

---

[73] Spinrad & Huang, *supra* note 46.

[74] *Id.*

[75] Kaercher & Cranor, *supra* note 50; Mike Kaercher & Taylor Cranor, *IRS Issues Sound Guidance on Taxation of Cryptocurrency Consistent with TLC's Recommendations,* Tax Law Center (June 21, 2023).

[76] *See* CRS, R45092, The 2017 Tax Revision (P.L. 115-97): Comparison to 2017 Tax Law (2018) (providing a summary of TJCA's provisions, including base broadeners).

[77] If all of the net tax cuts set to expire in 2017 are made permanent without any offsets, they will cost roughly $3.5 trillion over the next decade, representing roughly 1% of GDP. Households in the 95th-99th percentiles would reap the largest benefits and the top 1% would disproportionately benefit. Deese & Kamin, *supra* note 7, at 5. The Tax Law Center and other experts have written about how these tax cuts should be addressed more broadly. *See* Huang, *Testimony*, *supra* note 1; Chuck Marr, *2025 Tax Debate Begins, Offers Opportunity for Course Correction*, CBPP (March 7, 2023); Deese & Kamin, *supra* note 7.

[78] Huang, *Testimony, supra* note 1; Marr, *supra* note 58.

revenue over $29 million annually.[79] If this new limitation were reversed, and full expensing for R&E were restored in tandem, certain businesses would again be able to both claim deductions for investments *and* be able to deduct more of their interest costs on their borrowing. That combination would be especially valuable for the leveraged buyout ("private equity") industry that relies on being able to load up acquired companies with debt.[80] It would also be valuable for large multinational corporations that avoid taxes by making large interest payments to their foreign affiliates.[81] Undoing the limitation on interest deductions for large businesses would also further increase the federal tax system's tilt towards financing investments with debt rather than equity.[82] Innovation can be more effectively supported through other policies.[83]

If Congress decides that it nevertheless wishes to reverse part of the 2017 tax law's corporate base broadening, it should trade off a reduced base with a higher rate or other base broadening. That was the trade reflected in the 2017 tax law, and given revenue needs, undercutting the base without other base broadening or raising rates is an unacceptable combination.

Part II.2 also discusses how the GILTI minimum tax should be strengthened to protect the corporate tax base.

- Provisions that shrank the tax base in ways that give large tax cuts to wealthy filers and encourage tax avoidance should expire.[84] These include:

---

[79] The limitations on deducting interest expense under section 163(j) went into effect in 2018. Tax Cuts and Jobs Act, Pub. L. No. 115-97, § 13301, 131 Stat. 2054, 2117-21. The requirement to amortize research and experimental expenditures went into effect in 2022. *Id.* at § 13206, 131 Stat. 2111-13. There are also exceptions for certain expenses. *See* section 163(j)(5). Some lawmakers are proposing to reinstate a weaker limitation on interest expenses based on EBITDA. Doug Sword, *Senate, House Backers Try to Push 163(j) Relief Into Limelight,* Tax Notes (September 15, 2023).

[80] Michael Kaercher, *American Ingenuity: Promoting Innovation Through the Tax Code,* Testimony for the Committee on Small Business, Subcommittee on Economic Growth, Tax, and Capital Access (June 6, 2023).

[81] *Id.*

[82] *See* Treasury, Effective Marginal Tax Rates (EMTRs) on new investment under Current Law and Policy (November 2021). Analysts across the political spectrum have recognized this tax tilt towards debt financing as a problem, and some have proposed even stronger limitations on interest deductibility. See American Compass, *Rebuilding American Capitalism: A Handbook for Conservative Policymakers* 58 (2023) (proposing eliminating deductions for interest expense).

[83] *See* Kaercher, *supra* note 61.

[84] *See* Huang, *Testimony*, *supra* note 1; Marr, *supra* note 58; Deese & Kamin, *supra* note 7.

- *The section 199A "pass through" deduction,* a special lower rate on most income earned through pass-through business entities. If kept in place, it will cost $700 billion over 2026-2035.[85] More than half of its value goes to the highest-income one percent of filers, and a full quarter goes to the highest-income one out of every thousand tax filers.[86] Despite supposed guardrails, tax advisors have called section 199A a "gaping hole" in the code.[87] It is "the very worst kind of tax policy, picking winners and losers haphazardly in a complex tax provision, and then generating significant incentives for people to rearrange their businesses to try to get on the right side of the line."[88] The deduction did not provide any boost in economic activity in the two years following its enactment, research suggests.[89]
- *The doubled exclusion from estate and gift taxes.* The 2017 tax law doubled the amount that a wealthy couple can pass tax-free to their heirs from $11 million to $22 million (adjusted for inflation). Extending this would cost $125 billion between 2026 and 2033.[90] The doubled exclusion potentially *more than* doubles the amount of money it allows wealthy individuals to pass on tax-free. Individuals can make lifetime gifts of assets to donees, and those assets may appreciate over the donee's lifetime—and such gifts are also key to some of the most complex tax avoidance techniques used to push large fortunes out of the transfer tax base.[91]

---

85 Chuck Marr & Samantha Jacoby, *The Pass-Through Deduction is Tilted Heavily to the Wealthy, Is Costly, and Should Expire as Scheduled,* CBPP (June 8, 2023).

86 TPC, *Tax Benefit of the Deduction for Qualified Business Income, Baseline: Current Law, Distribution of Federal Tax Changes by Expanded Cash Income Percentile, 2022* (December 29, 2022).

87 Emily Horton, *Tax Planner: Drive Wealthy Clients Through "Gaping Hole" in Tax Code,* CBPP (May 31, 2018).

88 Samantha Jacoby, *Repealing Flawed "Pass-Through" Deduction Should Be Part of Recovery Legislation*, CBPP (June 1, 2021) (quoting David Kamin). Similarly, former JCT Chief of Staff Edward Kleinbard called it "Congress' worst idea ever." *Id.*

89 Lucas Goodman, et al., *How Do Business Owners Respond to a Tax Cut? Examining the 199A Deduction for Pass-Through Firms* 1-4 (National Bureau of Economic Research, Working Paper No. 28680, 2022).

90 CBO, Budgetary Outcomes Under Alternative Assumptions About Spending and Revenue Table 1 (May 2023).

91 *See, e.g.,* Jesse Drucker & Maureen Farrell, *A Lavish Tax Dodge for the Ultrawealthy Is Easily Multiplied,* New York Times (December 28, 2021); Barbara Bryniarski, *Helping a Client Benefit from an Intentionally Defective Grantor Trust*, Tax Adviser (November 11, 2021).

- *Individual base broadening should be strengthened.* The 2017 tax law made changes to the individual income tax structure, including a doubled standard deduction, additional limits on certain itemized deductions, and paring back the Alternative Minimum Tax (which was originally intended as a broader backstop to the too-narrow normal tax base).[92] These interacting changes limited the cost of itemized deductions but made some (such as the mortgage interest deduction) even more concentrated on the highest-income filers, and so likely less effective and efficient at achieving their purported policy aims.[93] The limitation on the State and Local Tax Deduction (SALT) has also been implemented in a way that encourages states to support their high-income filers to engage in aggressive and complicated tax avoidance using pass-through entities to avoid the cap, reducing its effectiveness and creating new disparities between types of businesses, filers, and states.[94] Depending on how lawmakers address expiring individual tax provisions more broadly, they may have an opportunity to improve the individual tax base in ways that reduce wasteful avoidance, raise revenues, and make any retained tax preferences more efficient and effective.

2. Address three glaring areas that combine a tax base that isn't broad enough with major tax non-compliance: (a) the non-taxation of income from extraordinarily large fortunes; (b) the non-taxation of certain foreign profits; and (c) pass-through taxation.

(a) Ensure income from extraordinarily large fortunes faces at least some tax and reduce preferences for income from wealth over work. Much of the income generated by wealth is currently carved out of the US tax base. Income from wealth can entirely disappear from the federal income tax base if it comes from assets (such as stocks and bonds) that have grown in value but have not been realized (e.g., sold)

---

[92] *See* CRS, *supra* note 57, at 8-19.

[93] *See* Howard Gleckman, *The TCJA Shifted the Benefits of Itemized Deductions to Higher-Income Households*, Forbes (October 16, 2018); TPC, *Briefing Book: How did the TCJA change the standard deduction and itemized deductions?* (May 2020).

[94] The 2017 tax law includes a $10,000 limitation on SALT deductions. Certain states have created "workarounds" by allowing partnerships and S corporations to pay state income taxes on behalf of partners or owners. *See* Richard Rubin, *The SALT Cap Has a $20 Billion Hole*, Wall Street Journal (August 27, 2023). This could be addressed with guidance or legislation. *See* Daniel Hemel, *The Passthrough Entity Tax Scandal* 26-28 (New York University Law and Economics Research Paper, No. 23-01, 2023).

during the lifetime of the owner.[95] Combined with exclusions and other holes in the estate and gift taxes, this can allow income from extraordinary fortunes to not be included in the US tax base over decades, lifetimes, and generations.[96] Other carve-outs for income from wealth include tax rates as low as zero percent.[97] This array of tax benefits for income from wealth goes overwhelmingly (and sometimes exclusively) to the already very wealthy and entrenches and exacerbates racial wealth disparities.[98]

There are many ways to bring more income from wealth into the US tax base.[99] A key priority should be ensuring that income from the gain in assets faces at least some income tax, and various proposals to address this problem are superior to current law.[100] For example, President Biden's proposal to treat unrealized capital gains as taxable income for the wealthiest people in the country would raise $437 billion over 2024-2033.[101]

(b) Ensure that less of the foreign income of large US multinationals escapes the US tax base. The cost to the public of subsidizing the foreign profits of US multinationals is about $60 billion annually.[102] That subsidy takes the form of excluding some of that income entirely from the US tax base and from lower tax rates on foreign profits (between zero and 10.5 percent) compared to the 21 percent tax rate on domestic profits.[103] This invites US multinationals to try to siphon profits out of the US tax base and out of the tax bases of other countries where they have customers or do business, and into low-taxed "tax haven" countries like Ireland and Bermuda. Multinationals

---

[95] *See* Harry L. Gutman, *Taxing Gains at Death,* Tax Notes Federal (January 11, 2021).

[96] *See* Lily L. Batchelder & David Kamin, *Taxing the Rich: Issues and Options* 3-7 (February 1, 2020) (unpublished manuscript).

[97] *Id.* at 6.

[98] *See id.*; Chuck Marr, Samantha Jacoby & Kathleen Bryant, *Substantial Income of Wealthy Households Escapes Annual Taxation Or Enjoys Special Tax Breaks*, CBPP (November 13, 2019); Chye-Ching Huang & Roderick Taylor, *How the Federal Tax Code Can Better Advance Racial Equity*, CBPP (July 25, 2019); Dorothy Brown, *The Whiteness of Wealth: How the Tax System Impoverishes Black Americans and How We Can Fix It* (2021).

[99] *See* Batchelder & Kamin, *supra* note 77.

[100] *See* Huang, *Building Back Better*, *supra* note 1, at 9-10.

[101] Treasury, *supra* note 11 at 82, 214.

[102] CRS, *supra* note 23, at 43.

[103] *See id.*, at 43-45; Jane G. Gravelle, CRS, IF11943, GILTI: Proposed Changes in the Taxation of Global Intangible Low-Taxed Income 1 (2021). The GILTI rate is scheduled to increase to 13.125% in 2026. Gravelle, *supra*, at 1.

report about 56% of their income in major tax havens, about the same share as they did before the 2017 tax law.[104]

Multinational tax non-compliance is usually less about outright tax evasion than corporations trying to use regulations and the courts to stretch the boundaries of their ability to move profits out of the US tax base, and an understaffed IRS can have limited ability to push back.[105]

Lawmakers can adopt reforms to include more of the foreign profits of US multinationals in the tax base. A key way would be to build on the GILTI provisions of the 2017 tax law. GILTI takes a sound basic approach of attempting to ensure that foreign profits of US multinationals are included in the US tax base by having to face at least some minimum level of tax. GILTI provided the blueprint for the 15 percent minimum tax that is now at the heart of the deal to address multinational tax avoidance by 143 countries and jurisdictions including the US.[106]

But the GILTI rate is too far below the tax rate on profits earned in the US, and, due to flaws in its design, the regime excludes too much foreign income that which leads to the perverse outcome that it can make the US the least attractive place to locate investments or profits from a tax perspective.

The US can plug these holes in its tax base by strengthening GILTI and other parts of its international tax regime, through such proposals as those in the Biden Administration's budget that would raise over $1 trillion between 2024 and 2033.[107] That would also bring the US into compliance with the Inclusive Framework deal that the EU, Japan, and other major trading partners are moving to implement.[108]

If the US does not ensure that this income is subject to some minimum

[104] Kimberly Clausing, Testimony Before the US Senate Committee on the Budget (April 18, 2023); Wendy Edelberg, Chye-Ching Huang & Rose Jenkins, *Six Economic Facts on International Corporate Taxation*, The Hamilton Project (June 2022).

[105] *See, e.g.*, Jesse Drucker & Jim Tankersley, *How Big Companies Won New Tax Breaks From the Trump Administration*, New York Times (December 30, 2019); Joseph Walker & Richard Rubin, *Amgen Fights IRS over $10.7 Billion Tax Bill*, Wall Street Journal (August 1, 2022).

[106] OECD, *Members of the OECD/G20 Inclusive Framework on BEPS* (June 9, 2023).

[107] Treasury, *supra* note 11 at 211.

[108] David Kamin, Rebecca Kysar, & Chye-Ching Huang, *A (Less Rocky) Path Forward on International Corporate Tax Reform*, Tax Law Center (December 16, 2022); Ernst & Young, *Japan Enacts 2023 Tax Reform Bill Including Legislation to Implement IIR to Align with OECD BEPS 2.0 Pillar Two* (March 30, 2023).

inclusion in tax base then, under the global agreement, other countries will, and will enjoy the benefit of that revenue.[109] There is no reason for the US to give up revenue that it could instead use to meet national priorities.

Reducing multinationals' ability to shift profits offshore can also help create a fairer competitive environment for US businesses that are unable or unwilling to use tax avoidance as a business strategy. Instead of sinking resources into a tax-avoidance arms race, companies will be able to focus more on customers, products, and innovation.

(c) Close holes in passthrough regimes. Over 50 percent of business profits now flow through "pass-through" entities rather than through corporations subject to the corporate income tax.[110] Research has found that over 60 percent of pass-through income earned by individuals flows to the top 1 percent of filers.[111] There are many deliberate and accidental holes in the tax base specifically involving pass-throughs that should be plugged. Repealing section 199A and addressing the pass-through workarounds in the SALT cap is discussed above.

The President's FY2024 budget proposes to close the holes in the Medicare payroll taxes and NIIT, raising $306 billion over ten years.[112] Another proposal in the President's budget would increase the rate on Medicare payroll, self-employment, and NIIT taxes for filers with incomes over $400,000 from 3.8 to 5 percent, raising $344 billion over ten years.[113] The proposal would also dedicate all NIIT revenues to the Medicare trust fund.[114]

---

109 Kimberly A. Clausing, *The Revenue Consequences of Pillar 2: Five Key Considerations*, Tax Notes (July 24, 2023).

110 Author's calculations using IRS, Corporation Income Tax Returns Complete Report 1-3 (2019); IRS, SOI Tax Stats – Partnership Statics by Entity Type Table 9b; IRS, SOI Tax Stats – Nonfarm Sole Proprietorship Statics, Business Receipts, Selected Deductions, and Net Income; IRS, SOI Tax Stats Individual Income Tax Returns Complete Report (Publication 1304), Table A, Row 57 (2019).

111 *See* Michael Cooper et al., *Business in the United States: Who Owns It, and How Much Tax Do They Pay?*, 30 Tax Policy and the Economy 91, 94 (2016). *But see* Natasha Sarin, Treasury, *The Case for a Robust Attack on the Tax Gap* (September 7, 2021) (suggesting that 35 percent of corrected partnership and S-Corporation income flows to those with a corrected adjusted gross income of $500,000 and over).

112 Treasury, *supra* note 11 at 214. *See also* Paul N. Van de Water, *President Biden's 2024 Budget Would Strengthen, Improve Medicare*, CBPP (May 3, 2023).

113 Treasury, *supra* note 11 at 214.

114 *Id.* at 75-76.

Lawmakers can also address other problems with partnerships—a form of pass-through controlling more than $30 trillion in assets and vastly outnumbering public firms.[115] Partnership taxation currently combines complexity, inconsistency in the system, and optionality. That means leeway for large partnerships to choose what revenue and expenses are counted by the partnership and how they are allocated between different partners. Reforms could seek to move results closer to economic reality, reduce known inconsistencies, and reduce optionality in ways that would make the regime more administrable.[116]

Passthroughs are also a key source of tax non-compliance, thought to account for $130 billion of unpaid owed taxes annually in the most recent tax gap estimates, a full 26 percent of the tax gap, and more than three times as large as corporate tax noncompliance.[117] IRS and academic research assumes that the share of the tax gap attributable to pass-throughs is about as concentrated among high-income filers as reported pass-through income.[118] But recent research suggests that passthrough tax evasion may be especially underestimated for high-income filers because of the difficulty the IRS currently has tracing partnership income to its true owners.[119]

Some partnerships are owned through circular structures of partnerships owning partnerships owning other partnerships,[120] or partnerships that "resemble 'spiderwebs' with groups of related entities and clusters of overlapping partners."[121] So, "complexity of partnership structures makes them an apt vehicle for business tax

---

[115] Emily Black et al., *The Spiderweb of Partnership Tax Structures* 1 (February 24,2023) (unpublished manuscript).

[116] For some examples of approaches to partnership reform, see Press Release, US Senate Committee on Finance, Wyden Unveils Proposal to Close Loopholes Allowing Wealthy Investors, Mega-Corporations to Use Partnerships to Avoid Paying Tax (September 10, 2021); Monte A. Jackel, *Is It (Finally) Time? Reforming Subchapter K*, Tax Notes Today Federal (March 29, 2021).

[117] IRS, *supra* note 3, at 11.

[118] John Guyton et al., *Tax Evasion at the Top of the Income Distribution* 28 (National Bureau of Economic Research, Working Paper No. 28542, 2021). This may understate the percentage of the pass-through tax gap attributable to the one percent, as noncompliance may be higher at the top of the income distribution. *Id.*

[119] *See* Guyton et al., *supra* note 99, at 26.

[120] Corey Husak, *The Sources and Size of Tax Evasion in the United States*, Center for Equitable Growth (May 14, 2021).

[121] Black et al., *supra* note 96 at 2.

planning."[122] Addressing non-compliance within this sector is therefore important for addressing tax under-reporting.

To sum up, lawmakers can improve the pass-through tax base and tax compliance in three main ways:

(a) Remove pass-through tax breaks and clean up underlying rules. As noted above, lucrative tax breaks for pass-throughs as well as complex underlying rules may not only lead to revenue lost directly, but also encourage aggressive tax avoidance that can step over into non-compliance as filers search for these tax savings.

(b) Ensure the IRS continues to have the resources needed to increase the number and quality of audits on partnerships and other pass-throughs. Increasing the coverage and quality of both operational and research audits can help both the IRS and lawmakers to understand other steps needed to secure the pass-through tax base. IRA funding has already enabled the IRS to establish a special work unit to focus on large and complex pass-throughs.[123104]

(c) Improve tools for understanding and addressing pass-through non-compliance, including closing holes in information reporting. Not only are pass-through regimes often complex, but much of the income that flows through pass-throughs is not subject to information reporting. Lawmakers can provide the IRS with information reporting tools that encourage voluntary compliance and allow the IRS to identify the most egregious forms of tax evasion using pass-throughs. One option is to strengthen the bipartisan Corporate Transparency Act (discussed below).

(3) Choose from a large menu of big and small options to address problematic avoidance/non-compliance. The Tax Law Center has compiled several dozen options to strengthen the tax base that we have either designed or analyzed in "Broadening the US Federal Tax Base." The Tax Law Center's development and analysis of these options draws on the deep tax practice, tax administration, and research expertise of our staff, and our networks of public interest minded tax lawyers, accountants, researchers, and market actors. We have proposed or analyzed these base broadening options in the course of our work to date including submitting proposals for consideration in the Green

---

[122] *Id.* at 5.

[123] Press Release, IRS, IRS to establish special pass-through organization to help with high-income compliance efforts; new workgroup to blend current employees and new hires to focus on complex partnerships, other key areas (September 20, 2023).

Book and the regulatory Priority Guidance Plan. Examples of base-broadening options included in this compilation[124] are:

Improving the bipartisan Corporate Transparency Act to identify tax evasion and other criminal activity using pass-throughs. Lawmakers took a sound bipartisan step by enacting the CTA in response to the Panama Papers leak, which highlighted the use of shell companies to hide wealth from tax and law enforcement agencies. The CTA establishes a registry of the ultimate owners of certain entities that is available to the IRS and other regulators. The registry covers many corporations and LLCs but does not currently include most general partnerships, trust arrangements, or other entities with no state filing requirement. The most egregious tax evasion linked with corruption, sanctions evasion and other criminal activities is likely to flow towards the pass-throughs and other entities left in the shadows, unless lawmakers act. The Tax Law Center has proposed paths forward.[125]

Repealing the tax exemption for in-kind redemptions of exchange-traded funds (ETFs): Under section 852(b)(6), if an ETF or other regulated investment company distributes appreciated securities or other property, no gain recognition is required. Section 852(b)(6) allows deferral and even complete avoidance of tax on gains in ways that investors investing independently and even through mutual funds cannot achieve. This allows for extreme forms of tax avoidance such as "heartbeat trades," in which investment banks partner with ETFs to cycle large stock portfolios into funds and then quickly out of them using in-kind redemptions to avoid capital gains tax. The flow of funds into ETFs is driven disproportionately by high-net-worth individuals. Congress should repeal the exemption in section 852(b)(6) for regulated investment companies that allows them to distribute appreciated property in kind to a redeeming shareholder without realizing capital gains. JCT estimates that closing this loophole would raise $205 billion over 10 years.[126]

---

[124] Many other compilations of potential base broadening options include Treasury's "Green Books," tax reform proposals, and CBO's "Budget Options." Ours focuses on options that the Tax Law Center has developed or analyzed recently in consultation with other experts and includes links to relevant Tax Law Center publications such as our Priority Guidance Plan submissions and analyses of proposed legislation.

[125] Sophia Yan, *How Strengthening the Corporate Transparency Act Can Help the IRS Follow the Money*, Just Security (April 12, 2022); Sophia Yan, *Budget Represents a Missed Opportunity to Promote Corporate Transparency Act Reforms*, Tax Law Center (April 19, 2023); Tax Law Center, Comment Letter on Beneficial Ownership Information Reporting Requirements (February 7, 2022).

[126] Sam Potter, Katherine Greifeld & Elaine Chen, *ETF Industry Risks Losing Key Tax Edge as Democrat Whets Knife*, Bloomberg (September 14, 2021).

Applying the wash sale rules to digital assets: Investors can currently use wash sales to harvest losses on digital assets without changing their investment portfolio. Long-standing rules in section 1091 prevent taxpayers from engaging in wash sales to harvest losses on stocks and securities. However, lawmakers have not modified section 1091 to apply to digital assets. Congress should close the loophole that allows digital asset investors to access this aggressive tax planning practice. Extending the wash sale rules to digital assets, along with other changes, including addressing related party transactions in the wash sale rules, would raise $23.5 billion over 10 years.[127]

Extending broker reporting to high-value art and antiquities transactions: The opaque art and antiquities market facilitates tax and sanctions evasion and money laundering.[128] Under section 6045, brokers must provide information reporting on the gross proceeds of and gain or loss on dispositions of certain assets, including stocks, securities, and digital assets. It does not, however, currently apply to art and antiquities.[129] The Tax Law Center proposes that Congress extend broker reporting to art and antiquities to address their role in enabling tax evasion.

Testimony Submitted to the Senate Budget Committee: "Medicare Forever: Protecting Seniors by Making the Wealthy Pay Their Fair Share," James C. Capretta, Senior Fellow, American Enterprise Institute September 27, 2023

Chairman Whitehouse, Ranking Member Grassley, and distinguished members of the committee, thank you for the invitation to participate in this hearing.

---

[127] Treasury, *supra* note 11 at 218.

[128] *See, e.g.*, Graham Bowley, *As Money Launderers Buy Dalís, U.S. Looks at Lifting the Veil on Art Sales*, New York Times (June 19, 2021); Permanent Subcommittee on Investigations, Committee on Homeland Security and Governmental Affairs, *The Art Industry and U.S. Policies that Undermine Sanctions* 35-37 (July 27, 2020).

[129] Section 6045 gives the Secretary of the Treasury sufficient authority to require brokers to report the gross proceeds of transactions involving art and antiquities, but the Secretary has not exercised that authority. *See* 6045(a).

The Medicare HI Signal

The headline focus of today's session is the impending depletion of reserves in the Medicare Hospital Insurance (HI) trust fund, which is of course a pressing concern requiring the attention of Congress.

The Medicare trustees projected in their latest annual report that the HI trust fund would run through its reserves in 2031.[130] If that were allowed to happen, incoming revenue could continue to pay for a portion of the costs of submitted claims for services, but it would not be sufficient to fully cover those expenses.

While Congress has never allowed the Social Security and Medicare trust funds to become fully depleted before stepping in with a fix, if it happened in the coming years it is possible that the remedy would be for the Centers for Medicare and Medicaid Services (CMS) to apply across-the-board cuts to prevent Medicare HI spending from exceeding incoming revenue. Hospitals would be certain to see such a step as a serious threat to their ability to provide high-quality care to the program's beneficiaries.

Given the potential harm trust fund exhaustion might cause, addressing the HI shortfall expeditiously is, of course, very important, but it would be a mistake to see fixing this problem as all that needs to be done to make Medicare sustainable.

The imbalance between HI spending and outgo is actually a manifestation of a larger problem, which is the widening gap between Medicare's *total* costs, for both HI (also called part A) *and* Supplementary Medical Insurance (also called part B), and the receipts (taxes and premiums) collected to pay for both trust funds' expenses. Moreover, it no longer makes sense to treat Medicare as two separate insurance plans (or three with inclusion of the drug benefit), as that is not how most Americans experience health coverage outside of the Medicare context.

Figure 1 replicates the key projection data for all of Medicare's costs and receipts from the 2023 trustees' report, shown as a percentage of Gross Domestic Product (GDP), from the program's inception in the mid-1960s through the projection period covering the next 75 years. The core problem is

---

130 "2023 Annual Report of the Boards of Trustees of the Federal Hospital Insurance and the Federal Supplementary Medical Insurance Trust Funds," The Boards of Trustees of Federal Hospital Insurance and the Federal Supplementary Medical Insurance Trust Funds, March 31, 2023, https://www.cms.gov/oact/tr/2023.

the rapid growth of total Medicare spending, driven by an aging population and escalating costs for services.[131]

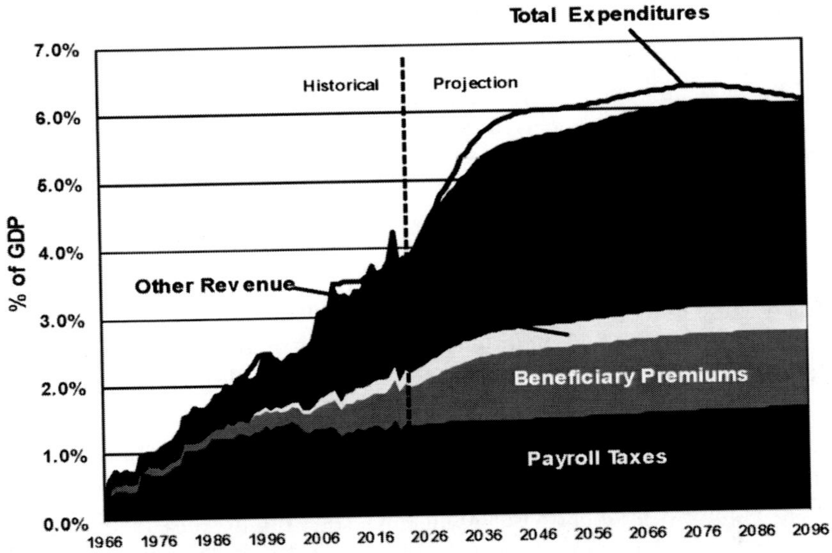

Source: Medicare Trustees (2023).

Figure 1. Total Medicare Spending and Sources of Financing.

In 1990, total program spending equaled 1.9 percent of GDP; three decades later, it had reached 4.0 percent of GDP. Medicare's trustees expect costs will reach 4.9 percent of GDP in 2030 and 6.0 percent in 2050.[132]

What is most striking about this figure is the increase in general revenue transfer to Medicare over time.

The initial versions of Medicare legislation focused on HI, which was modeled on Social Security, with a trust fund and a payroll tax on workers to cover its costs. The addition of Supplementary Medical Insurance (SMI) came late in the legislative process and was offered as a way of covering

[131] These projections may be too optimistic, according to the actuaries who produce estimates of future Medicare spending and receipts, because they assume a perpetual widening between what is paid for services by Medicare relative to commercial insurance, driven by payment limits enacted by Congress in 2010 and 2015. See "Projected Medicare Expenditures under an Illustrative Scenario with Alternative Payment Updates to Medicare Providers," John D. Shatto and M. Kent Clemens, Centers for Medicare and Medicaid Services, March 31, 2023, https://www.cms.gov/files/document/illustrative-alternative-scenario-2023.pdf.

[132] 2023 Trustees' Report.

physician fees through a voluntary program (participation in HI is mandatory in the same way it is for Social Security as nearly all workers are required to pay the payroll tax).

At enactment, the intention was to finance half of SMI spending from beneficiary premiums, with the other half covered by transfers from the general fund of the Treasury. Over time, the share covered by premiums was allowed to fall to 25 percent, which is where it remains. The other 75 percent of expenses paid from SMI -for physician services, prescription drugs, and other ambulatory care -comes from the general fund of the Treasury, which is just another way of saying other sources of revenue for the federal government, including other taxes and the proceeds from selling debt instruments.

The transfers from the Treasury to Medicare SMI are not capped; they occur automatically and are set at levels which ensure the SMI trust fund is perpetually solvent. Thus, Congress is never asked to "rescue" SMI because the trust fund is never in danger of being depleted.

But that does not mean it imposes no economic burden on taxpayers. As shown in Figure 1, the transfers to SMI are substantial, and escalating rapidly. The 2023 Trustees' report estimates the transfers to SMI will total $6.6 trillion over the next decade alone. By 2050, the annual transfer will equal 2.8 percent of GDP, up from about 0.5 percent in 1990.

Again, these funds must come from taxpayers at some point, either immediately in the form of current taxes, or in the future as tax collections to pay off the debt that was incurred to keep paying benefits in previous years.

Spending Not Covered by Taxes or Premiums

The Department of the Treasury releases an annual statement assessing the financial status of the entire federal government which relies on accrual accounting to present as much of the data as is practical. The accrual method is useful when comparing long-term benefit obligations with the expected revenue to pay for them because it converts future streams of spending and taxes into present values. The difference between the totals is the unfunded liability.

For Medicare, the trend is what is most alarming. As shown in Table 1, in the most recent report from February 2023 reveals Medicare has unfunded liabilities of $52.5 trillion as of 2022 when the general fund transfer to SMI are removed as sources of funding (because there is no dedicated taxes behind them). As of 2016, the unfunded liability estimate was $20.0 trillion less.[133] The implication is that Medicare is adding new benefit commitments at a rate that far exceeds its funding sources. It should be noted that it is unrealistic to entirely displace the general fund transfers with new taxes, so Medicare's unfunded liabilities using this definition will always be substantial. The concern is that the trend shows the burden is growing rapidly.

Table 1. Medicare's accrued unfunded liabilities ($ trillions)

	2016	2017	2018	2020	2022
Open Group Method	32.5	33.5	37.7	45.7	52.5

Source: Department of the Treasury (2023 and 2021).

Table 2. Overview of key federal budget aggregates (historical and projected)

			% of GDP		
	1980	2000	2022	2030	2050
Social Security	4.2	4.0	4.8	5.8	6.2
Medicare (Gross)	1.3	2.2	3.9	4.5	6.9
Defense	4.8	2.9	3.0	--	--
Rest of Gov't	9.0	6.8	11.5	10.2	9.1
Net Interest	1.9	2.2	1.9	3.2	6.1
Total Spending	21.2	17.7	25.1	23.7	28.3
Total Revenues	18.5	20.0	19.6	18.1	18.9
Annual Surplus (+) or Deficit (-)	-2.6	+2.3	-5.5	-5.6	-9.4
Federal Debt	25.5	33.7	97.0	108.3	168.7

Source: CBO (Historical Tables and Long-Term Projections).

The growing gap is a major reason the full federal budget has a deteriorating outlook, as reflected in data published by the Congressional Budget Office (CBO) and summarized in Table 2.[134] With the revenue dedicated to Social Security and Medicare falling behind spending growth,

---

133 "Financial Report of the United States Government: Fiscal Year 2022," Department of the Treasury, February 16, 2023, https://www.fiscal.treasury.gov/files/reports-statements/financial-report/2022/02-16-2023-FR-(Final).pdf and "Financial Report of the United States Government: Fiscal Year 2020," Department of the Treasury, March 25, 2021, https://fiscal.treasury.gov/files/reports-statements/financial-report/2020/fr-03-25-2021-(final).pdf. The unfunded liability calculation presented here is based on the open group method, which includes all current and future participants in the Medicare program.

134 See "Historical Tables" and "Long-Term Budget Projections," Congressional Budget Office, https://www.cbo.gov/data/budget-economic-data#2.

federal debt is forecast to rise to nearly 170 percent of GDP in 2050. At the end of 2008, it was 40 percent of GDP.

Reforms

Congress should view HI's challenges as an indication that the broader program needs to be updated and reformed. After all, hospital care does not occur without the patient also getting attention from a physician. Many other services and treatments are also usually provided to the patient both before and after an admission occurs. A narrow focus on hospital and other institutional costs risks perpetuating a fragmentation within Medicare that is outdated.

The following are broad recommendations for proceeding with changes to Medicare to address the program's financial challenges.

1) *Address Both the Revenue and Spending Sides of the Equation (and Seek Bipartisan Support)*. Medicare's finances will be improved most by updating both sides of the financial equation. With an aging population, it is appropriate for Congress to revisit the taxes used to pay for the program. At the same time, there is also room for making Medicare more efficient in the coming years. Finding the right balance also might help build a bipartisan coalition in support of the legislation, which would foster public acceptance and strengthen long-term program stability.
2) *Define a Standardized and Less Fragmented Benefit*. When Medicare was enacted, in 1965, it was modeled on the prevailing private insurance plans of that time, which often provided separate coverage for hospitalizations and physician services. Medicare did so too, and Congress also established separate cost-sharing rules for its two parts. It also paid for HI with payroll taxes and B with premiums and general fund transfers. Initially, Medicare did not cover prescription drugs, nor did it limit what beneficiaries must pay out-of-pocket on an annual basis (a so-called "catastrophic cap").

   In the intervening decades, the basic structure of Medicare did not change, but workarounds were created to address the program's limitations. Seniors bought supplemental plans, and HMOs were introduced to provide a more integrated plan (with less cost-sharing) for the beneficiaries. In 2003, Congress added a new part to the program -D -for prescription drugs.

It is time to bring Medicare's benefit design into line with the standards of today's insurance plans. There should be one cost-sharing structure and a limit on out-of-pocket costs. Drugs can be covered separately for the time being, but, in time, part D should be folded into the larger plan too. This redesign would lessen the need for supplemental coverage and can be accomplished on a budget-neutral basis.

3) *Improve the Choice Structure for Beneficiaries.* Medicare's original two-part structure and the program's evolution since enactment have made it difficult for the beneficiaries to accurately assess their options. When eligible persons enroll in part A, typically at age 65, they also can voluntarily enroll in parts B (for physician and ambulatory care) and D (for prescriptions) by agreeing to pay monthly premiums covering a portion of the costs. They also can enroll in a Medicare Advantage (MA) plan or buy a supplemental policy (Medigap) wrapped around the traditional fee-for-service (FFS) benefit.

Adding to the complexity is the lack of a single, coordinated enrollment system. Under current processes, it is not a simple matter to compare the all-in financial implications of the various combinations of coverage. Many beneficiaries end up relying on brokers even though they are paid most often by private insurance plans seeking to gain an advantage in the market.

Improving the program and lowering its costs should include simplification of the enrollment process so that beneficiaries can readily identify low-cost and high-value options.

Beneficiaries should be presented with the full range of their benefit options through one government-administered enrollment portal that makes it less necessary for beneficiaries to rely on outside parties to help them make their choices. Through it, they should be able to compare competing approaches for delivering covered services on an apples-to-apples across the three main benefit components, as shown in Figure 2. Standardization of the benefits is crucial (including for the supplemental options) to ensure ready premium comparisons.

Required Medicare-Covered Services	Prescription Drug Coverage	Supplemental Coverage
Traditional FFS	Stand-Alone Part D Plans	Reformed Medigap Options
ACOs	Stand-Alone Part D Plans	ACO-Affiliated Medigap
Medicare Advantage Plans	MA-Affiliated Part D Coverage (MA-PD)	MA-Sponsored Optional Supplements

Source: Author.

Figure 2. Restructured Choices for Medicare Beneficiaries.

Accountable Care Organizations (ACOs) -now a subpart of FFS -should become a coverage option that is distinct from both FFS and MA. ACOs differ from MA plans in that they are organized and run by the hospitals and physician groups providing care to patients, not insurance companies. Some Medicare beneficiaries may be comforted by this distinction. ACOs also are not traditional FFS because they need to have systems in place for coordinating care across settings and disciplines.

4) *Promote Premium Competition*. CBO has confirmed that strong competition among the coverage options can lower costs for the government and the beneficiaries, but reform of the payment system is required to achieve these results.
   MA plans already submit competitive bids under current law, but those bids are considered in relation to benchmarks tied in part to historical cost rates that may not accurately reflect what spending would be with efficient care provision. Further, FFS does not participate in the bidding process in that its enrollees pay the same premium irrespective of the relative cost of FFS to other plans.

Fair competition requires the submission of bids from MA plans, ACOs, and FFS for the same set of *standardized* benefits, as defined in law for a reformed Medicare benefit package. FFS's bid would be calculated by the government based on the cost per-beneficiary in each market. The government should also reform its risk adjustment methodology to ensure the competition is based on efficient care delivery and not differences in the ability of plans to identify risk factors.

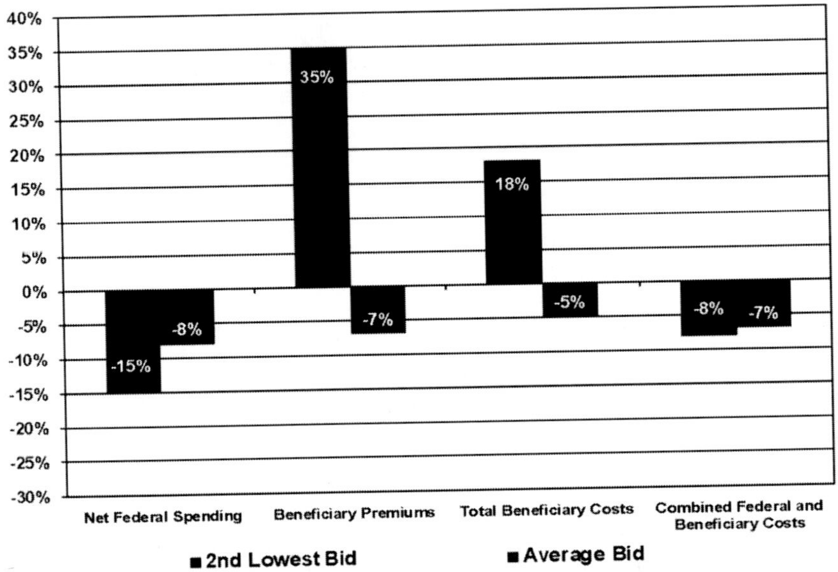

Source: CBO (2017).

Figure 3. Premium Support Effects on Program and Enrollee Costs.

The government's contribution toward coverage (its "premium support") would be based on the submitted bids. CBO has estimated that if the government set its contribution based on the average bid, there would be savings both for the government and the beneficiaries, as shown in Figure 3. The government's costs would fall by 8 percent, and the beneficiaries would pay 5 percent less in out-of-pocket costs and premiums.

CBO's assessment confirms that competition would lower costs by encouraging migration toward more efficient coverage options. It also suggests that the competition likely would slow cost growth in future years by encouraging the development and adoption of cost-reducing technologies that improve the efficiency of care delivery.[135]

5) *Promote Provider Price Competition in FFS.* Premium support is not the only means by which stronger market discipline can be introduced into Medicare. Enrollees in FFS can be encouraged to select low-cost and high-quality service providers too.

135 "A Premium Support System for Medicare: Updated Analysis of Illustrative Options," Congressional Budget Office, October 2017. https://www.cbo.gov/system/files/115th-congress-2017-2018/reports/53077-premiumsupport.pdf.

For this to occur, Medicare will need to become a leader in using transparent pricing for standardized services to foster strong competition among providers. Not all medical care is amenable to such a system, but some is (perhaps 40 percent).[136]

Hospitals and physicians today have weak incentives to post clear pricing for their services, and the complexity of medical care makes price comparisons difficult for patients when multiple line items are billed for a full episode of care.

Medicare could promote strong provider competition by requiring participating facilities and practitioners to disclose their prices for standardized interventions including common procedures, diagnostics, and management of chronic diseases.[137] Further, this requirement should force those providing services to work with each other to provide one, all-in price. It is essential that what is being priced be standardized and encompass all that is needed to properly take care of the affected patients.

An additional requirement is an incentive for the program's enrollees to select lower-priced options. Medicare could do this by calculating benchmarks based on prevailing FFS rates for the list of standardized interventions. Beneficiaries opting for lower-priced providers should get to keep some of the savings (perhaps 50 percent). In some cases, the financial benefit could be substantial, which would create strong incentives for the providers to compete aggressively.

6) *Reform the Trust Funds*. Medicare's trust funds need updating too. With a combined HI and SMI benefit package, the trust funds should be assessed as a unified whole rather than separately. That could be done in several ways.

A crucial first step should be to recalibrate the basis for general fund support of the program's spending obligations, with a view to limiting the amounts to what Congress deems to be affordable. Trust funds only work as political signals if their receipts are limited in some way and are defined to

---

136 "Estimating the Potential Savings Health Care Savings of Reference Pricing," American Academy of Actuaries, November 2018, https://www.actuary.org/sites/default/files/files/publications/ReferencePricing_11.2018.pdf.

137 For an explanation of the benefits of reference pricing, see "Reference Pricing Changes the 'Choice Architecture' of Health Care for Consumers," James C. Robinson, Timothy T. Brown, and Christopher Whaley, *Health Affairs*, March 2017, https://www.healthaffairs.org/doi/pdf/10.1377/hlthaff.2016.1256.

ensure affordability over time. That is most definitely not the case currently with SMI, with the government's contribution to SMI expected to rise to levels that will push federal debt well above what would be sustainable or advisable.

One option would be to tie the government's contribution to what was paid in a reference year and then index that amount to the rate of growth in the national economy when determining future transfers. This change would ensure that current and future taxpayers contribute the same amount of their combined incomes each year toward ensuring adequate health services for the nation's elderly and disabled citizens.

There are a number of ways to combine HI and SMI into a combined measure of financial sustainability. The objective should be to ensure that shortfalls in SMI are combined with those projected for HI so that reductions in spending or increases in taxes for either part would bolster the finances of the entire program.

7) *Authorize Automatic Adjustments to Ensure Permanent Stability.* As part of a plan to improve Medicare's financial outlook, Congress should build into the program provisions, which will automatically ensure stability even if the projections used when calibrating the initial reforms prove to be too optimistic. Future gaps in funding could be closed by authorizing the executive branch to gradually make adjustments in key program parameters to ensure spending stays even with receipts over the long term. The adjustments could adhere to a framework that Congress approves, with a split between new revenue and spending restraint that conforms to the wishes of the legislature.

Building automatic adjustments into Medicare (and also Social Security) would transform the federal government's long-term budget outlook by making it far less likely that a debt crisis will ever occur. If a gap were to emerge in either of the major programs, pre-determined changes could restore balance and prevent benefit obligations from ever outrunning the revenue needed to pay for them.

Conclusion

Medicare is one of the federal government's most important programs because of the access to medical services it provides to its participants. The program's financial status should be improved to ensure those benefits are secure for both current beneficiaries and future generations. As the needed changes will take time to implement, Congress should begin to develop and consider the necessary legislation as soon as possible.

Related Material

US Health Policy and Market Reforms: An Introduction, James C. Capretta, AEI Press (2022), https://www.aei.org/research-products/book/us-health-policy-and-market-reforms-an-introduction/.

"Medicare's Supplementary Medical Insurance Fund: A Growing Burden on Taxpayers," James C. Capretta, *Health Affairs Forefront*, June 6, 2023, https://www.healthaffairs.org/content/forefront/medicare-s-supplementary-medical-insurance-fund-growing-burden-taxpayers.

"Medicare's Price Regulations: How the Government Determines What Is Pays for Medicare Care," James C. Capretta and David N. Bernstein, Economic Perspectives, American Enterprise Institute, September 2023, https://www.aei.org/wp-content/uploads/2023/09/Medicares-Price-Regulations-How-the-Government-Determines-What-It-Pays-for-Medical-Care.pdf.

"Price Transparence 2.0: Helping Consumers Identify and Select Providers of High-Value Medical Services," James C. Capretta and David N. Bernstein, Economic Perspectives, American Enterprise Institute, January 2023, https://www.aei.org/wp-content/uploads/2023/01/Price-Transparency-2.0.pdf.

"Medicare as a Catalyst for Competitive Reforms," James C. Capretta, in *American Renewal: A Conservative Plan to Strengthen the Social Contract and Save the Country's Finances*, Paul Ryan and Angela Rachidi, eds., AEI Press (2022), https://americanrenpr.wpengine.com/wp-content/uploads/2022/11/AR-final.pdf.

"Fiscal Rules for Social Security and Medicare: Would Accrual Accounting Help?," James C. Capretta, in *Public Debt Sustainability: International Perspectives*, Barry W. Paulson, John Merrifield, and Steven H. Hanke, eds., Lexington Books, 2022.

Charles E. Grassley
United States Senator

Questions for the Record
From: Ranking Member Chuck Grassley
To: Mr. James Capretta
"Medicare Forever: Protecting Seniors by Making the Wealthy Pay Their Fair Share"
September 27, 2023
Senate Budget Committee

Question #1
The Centers for Medicare and Medicaid Services (CMS) actuary has analyzed Medicare and Social Security Fair Share Act. However, the CMS actuary cannot "independently assess the reasonability of the revenue estimates" for the proposal. The nonpartisan Joint Committee on Taxation and the Congressional Budget Office (CBO) have not publicly scored the proposal. The Tax Foundation finds that the bill's capital gains tax hike is a revenue loser, and the overall bill would cost over 700,000 jobs, and lower GDP. Should we question the revenue projections that the CMS actuary cannot validate? What impact does a marginal effective tax rate of 54.4 percent on wages and 37.4 percent on capital gains and dividends have on the economy?

Answer to Question #1:

The economic effects of the proposed tax changes advanced in the Social Security and Medicare Fair Share Act are likely to be of sufficient size that they should be analyzed by CBO and Joint Committee on Taxation. As is often the case with large changes in tax and spending policies, there are likely to be effects on the economy that require careful review. On the one hand, the proposal would substantially narrow future budget deficits by increasing revenue, which might increase private capital investment and long-term growth. On the other hand, the tax increases could lower after-tax returns to labor and capital, which might dampen growth. The net effect of these changes is hard to predict and should be the subject of a review by the scorekeeping agencies working for Congress. There is little doubt, however, that the tax increases also would improve the solvency of the HI trust fund rather substantially, even if some economic effects would lessen the amount of net revenue that is collected from them.

Question #2
Value-based purchasing efforts are certainly important to bending the cost-curve of our nation's health care spending, including in the Medicare program. Former Centers for Medicare and Medicaid Innovation (CMMI) Director, Brad Smith, has written that "the vast majority of the Center's models have not saved money, with several on pace to lose billions of dollars." Furthermore, CBO has consistently stated, "the most recent evidence indicates that ACOs have achieved only modest savings for Medicare after accounting for the shared savings bonuses they received." Is there evidence of accountable care organizations (ACOs) advanced payment

models and/or Medicare Access and CHIP Reauthorization Act (MACRA) bending the Medicare total cost of care curve? If so, what is the evidence?

Answer to Question #2:

In a recently released report, CBO analyzed the budgetary effects of the Center for Medicare and Medicaid Innovation (CMMI). The agency found that from 2011 to 2020, CMMI increased net spending by the Medicare program by a modest amount. At enactment, CBO projected that CMMI would decrease overall spending.[1]

As I indicated during the hearing, I support the inclusion of a provider-run managed care option within Medicare. ACOs can fill that role and have shown some potential as entities capable of delivering better quality care at a lower overall cost. However, as of today, they remain too tied to the existing fee-for-service system. Congress should consider amending Medicare to allow ACOs to compete directly with Medicare Advantage by allowing the beneficiaries to opt into them based on the premiums they would charge for covered services.

Question #3
Earlier this year, I asked CBO to issue a budget spotlight on the use of Medicare Improvement Fund and Medicaid Improvement Fund. Have these improvement funds been used for their intended purpose to make improvements in the programs?

Answer to Question #3:

The Medicare and Medicaid Improvement Funds were created in 2008 to make changes in the fee-for-service insurance model that enhance the quality of the services provided to program beneficiaries. In reality, however, these funds have served as accounts into which Congress can "park" excess savings created for later use.

In the case of the Medicare Improvement Fund, the account's balance has been amended by Congress 29 times since 2008.[2] Some of the amendments have placed money into the account, while others have reduced the available funds in the account to pay for other congressional priorities. The account has never been used for its original statutory purpose.

Question #4
The Medicare Trustees have issued seven consecutive "Medicare Funding Warnings," including in the 2023 Trustees Report. What is required of the President when these warnings are issued and has President Biden met that requirement?

---

[1] "Federal Budgetary Effects of the Activities of the Center for Medicare and Medicaid Innovation," Congressional Budget Office, September 2023, https://www.cbo.gov/system/files/2023-09/59274-CMMI.pdf and "Letter to House Speaker Nancy Pelosi," Congressional Budget Office, March 20, 2010, https://www.cbo.gov/sites/default/files/111th-congress-2009-2010/costestimate/amendreconprop.pdf.
[2] "The Medicare and Medicaid Improvement Funds: Budgetary History and Projections," Congressional Budget Office, April 2023, https://www.cbo.gov/system/files/2023-04/59055-Improvement-Funds.pdf.

Answer to Question #4:

Congress established the process for issuing Medicare funding warnings in the Medicare Modernization Act (MMA) of 2003. The intention was to raise awareness and incentivize legislative responses to limit the program's dependence on general revenue transfers to no more than 45 percent of the program's total revenue. If the general revenue transfers (present or future) are expected to be above 45 percent over a series of years, the president is supposed to develop and submit a plan to Congress to eliminate the breach.

However, in the years since the law's enactment, only President George W. Bush submitted a plan pursuant to the requirements of the legislation. One reason for the noncompliance seems to be that the executive branch does not believe Congress has the constitutional authority to force a president to submit a corrective plan that meets the requirements established by Congress.[3]

---

[3] "Medicare Trigger," Congressional Research Service, February 4, 2020, https://crsreports.congress.gov/product/pdf/RS/RS22796/27#.

AARP
STATEMENT FOR THE RECORD
for the

UNITED STATES SENATE
COMMITTEE ON THE BUDGET
on

MEDICARE FINANCIAL STABILITY AND
THE FUTURE OF MEDICARE SOLVENCY

September 27, 2023
Washington, DC

AARP, which advocates for the more than 100 million Americans age 50 and older, appreciates the Senate Committee on the Budget's effort to examine the Medicare Part A Hospital Insurance Trust Fund and the future of Medicare financing. Medicare faces long-term financial challenges that must be addressed. The 2023 Medicare Trustees' Report estimates that the Hospital Insurance (HI) Trust Fund, which funds Part A and is mainly financed by payroll taxes, will be fully solvent until 2031. While another 8 years is a long time compared to historic solvency projections, that date is constantly in flux. Continued increases in medical costs, rapid changes in medical technology, and a growing population — which will add 21 million enrollees to the program by 2030 — require that we consider policies to secure Medicare's financial sustainability. Medicare must remain a strong, broadly supported social insurance program so that it can continue to provide critically needed benefits to protect current and future generations.

It should be noted that HI Trust Fund insolvency does not mean Medicare is 'going broke' or will be out of money; rather, it means that Medicare will not be able to *fully* pay for the services financed by Part A. Current projections indicate that in 2031 the Trust Fund will still be able to cover 89 percent of Part A billed services. It is also noteworthy that Medicare Part B and Part D will continue to be fully funded by the Supplemental Medical Insurance (SMI) Trust Fund, which is financed through general revenues and premiums. While we must strive to avoid HI insolvency, this must be done through responsible reforms rather than reductions to Medicare benefits and eligibility.

As described in AARP's *Medicare Financial Outlook: What Do Trust Fund Solvency Projections Mean?*,[1] throughout Medicare's history, Congress has enacted numerous policy changes that have affected the Trust Fund by reducing Medicare's spending compared with previous projections. Other policy changes have repeatedly extended the Trust Fund's solvency by expanding the Trust Fund's revenue. Policymakers should again look to similar policy approaches to address current solvency challenges.

Past experience shows that a combination of policy interventions – rather than one single solution – can substantially improve Trust Fund solvency. For example, the Balanced Budget Act of 1997 reduced spending growth by decreasing the annual updates to hospital payments, modifying payment methods for home health care and skilled nursing facilities, and shifting some home health spending from Part A to Part B. In addition, the Act increased Trust Fund income from payroll taxes. As a result, the 1998 Medicare Trustees' Report projected solvency period increased by 6 years compared to the prior year's report.

In a more recent example, the Trustees increased the estimated Part A solvency period by 12 years, reflecting numerous changes enacted in the 2010 Affordable Care Act. These changes reduced spending growth for hospitals and other Part A services and increased Trust Fund revenue by establishing a higher payroll tax on earnings over a specified amount beginning in 2013.

As has always been the case, sustaining Medicare for the future will require continued attention to reducing unnecessary spending, addressing quality of care improvements, and ensuring adequate revenue. One potential solution is the continued testing and implementation of new payment innovations and person-centered care pilots and demonstrations. These efforts have the potential to identify new

[1] Komisar, Harriet. *Medicare Financial Outlook: What Do Trust Fund Solvency Projections Mean?* Washington, DC: AARP Public Policy Institute. May 2020. https://doi.org/10.26419/ppi.00102.001

approaches that, when scaled, could reduce unnecessary spending and slow spending growth. Scaling such approaches could improve the solvency outlook over time.[2] Still, other policy changes may be needed to strengthen the Part A Trust Fund for the future.

Another action Congress can take right now to improve the Medicare program's finances is to continue addressing high prescription drug prices. Fully implementing prescription drug reforms, like those contained in the Inflation Reduction Act, as well as adopting new reforms, would save nearly all Medicare beneficiaries money in their out-of-pocket expenses and save the Medicare program billions of dollars each year. Lower drug prices, and the better health outcomes and reduced hospitalizations that result from improved medication adherence, would benefit both the HI and SMI Trust Funds.[3]

Congress can also improve Medicare's program-wide finances by addressing excess payments to private Medicare Advantage (MA) plans. AARP believes Medicare payments should be neutral with respect to Medicare coverage options. Congress should set and maintain benchmarks upon which MA plan payments are based so they are more in line with Original Medicare costs. Further, as MedPAC has recommended, Congress should periodically evaluate the impact of the MA reimbursement methodology to ensure reasonable private health plan participation in the Medicare program and appropriate Medicare payments to participating plans.

Beyond these immediate improvements, a wide variety of incremental changes in Medicare policy could extend the Trust Fund's solvency. History shows that relatively small payment modifications to slow spending growth can have a significant positive impact on the Trust Fund. Congress should consider revisiting previous policies that increased Trust Fund revenue, including raising new revenue or redirecting revenue from existing sources.

Medicare continues to provide critical health coverage for older Americans, and measures to address Medicare's long-term financial outlook are necessary to protect access to high quality care and prevent simply shifting costs to current and future Medicare beneficiaries. We urge you to work together on the necessary combination of policies to the program's finances and payments to maximize the value of every dollar spent.

Thank you for the opportunity to provide AARP's perspective on improving Medicare's current and future finances. We look forward to working with you to address this important issue and ensure continued access to affordable health benefits for older Americans.

[2] Lind, Keith. *Savings Expected from Slowdown in Medicare Spending*. Washington, DC: AARP Public Policy Institute. February 2017.

[3] https://www.cbo.gov/publication/58850

September 27, 2023

The Honorable Sheldon Whitehouse
Chair, Committee on Budget
United States Senate
Washington, D.C. 20510

Dear Mr. Chairman:

On behalf of the 1.4 million members of the American Federation of State, County and Municipal Employees (AFSCME), I write to express our support for the Medicare and Social Security Fair Share Act (S. 1174). I request that this letter be included in the record of the September 27 hearing on "Medicare Forever: Protecting Seniors by Making the Wealthy Pay Their Fair Share."

Medicare and Social Security are vital to Retirement Security

For nearly six decades Medicare has given peace of mind to seniors because they know they can see a doctor, go to the hospital, and get the health care they need when they need it. Medicare provides health care and economic security through health insurance coverage to 65 million people in the U.S., including 57 million older adults and nearly 8 million younger adults with disabilities.

Since 1935, Social Security helps workers to earn a benefit to allow them to retire with dignity, provide for their spouse and dependent children when they die and to have insurance in case a disabling long-term illness or injury strikes before they retire. About 66 million people, or about 1 in every 5 U.S. residents, collected Social Security benefits in February 2023. Social Security reduces poverty dramatically among older adults. Without Social Security, the poverty rate for those aged 65 and over would meet or exceed 40% in one-fourth of states; with Social Security, it is less than 10% in over two-thirds of states. Social Security lifts more than 1 million older adults above the poverty line in California, Florida and Texas, and over half a million in Illinois, Michigan, New York, North Carolina, Ohio and Pennsylvania.

The Medicare and Social Security Fair Share Act helps preserve these two vital programs for the next generation while safeguarding benefits. AFSCME supports S. 1174 because it would extend the solvency of the trust funds for both Medicare and Social Security by more than 75 years. The bill does this by requiring taxpayers with over $400,000 in income to contribute their fair share to Social Security and to contribute more to the Medicare Hospital Insurance fund. The bill also closes loopholes that allow taxpayers making more than $400,000 to disguise their earned income to evade their fair share of taxes.

These proposed changes are needed to make sure the bedrock programs of Social Security and Medicare are here for this and future generations.

Sincerely,

Edwin S. Jayne

Edwin S. Jayne
Director of Federal Government Affairs

Alliance for Retired Americans®

President
Robert Roach, Jr.

Secretary-Treasurer
Joseph Peters, Jr.

STATEMENT FOR THE RECORD
SUBMITTED TO THE SENATE COMMITTEE ON THE BUDGET

MEDICARE FOREVER. PROTECTING SENIORS BY MAKING THE WEALTHY PAY THEIR FAIR SHARE

September 27, 2023

ALLIANCE FOR RETIRED AMERICANS
815 16TH STREET, NW
WASHINGTON, DC 20006
www.retiredamericans.org

The Alliance for Retired Americans appreciates the opportunity to submit comments to the Senate Committee on the Budget to share our views on the hearing entitled "*Medicare Forever: Protecting Seniors by Making the Wealthy Pay Their Fair Share.*" We thank Committee Chairman Whitehouse and Ranking Member Grassley for holding this hearing, and are most appreciative of the witnesses for providing insightful testimony.

Founded in 2001, the Alliance is a grassroots organization representing more than 4.4 million retirees and seniors nationwide. The Alliance and its 39 state chapters work to advance public policy that strengthens the health and retirement security of older Americans.

For decades, Medicare has been our nation's largest and most successful health insurance system, serving the health needs of nearly 57 million older Americans and 8 million beneficiaries with disabilities. Since 1965, Medicare has been the most financially efficient health care system in the U.S., delivering guaranteed coverage to millions who would otherwise have to forego health insurance later in life. Like Social Security, Medicare benefits are earned over a lifetime of work and are an essential component of a secure retirement.

The Alliance strongly believes that to continue to provide retirement security for current and future generations, Congress needs to strengthen and expand Medicare benefits. One outstanding proposal that would go a long way towards accomplishing this is Senator Whitehouse's bill, S. 1174, "The Medicare and Social Security Fair Share Act," which extends Medicare solvency indefinitely while simultaneously augmenting fairness in the tax system by increasing the share that taxpayers earning over $400,000 in income contribute, regardless of the source of their income since the tax applies to wages, self-employment and investment income.

And while many in Congress, as exemplified by the House Republican Study Committee's FY 2023 budget entitled The Blueprint to Save America, continue their efforts to devise plans to make cuts to Medicare and Social Security, Senator Whitehouse's bill shores up Medicare's financing, thus protecting Americans' earned benefits without cuts for beneficiaries.

In an effort to shore up Medicare's finances, Senator Whitehouse's Medicare and Social Security Fair Share Act would:

- **Preserve Medicare and Social Security while safeguarding benefits.**
  - Extend both Medicare and Social Security solvency indefinitely.
- **Require taxpayers with over $400,000 in income to contribute a fairer share to Medicare and Social Security.**
  - Ensure that no matter the source of their income, high-earning taxpayers contribute 5 percent of their incomes to Medicare.

- **Require taxpayers with incomes above $400,000 to contribute more to Medicare and close a loophole in the law that favors high earners, as proposed by President Biden.**
    - Increase the rate for income above $400,000 by 1.2 percent and dedicate the revenue to Medicare.
    - Ensure that wealthy owners of pass-through businesses like hedge funds and private equity firms with more than $400,000 in annual income cannot avoid Medicare taxes.

Alliance for Retired Americans members are frustrated that instead of enacting common sense changes like those outlined in Senator Whitehouse's legislation, many members of Congress are advocating for drastic changes that threaten Medicare and Social Security and the benefits that Americans of all ages have earned. Proposals include the creation of special commissions or panels to make decisions that adversely affect beneficiaries without the benefit of public input or increasing the full retirement age for which beneficiaries can claim the benefits they have earned over a lifetime of work to collect Social Security. The Alliance opposes any and all attempts to reduce benefits or enact proposals that would lead to the reduction of Medicare and/or Social Security benefits.

The time to strengthen and expand Medicare and Social Security is now, and the Alliance stands in strong support of Chairman Whitehouse's proposal to extend the system's solvency. On behalf of our more than 4.4 million members, the Alliance deeply appreciates the opportunity to submit testimony on this vitally important issue.

Medicare Rights Center, Statement for the Record, Submitted to the U.S. Senate Committee on Budget, Regarding the September 27, 2023, hearing "Medicare Forever: Protecting Seniors by Making the Wealthy Pay Their Fair Share"

The Medicare Rights Center (Medicare Rights) appreciates this opportunity to submit a statement for the record on the September 27, 2023, hearing of the U.S. Senate Committee on Budget, titled "Medicare Forever: Protecting Seniors by Making the Wealthy Pay Their Fair Share." Medicare Rights is a national, nonprofit organization that works to ensure access to affordable and equitable health care for older adults and people with disabilities through counseling and advocacy, educational programs, and public policy initiatives. Each year, Medicare Rights provides services and resources to nearly three million people with Medicare, family caregivers, and professionals.

Medicare is a vital, life-saving program that protects the health and well-being of over 63 million older adults and people with disabilities.[138] To strengthen the program for current and future beneficiaries, we support responsibly bolstering Medicare's financing in ways that maintain the

[138] Centers for Medicare & Medicaid Services, "CMS Releases Latest Enrollment Figures for Medicare, Medicaid, and Children's Health Insurance Program (CHIP)" (December 21, 2021), https://www.cms.gov/newsroom/news-alert/cms-releases-latest-enrollment-figures-medicare-medicaid-and-childrens-health-insurance-program-chip.

program's universality, safeguard current benefits and cost protections, and modernize coverage to meet the evolving, diverse, and whole-body needs of beneficiaries.

While this will require a holistic approach that contemplates both savings and revenues, the focus of today's hearing, and therefore our statement, is on the latter. We look forward to future opportunities to discuss cost containment, such as improving Medicare Advantage payment accuracy[139] and reigning in certain provider, setting, and service expenses.

Existing Revenue Levers

Currently, Medicare Part A is funded through the Hospital Insurance (HI) trust fund. As its name suggests, the HI trust fund helps pay for inpatient hospital care for people with Medicare. In addition, it helps cover hospice, skilled nursing facility care, and home health services that follow a qualifying hospital stay.[140]

Medicare Tax

The HI trust fund is financed primarily by a dedicated payroll tax of 2.9% on covered earnings. Though it is divided equally between employers and employees, with each paying 1.45%, many economists believe the employer share of the tax is ultimately paid by the employee in the form of reduced compensation.[141]

Additional Medicare Tax

Due to changes in the Affordable Care Act (ACA), wages above a certain threshold ($200,000 for individuals, $250,000 for couples) are now subject to an additional HI payroll tax of 0.9%.[142] There is no employer-employee split, bringing the effective Medicare payroll tax rate for these households to 3.8%.

---

139 Medicare Rights Center, "Medicare Advantage 101" (July 2023), https://www.medicarerights.org/policy-series/medicare-advantage-101.

140 The Boards of Trustees, Federal Hospital Insurance and Federal Supplementary Medical Insurance Trust Funds, "2023 Annual Report" (March 31, 2023), https://www.cms.gov/oact/tr/2023.

141 Congressional Research Service, "Payroll Taxes: An Overview of Taxes Imposed and Past Payroll Tax Relief" (April 4, 2022), https://crsreports.congress.gov/product/pdf/R/R47062.

142 Internal Revenue Service, "Questions and Answers for the Additional Medicare Tax" (last accessed September 22, 2023), https://www.irs.gov/businesses/small-businesses-self-employed/questions-and-answers-for-the-additional-medicare-tax.

Net Investment Income Tax

Also introduced within the context of the ACA, the Net Investment Income Tax (NIIT) is a 3.8% tax on certain types of nonwage income, such as dividends and capital gains, for individuals making $200,000 a year ($250,000 for couples).[143] Despite being described as an "unearned income Medicare contribution" and originally designed to operate as such, it does not actually fund Medicare.[144]

Potential Solutions

Redirect NIIT Revenues

That NIIT revenues go to the general fund and not the HI trust fund is widely considered the result of a legislative drafting error and procedural limitations.[145] Correcting this misallocation is a long overdue intervention that could considerably improve Medicare's financial outlook.

The NIIT generates billions of dollars each year, yielding nearly $60 billion in 2021 alone.[146] Redirecting its future proceeds could grow the HI trust fund by $350 billion over ten years, alleviating more than half of its Congressional Budget Office (CBO)-estimated shortfall.[147] Transferring the present value of the NIIT's past proceeds would shore up the trust fund even further, by an additional $200 billion.

Among the revenue raisers outlined herein, properly allocating NIIT dollars to the HI trust fund is a commonsense first step. It would improve Medicare sustainability by ensuring an existing tax is operating as intended, leaving payment obligations untouched.

---

143 Internal Revenue Service, "Questions and Answers on the Net Investment Income Tax" (last accessed September 22, 2023), https://www.irs.gov/newsroom/questions-and-answers-on-the-net-investment-income-tax.

144 P.L. 111-152.

145 Leonard E. Burman, "ACA and the Perils of Reconciliation" (March 13, 2017), https://www.taxpolicycenter.org/taxvox/aca-and-perils-reconciliation.

146 Congressional Research Service, "The 3.8% Net Investment Income Tax: Overview, Data, and Policy Options" (June 30, 2023), https://crsreports.congress.gov/product/pdf/IF/IF11820.

147 Paul N. Van de Water, "Strengthening Medicare Financing" (December 14, 2020), https://www.cbpp.org/research/health/strengthening-medicare-financing.

Close Tax Loopholes

As noted above, many higher-income households are subject to a 3.8% Medicare tax on their wage income and a 3.8% NIIT on their net investment income. However, owners of pass-through businesses like S-corporations and limited partnerships can bypass these taxes by classifying some of their income as "distributed profits" instead of "salary."

As the experts at the Institute on Taxation and Economic Policy explain, this creates significant opportunities for tax avoidance that negatively impact Medicare financing: "If a partner of a law firm earns $10 million through their practice, they do not need to claim all that income as salary. Instead, they could claim just $200,000 as their salary and the rest as distributed profits. In this simplified scenario, they would save over $200,000 in health care taxes."[148]

There are several ways to address this, in whole or in part.[149] For example, broadening the Medicare and NIIT tax bases to cover the pass-through income for some higher-income taxpayers, such as individuals making over $400,000 per year and couples making over $500,000, combined with a redirection of NIIT proceeds to the HI trust fund, would raise over $200 billion through 2031, reducing the HI deficit by over 80% based on CBO projections.[150]

Closing this egregious loophole improves Medicare's finances by solving an existing problem with an existing tax. It is the next logical revenue-raising step after correcting the NIIT. We strongly urge policymakers to take such an iterative approach—to ensure all tax incentives are aligned and all proceeds are appropriately collected and directed—before contemplating any changes to individual tax rates.

Raise the Payroll Tax Rate

At the same time, we recognize the likely need for broader tax changes. As Dr. Moon has written previously, "[w]hen Medicare was enacted, it was expected that payroll tax rates would need to rise over time to meet the needs of a growing population of older adults and pay for care that was likely to

---

148 Joe Hughes, "Key Reform in Build Back Better Act Would Close Loophole Used by the Rich To Avoid Funding Healthcare" (November 18, 2021), https://itep.org/key-reform-in-build-back-better-act-would-close-loophole-used-by-the-rich-to-avoid-funding-healthcare/.

149 Karen C. Burke, "Exploiting the Medicare Tax Loophole" (June 17, 2018), https://papers.ssrn.com/sol3/papers.cfm?abstract_id=3041694.

150 Committee for a Responsible Federal Budget, "CBO Updates Major Trust Fund Baselines" (June 1, 2022), https://www.crfb.org/blogs/cbo-updates-major-trust-fund-baselines.

become more expensive."[151] However, "[t]he basic payroll tax rate that funds Part A of Medicare has remained constant since 1987 despite a doubling of the population served and a doubling of per capita spending."[152] Despite being conceptualized as dynamic, Medicare taxation has been too static for too long, to the program's detriment.

Manageable solutions are still possible. Modeling shows relatively small increases to the Medicare tax rate could generate substantial revenue. However, advance planning is necessary to minimize any potential disruptions. For example, immediately raising the Medicare payroll tax rate by one percentage point—from 1.45% to 1.95% for both employees and employers—would add $1 trillion to the HI trust fund over the next 10 years. But such an abrupt shift may be difficult for many households to absorb, creating challenging circumstances for taxpayers and the economy.[153] While gradually phasing in such a shift would likely be easier to manage, it would only raise about half as much, roughly $400 billion, over the same time frame.[154] Both strategies would zero out the 10-year HI financing gap the Trustees currently project ($390 billion), but that may not always be true. The longer we wait to act, the bigger hole we'll have to fill, and the fewer tools we'll have.

Any payroll tax increases must be broad-based, modest, and phased-in to prevent a worsening of income inequality or financial insecurity. They must also be part of a beneficiary-centered, comprehensive approach that includes the revenue raisers discussed above as well as important program efficiencies.

Conclusion

Medicare sustainability is a critical issue for millions of Americans. The program's financing challenges are well known,[155] as are many of the

---

[151] Marilyn Moon, "Ensuring Medicare's Future Will Require New Revenue" (January 28, 2021), https://www.commonwealthfund.org/blog/2021/ensuring-medicares-future-will-require-new-revenue.

[152] *Id.*

[153] Gordon B. Mermin, et al. "Options for Increasing Medicare Revenues" (February 1, 2023), https://www.taxpolicycenter.org/publications/options-increasing-medicare-revenues/full.

[154] Marilyn Moon, "Ensuring Medicare's Future Will Require New Revenue" (January 28, 2021), https://www.commonwealthfund.org/blog/2021/ensuring-medicares-future-will-require-new-revenue.

[155] Juliette Cubanski and Tricia Neuman, "What to Know about Medicare Spending and Financing" (January 19, 2023), https://www.kff.org/medicare/issue-brief/what-to-know-about-medicare-spending-and-financing/.

solutions. This reality must not be used as an excuse to cut benefits, increase out-of-pocket costs, or otherwise undermine access to care in the name of "urgency." Now is the time for measured policies, not brash rhetoric.

As Dr. Moon has explained: "The Medicare Part A trust fund was intended to warn policymakers when changes were needed to sustain this crucial program for future generations. It should spur a debate on how best to protect the program rather than as a mandate for cutting this crucial benefit…"[156]

We agree. The Medicare Rights Center looks forward to thoughtful conversation on improving the program and its financial footing.

Date: September 18, 2023
From: Paul Spitalnic, ASA, MAAA
Chief Actuary, Centers for Medicare & Medicaid Services
Subject: Impact of the Medicare and Social Security Fair Share Act on the Solvency of the Hospital Insurance Trust Fund

The 2023 Medicare Trustees Report, which was released on March 31, 2023, projected that the Hospital Insurance (HI) trust fund would be depleted in calendar year 2031. The Medicare and Social Security Fair Share Act was introduced in the Senate on April 18, 2023 and in the House of Representatives on July 11, 2023. This proposed bill contains two provisions that have a direct impact on the HI trust fund:

- Sections 2 and 3—Increase the additional Medicare tax rates for employment taxes under the Self-Employment Contributions Act and the Federal Insurance Contribution Act by 1.2 percentage points for taxpayers with modified adjusted gross income (MAGI) above the unindexed thresholds of $400,000 for a single filer and $500,000 for a married couple filing jointly.
- Section 4—Expand the tax on net investment income (NII) as defined in the Affordable Care Act to cover earnings from active S corporation holders and active limited partners. Apply a 5.0-percent tax on this expanded definition of NII, payable to the HI trust fund with specified thresholds, effective for 2024 and later. The NII tax would apply to

156 Marilyn Moon, "Ensuring Medicare's Future Will Require New Revenue" (January 28, 2021), https://www.commonwealthfund.org/blog/2021/ensuring-medicares-future-will-require-new-revenue.

the lesser of NII and the excess of MAGI above the unindexed thresholds of $400,000 for a single filer and $500,000 for a married couple filing jointly.

The Office of the Chief Actuary at the Social Security Administration provided estimates for the additional HI revenue that would result from these provisions.[157] The CMS Office of the Actuary estimates that if this proposed bill were enacted, the additional revenue would extend the solvency of the HI trust fund throughout the 75-year projection period included in the 2023 Medicare Trustees Report. Similarly, the additional revenue would eliminate the actuarial deficit of 0.62 percent of taxable payroll over this same period and would result in a 75-year surplus of 0.38 percent of taxable payroll.

In calendar year 2024, total non-interest income for the HI trust fund, including the additional revenue from this proposal, would be 17 percent higher than under the intermediate assumptions in the 2023 Medicare Trustees Report, and it would rise steadily to 36 percent higher by the end of the 75-year period.

Figure 1 illustrates the projected HI trust fund ratio through 2070 under current law and under the assumption that the proposal is enacted. The trust fund ratio is defined as the trust fund reserves at the beginning of the year expressed as a percentage of annual expenditures during the year. Assuming enactment of the proposal, and under the intermediate assumptions of the 2023 Medicare Trustees Report, this ratio is expected to continue to increase significantly, and the trust fund is expected to be able to pay scheduled benefits in full and on time throughout the 75-year projection period.[158]

Under current law, the percentage of expenditures covered by non-interest income is projected to decrease from 89 percent in 2031, after depletion of the trust fund reserves, to 81 percent in 2047 and then to increase to about 96 percent by 2097. Assuming enactment of the proposal, non-interest income is projected to cover 118 percent of expenditures in 2024, to gradually decrease to 97 percent of expenditures in 2041, and then to increase to roughly 130 percent of expenditures by 2097.

The Trustees measure the long-range actuarial status of the HI trust fund by comparing, on a year-by-year basis, the non-interest income (from payroll

---

[157] The Office of the Actuary at CMS did not independently assess the reasonability of the revenue estimates for the stated provisions. More information on the Medicare and Social Security Fair Share Act, including the impact on the Old Age, Survivors, and Disability Insurance Trust Funds, can be found here.

[158] The trust fund ratio is projected to exceed 800 percent by the end of the 75-year period.

taxes, taxation of benefits under the Old Age, Survivors, and Disability Insurance program, premiums, general fund transfers for uninsured persons, and monies derived from the fraud and abuse control program) with the corresponding incurred costs, expressed as percentages of taxable payroll.[159] These percentages are referred to as income rates and cost rates, respectively.

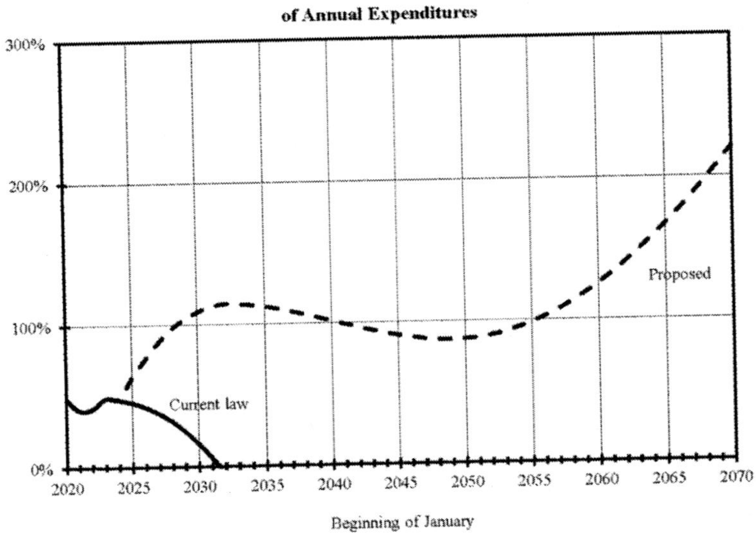

Figure 1. HI Trust Fund Balance at Beginning of Year as a Percentage of Annual Expenditures.

Figure 2 shows the year-by-year non-interest income and costs as a percentage of taxable payroll under current law, as well as the income rate reflecting enactment of the proposal. Based on the intermediate assumptions, cost rates will continue to exceed income rates in all years starting in 2024 under current law. However, if this proposal were to be enacted, then the income rate would be higher than the cost rate through 2033, drop lower through 2049, and be higher again throughout the remainder of the 75-year projection period.

While year-by-year comparisons of revenues and costs are necessary to measure the adequacy of HI financing, the financial status of the trust fund is often summarized, over a specific valuation period, by a single measure known as the actuarial balance. The actuarial balance of the HI trust fund is defined

---

159 Taxable payroll is the total amount of wages, salaries, tips, self-employment income, and other earnings subject to the HI payroll tax.

as the difference between the summarized income rate for the valuation period and the summarized cost rate for the same period.

The summarized income rates, cost rates, and actuarial balance are based upon the present values of future income, costs, and taxable payroll. The Trustees calculate the present values, as of the beginning of the valuation period, by discounting the future annual amounts of income and outgo using the projected effective rates of interest credited to the HI trust fund for the first 10 years and transition to the ultimate interest rate assumption by year 15. They then determine the summarized income and cost rates over the projection period by dividing the present value of income and cost, respectively, by the present value of taxable payroll. The difference between the summarized income rate and cost rate over the long-range projection period (after an adjustment to take into account the fund balance at the valuation date and a target trust fund balance at the end of the valuation period) is the actuarial balance.

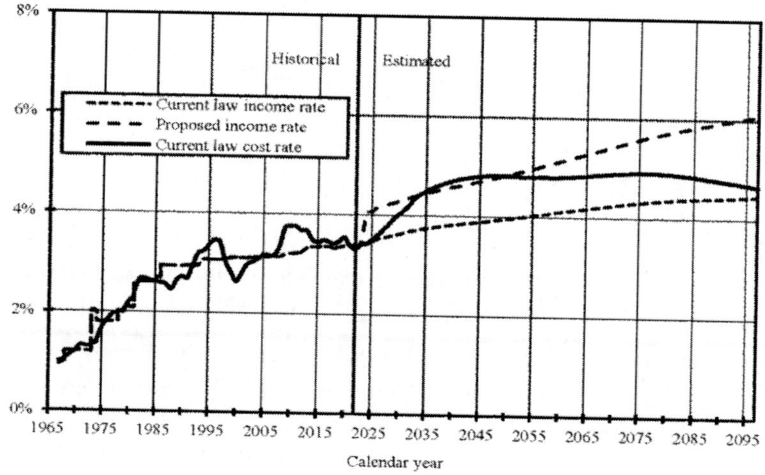

Figure 2. Estimated HI Cost and Income Rates as a Percentage of Taxable Payroll.

The summarized cost rate includes the cost of maintaining a trust fund balance at the end of the period equal to the following year's estimated costs. While a zero or positive actuarial balance implies that the end-of-period trust fund balance is at least as large as the target trust fund balance, there is no such implication for the trust fund balance at other times during the projection period.

Should this proposal be enacted, the actuarial balance for the HI program over the 75-year projection period would be improved by 1.00 percent of taxable payroll—from an actuarial deficit of 0.62 percent of payroll under current law to a positive actuarial balance of 0.38 percent of taxable payroll under the proposal.

Table 1. HI actuarial balances under current law and proposal

	Current Law	Proposed
Valuation periods:[1] 25 years, 2023–2047: Summarized income rate	3.77	4.46
Summarized cost rate	4.48	4.48
Actuarial balance	−0.70	−0.02
50 years, 2023–2072: Summarized income rate	3.92	4.77
Summarized cost rate	4.63	4.63
Actuarial balance	−0.70	0.14
75 years, 2023–2097: Summarized income rate	4.05	5.06
Summarized cost rate	4.67	4.68
Actuarial balance	−0.62	0.38

[1]Income rates include beginning trust fund balances, and cost rates include the cost of attaining a trust fund balance at the end of the period equal to 100 percent of the following year's estimated expenditures.

Note: Totals do not necessarily equal the sums of rounded components.

The Medicare Trustees Report includes several references to illustrative alternative scenario projections[160] that reflect the assumption that certain price-reducing features of current law are not fully adhered to throughout the projection period. Under this scenario, the HI trust fund is projected to be depleted in 2031, and the long-range actuarial balance is estimated to be −1.46 percent of taxable payroll. However, if this proposal were to be enacted, the trust fund would be depleted in 2052 under the illustrative alternative scenario, and roughly 92 percent of expenditures would be covered by non-interest income in that year. In addition, the 75-year actuarial balance would be an estimated −0.46 percent of taxable payroll.

[160] https://www.cms.gov/files/document/illustrative-alternative-scenario-2023.pdf.

September 20, 2023

The Honorable Sheldon Whitehouse
Chairman, Senate Committee on the Budget
624 Dirksen Senate Office Building
United States Senate
Washington, D.C. 20510

The Honorable Brendan Boyle
Ranking Member, House Budget Committee
204 Cannon House Office Building
United States House of Representatives
Washington, D.C. 20515

Dear Senator Whitehouse and Representative Boyle:

On behalf of the millions of members and supporters of the National Committee to Preserve Social Security and Medicare, I write to endorse your legislation, the "Medicare & Social Security Fair Share Act." The National Committee commends you for introducing this legislation, which ensures 75-year solvency for the Old-Age and Survivors (OASI) and the Disability Insurance (DI) Social Security Trust Funds, and the Hospital Insurance (HI) Medicare Trust Fund. Your bill should give all Americans confidence that Social Security and Medicare will be there for them when they need these critical programs.

The "Medicare & Social Security Fair Share Act" strengthens Social Security's financial foundations by increasing revenue dedicated to support the program through an extension of the payroll tax to the wages and unearned income of taxpayers in excess of $400,000. Over time, the provision establishing a new wage threshold for payroll taxes would completely eliminate the cap on Social Security taxes. Applying payroll taxes to unearned income better reflects the evolution of income for our nation's workforce, as higher-income workers receive increasingly smaller portions of their income from wages. While the National Committee supports both of these provisions, we believe that providing additional Social Security benefits for the enhanced contributions would better preserve the earned nature of the Social Security program.

Social Security has been a bedrock program protecting the financial security of American workers in the case of retirement, disability or death. However, Social Security benefits have not been improved in over half a century and some of their value has eroded over the years. We believe the solvency extensions in your legislation would be greatly enhanced if they were paired with benefit improvements that meet the needs of today's workers and beneficiaries.

In addition, your bill extends the solvency of the Medicare Hospital Insurance (HI) fund by increasing the Net Investment Income Tax (NIIT) by 1.2 percent (to 5 percent) for taxpayers over $400,000 in income. Your bill also closes the current loophole that allows the owners of pass-through businesses like hedge funds, private equity firms, and certain oil and gas companies to avoid Medicare taxes by requiring such taxpayers earning over $400,000 to contribute to Medicare and Social Security on their pass-through business income.

The National Committee generally supports the provisions included in your bill and endorses the "Medicare & Social Security Fair Share Act." This bill represents a bold and forceful step on behalf of seniors and all Americans by strengthening and safeguarding Social Security for future beneficiaries. We look forward to working with you on this important legislation.

Sincerely,

Max Richtman

Max Richtman
President and CEO

September 21, 2023

Senator Sheldon Whitehouse
Chair, Budget Committee
United States Senate

Dear Senator Whitehouse:

I am honored to share this testimony for the Budget Committee Hearing, "Medicare Forever: Protecting Seniors by Making the Wealthy Pay Their Fair Share." that you will be chairing on September 27, 2023. As Director of the Rhode Island Geriatric Education Center (RIGEC) at the University of Rhode Island (URI), I am extensively involved in developing and offering geriatric education programs to healthcare and human service professionals caring for older adults in our state. Through the experiences of the professionals with whom we work, I can offer important insights into the meaning and significance of the Medicare program for older adults.

Based at URI, RIGEC is funded by the Health Resources and Services Administration (HRSA) as a consortium of academic, clinical, and community-based partners providing interprofessional geriatrics education and training to prepare healthcare and human service professionals, faculty, students, and caregivers to better meet the physical, functional, and psychosocial needs of older adults. RIGEC's goal is to improve health outcomes for older adults by integrating geriatrics into primary care delivery systems and engaging patients, families, and caregivers in these efforts.

Older people report that their health is the most important factor in their ability to live independently and ensure they can do what is important to them. For this reason, Medicare is not just another program for older adults, it is the linchpin of their lives. The provision of both preventive and direct care services is an essential foundation of their well-being. However, there are gaps and problems in coverage that need to be addressed, and the following examples will illustrate these challenges.

Dental care.

Routine dental care is essential for older adults' health, due to the strong relationship between oral health and overall physical health. However, Medicare benefits for oral health care are incomplete and do not include essential services such as dentures. Unaddressed dental issues can cause more serious and expensive health problems later.

Impact of out-of-pocket costs

Older adults often find themselves having to delay annual exams or physician visits due to substantial out-of-pocket costs, even for those with supplemental insurance. This includes care by specialists. Care that is delayed or not received has substantial negative effects on quality of life and ultimately increases overall program costs.

Pharmaceuticals

Older adults must purchase a Part D pharmaceutical plan to cover part of their medication costs. Plans change the tier of each drug during the year, so older adults are paying exorbitant fees for some of their necessary drugs. This happens prior to and during the "donut hole."

Skilled nursing care coverage

Older adults and their families mistakenly believe that Medicare covers care in a skilled nursing facility. This is particularly a problem when an older adult is held at a hospital in a "diagnostic" room instead of an in-patient room for three days and subsequently discharged to a skilled nursing facility, where they discover that they do not qualify for Medicare coverage.

In sum and in summary, RIGEC's many years of experience in geriatric healthcare workforce development have clearly demonstrated that Medicare is an essential program for older adults that needs to be strengthened and extended to other benefits, not reduced in funding. It is the foundation of the wellbeing of older adults that makes all other aspects of their lives possible and meaningful.

Sincerely,

Phillip G. Clark, ScD
Professor and Director

Senior Agenda Coalition of RI

70 Bath Street, Providence, RI 02908

Phone: (401) 451-8158 • Email: Cynthia.Coyne@senioragendari.org

www.senioragendari.org

Cynthia A. Coyne
Executive Director

September 15, 2023

Hon. Sheldon Whitehouse
Chairman, Committee on the Budget
United States Senate
Washington, D.C. 20510

Dear Senator Whitehouse:

On behalf of the members of the Senior Agenda Coalition of Rhode Island, I appreciate the opportunity to comment on the need to ensure Medicare and Social Security solvency.

Medicare provides critical healthcare funding for almost one-quarter million older Rhode Islanders and adults with disabilities. By doing so, it provides a vital part of their financial security knowing they will be able to receive needed healthcare and not be faced with crushing health care costs due to illness or accidents.

Rhode Islanders contribute to Medicare throughout their working careers knowing their contributions support the healthcare needed by both present and future beneficiaries. And people make life plans based on the belief that the Social Security benefits they have been told they may anticipate will be there for them. If anticipated benefits are reduced for those at or nearing retirement age, there is simply no time or opportunity to make alternative plans. Benefits may be lost forever, and persons must simply find a way to adapt to less income most likely resulting in a reduced standard of living.

In commenting on Medicare, one of our active and engaged members, 90-year-old named Bob, described the importance of Medicare to him by stating, "Medicare was a financial 'partner' in my intestinal and eye operations."

The security of health care coverage extends beyond simply the member receiving benefits. As Maureen, another member of our Coalition states: "As cancer survivors, my husband and I depend upon Medicare being there to pay for our healthcare needs as we advance in age with its often-unanticipated health challenges and the potential for cancer to come back. Medicare is equally important for the hundreds of thousands of family caregivers of our older adults. I cared for my mother who died at 97 and know how important it was for her to have Medicare the several times she needed acute care and follow-up rehab. And, I want Medicare to continue to be strong to give assurance to my middle-aged children that Medicare will be for them as they approach their older years."

In closing, please know we are grateful for your continued support of our older adult population in Rhode Island. We are committed to working with you to protect Social Security and ensure Medicare solvency.

Sincerely,

Cynthia A. Coyne

Cynthia A. Coyne

Rhode Island Alliance for Retired Americans®

September 5, 2023
Committee on the Budget
U.S. Senate
Washington, DC 20510

Dear Chairman Whitehouse and members of this Committee,

My name is John A. Pernorio, I am the President of the 5,000-member Rhode Island Alliance for Retired Americans. We are a chartered member of the 4-million-member Alliance for Retired Americans.

I'm a 79-year-old resident of North Providence, RI. I have participated in Medicare since 1992 when I became totally disabled due to a work-related injury. This is my statement on why Medicare needs to be expanded, not reduced.

WHAT DOES MEDICARE MEAN TO ME?

If I didn't have Medicare, with my small pension and Social Security check, I would be financially ruined. Over these many years since my spinal cord injury, I have required many surgical procedures that have necessitated me to have skilled nursing, physical and occupational therapy **with no co-payments**. **That alone saves me $320.00 a month in co-payments**. One occurrence in particular happened in November of 2018 when I was rushed to the hospital with a Gallbladder attack that required emergency surgery. Because I live alone with my neurological condition, after the surgery, I was sent to a skilled nursing facility for one month. From there I was transferred to a rehabilitation hospital where I spent another month. While at the rehabilitation hospital, it was discovered that I had a large hernia. I was then transferred to another skilled nursing facility for 5 days until the hernia surgery was scheduled. After the surgery, I was admitted to that hospital for three days and was then transferred to another rehabilitation hospital for ten days. In March of 2019 I was finally discharged to return home.

To recap this, from November of 2018 to March of 2019, those three and one-half months I spent in two hospitals, two skilled nursing facilities, and two rehabilitation hospitals cost me **nothing**. If it wasn't for Medicare's Part A, hospitalization and Part B, medical services, I don't know how I would have afforded just this one episode in my life.

WHAT HAS MEDICARE ALLOWED ME TO DO?

Because I am home bound, Medicare has allowed me to live independently in my home with in-home medical health services like skilled nursing, physical and occupational therapy. Again, with **no** twice a week $40.00 co-payment per visit. Medicare Parts A, B & D have given me the protection from financial ruin and because I would not have been able to afford the medical services I have received since 1992. The three and one-half months I wrote **above cost me not one penny, zero, zilch, naught**.

Besides that one incident, and because of the progression of my paralysis, I have been confined to a power wheelchair for the last seven years. With Medicare's Durable Medical Equipment (DME), I am now in my second powerchair at no cost to me.

WHAT IF BENEFITS WERE REDUCED?

Medicare costs me $194.90 from my Social Security check and I pay another $290.00 for my Medicare Supplement for a total of $484.90 a month. That is a big bite from my monthly income but I consider that a small price to pay for the medical protection Medicare affords me.

If Medicare benefits are reduced, then millions of senior citizens like myself, could not afford the medical services we now receive.

My story is just one of the millions of stories from senior citizens that are in worse condition than myself.

Prior to Medicare's inception, roughly 35% of seniors didn't have basic insurance coverage, a situation that's unthinkable today. Medicare is a lifesaver for millions, plain and simple, without it, many would die. If anything, it needs to be expanded, not reduced.

Respectfully Submitted,

John A. Pernorio

John A. Pernorio, President
Rhode Island Alliance for Retired Americans

Rhode Island Alliance *for* Retired Americans 94 Cleveland Street • North Providence, RI • 02904-3525
Phone: 401-722-2622 • Fax: 401-722-2622 • riarajap@hotmail.com • www.ri-ara.org

Tax Foundation's Analysis of the "Medicare and Social Security Fair Share Act"

Static Revenue (Billions of Dollars)	2024	2025	2026	2027	2028	2029	2030	2031	2032	2033	2024 - 2033
Impose 12.4% Social Security Tax on wage income over $400,000 and levy on self-employment income	$105.5	$110.1	$114.6	$118.5	$123.0	$127.7	$132.5	$137.5	$142.6	$147.7	$1,259.6
Raise Net Investment Income Tax from 3.8% to 17.4% (12.4% for Social Security and 5% for combined Medicare tax) on income over $500K Joint/$400K Single	-$64.7	-$64.0	-$62.4	-$66.5	-$67.1	-$69.7	-$72.5	-$75.4	-$78.3	-$81.5	-$702.1
Increase Additional Medicare Tax from 0.9% to 2.1% on wage and self-employment income over $400,000	$15.7	$16.2	$16.3	$17.9	$18.5	$19.3	$20.1	$21.0	$21.8	$22.7	$189.4
Total	$56.5	$62.3	$68.5	$69.9	$74.5	$77.2	$80.1	$83.0	$86.1	$88.8	$747.0

Dynamic Revenue (Billions of Dollars)	2024	2025	2026	2027	2028	2029	2030	2031	2032	2033	2024 - 2033
Impose 12.4% Social Security Tax on wage income over $400,000 and levy on self-employment income	$72.8	$77.0	$77.2	$78.5	$81.3	$83.1	$85.5	$88.5	$91.9	$93.9	$829.7
Raise Net Investment Income Tax from 3.8% to 17.4% (12.4% for Social Security and 5% for combined Medicare tax) on income over $500K Joint/$400K Single	-$66.0	-$67.2	-$67.3	-$73.4	-$75.7	-$80.1	-$84.6	-$89.3	-$93.5	-$96.1	-$793.2
Increase Additional Medicare Tax from 0.9% to 2.1% on wage and self-employment income over $400,000	$11.5	$11.7	$11.1	$12.3	$12.7	$15.4	$16.2	$16.9	$17.6	$15.8	$141.2
Total	$18.4	$21.4	$21.1	$17.3	$18.3	$18.4	$17.1	$16.2	$16.0	$13.6	$177.7

Distributional Effects (Percent Change in After-Tax Income)	2024, Conventional	2033, Conventional	Long-Run, Dynamic
0% - 20.0%	0%	0%	-0.8%
20.0% - 40.0%	0%	0%	-0.8%
40.0% - 60.0%	0%	0%	-0.8%
60.0% - 80.0%	0%	0%	-0.7%
80.0% - 100%	-0.1%	-0.1%	-0.8%
80.0% - 90.0%	0%	0%	-0.7%
90.0% - 95.0%	0%	0%	-0.7%
95.0% - 99.0%	-0.1	-0.1	-0.8%
99.0% - 100%	-0.1%	-0.3%	-1.0%
Total for All	Less than -0.05%	-0.1%	-0.8%

Economic Effects (Long-Run)	
Gross Domestic Product (GDP)	-1.0%
Gross National Product (GNP)	-1.0%
Full-Time Equivalent Jobs	-711,000
Wage Rate	-0.3%
Capital Stock	-1.4%

Source: Tax Foundation General Equilibrium Model, September 2023

TheUpshot

A Huge Threat to the U.S. Budget Has Receded. And No One Is Sure Why.

By Margot Sanger-Katz, Alicia Parlapiano and Josh Katz Sep. 4, 2023

For decades, runaway Medicare spending was the story of the federal budget.

Now, flat Medicare spending might be a bigger one.

Something strange has been happening in this giant federal program. Instead of growing and growing, as it always had before, spending per Medicare beneficiary has nearly leveled off over more than a decade.

The trend can be a little hard to see because, as baby boomers have aged, the number of people using Medicare has grown. But it has had enormous consequences for federal spending. Budget news often sounds apocalyptic, but the Medicare trend has been unexpectedly good for federal spending, saving taxpayers a huge amount relative to projections.

"Without a doubt, this is the most important thing that has happened to the federal budget in the last 20 years," said David Cutler, a professor of health policy and medicine at Harvard, who helped the Obama White House develop the Affordable Care Act.

The reason for the per-person slowdown is a bit of a mystery. Scholars have been arguing about it for years, but no one seems sure enough to confidently predict whether it is likely to stick around for much longer.

Some of the reductions are easy to explain. Congress changed Medicare policy. The biggest such shift came with the Affordable Care Act in 2010, which reduced Medicare's payments to hospitals and to health insurers that offered private Medicare Advantage plans. Congress also cut Medicare payments as part of a budget deal in 2011.

But most of the savings can't be attributed to any obvious policy shift. In a recent letter to the Senate Budget Committee, economists at the Congressional Budget Office described the huge reductions in its Medicare forecasts between 2010 and 2020. Most of those reductions came from a category the budget office calls "technical adjustments," which it uses to describe changes to public health and the practice of medicine itself.

Older Americans appear to be having fewer heart attacks and strokes, the likely result of effective cholesterol and blood pressure medicines that became cheap and widely used in recent years, according to research from Professor Cutler and colleagues. And drug makers and surgeons haven't developed as many new blockbuster treatments recently — there has been no new Prozac or angioplasty to drive up spending. (Medicare is currently barred by statute from covering the new class of expensive anti-obesity drugs.)

Parts of the health system appear to have become more efficient, as medical providers have been more cautious about adopting new therapies without much evidence, and more care has shifted outside hospitals into cheaper settings.

If the spending trajectory had continued

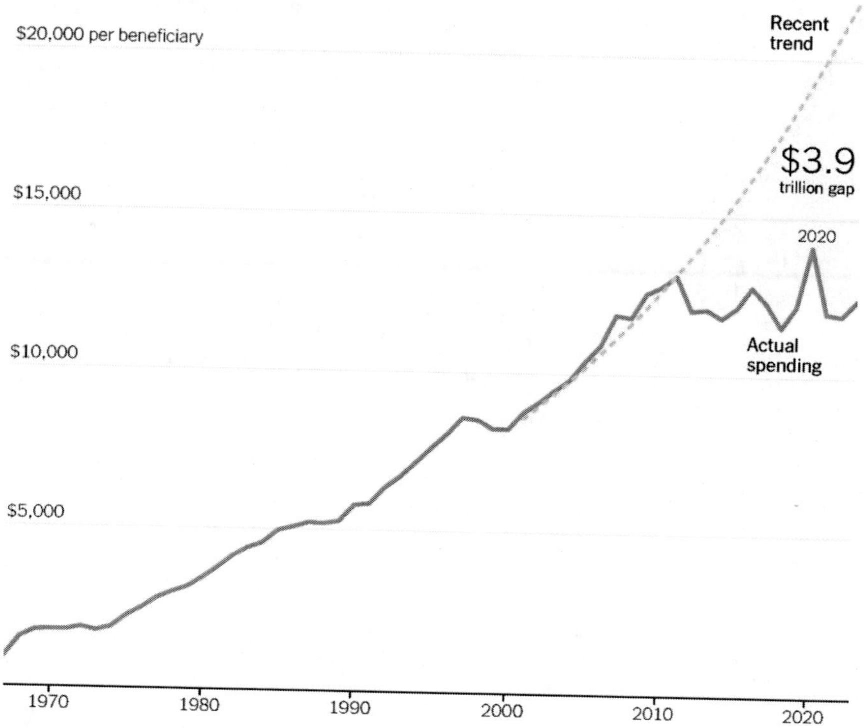

Sources: New York Times analysis of data from the Congressional Budget Office, the White House Office of Management and Budget, and the Medicare board of trustees. • Note: Mandatory Medicare outlays adjusted for inflation using the G.D.P. price index.

"What I've been arguing for more than a decade now is something that's very difficult to quantify but is nonetheless real," said Melinda Buntin, who measured the trend as a deputy assistant director at the Congressional Budget Office, and now studies it as a professor at Johns Hopkins. Professor Buntin says the direction of recent federal policies and choices by private insurers have caused doctors, nurses and hospital administrators to become more cost-conscious.

That budgetary good news isn't all good news for people with Medicare. Reductions in heart attacks and strokes have had big benefits for public health, but the paucity of major medical breakthroughs has been accompanied by slowing improvements in life expectancy for seniors. The cost containment strategies in hospitals may mean patients have been denied the treatments of their choice.

Medicare may even wind up saving money because of Covid-19 — because the older Americans who died from the disease tended to have other illnesses that would have been expensive to treat if they had survived, according to an analysis from the Medicare actuary.

If Medicare spending had grown the way it had for much of its history, federal spending would have been $3.9 trillion higher since 2011, and deficits would have been more than a quarter larger, according to an Upshot analysis. The difference is more than could be saved by raising the eligibility age for Social Security or converting Medicaid into a block grant, controversial proposals raised by legislators concerned about the federal debt.

It's so much money that almost no major legislation passed during this period comes close in scale. Even some major deficit reduction proposals, like the one known as Simpson-Bowles, aren't much bigger. The Trump tax cuts cost an estimated $2 trillion over 10 years. The recent deficit reduction deal passed by Congress will save a relatively modest trillion dollars in comparison. A new Medicare policy that will allow it to negotiate on the prices of some prescription drugs is expected to save just under $100 billion over a decade.

"There is basically no recent history of the kind of actual budgetary savings similar to what we have seen with the Medicare spending slowdown," said Joshua Gordon, the director of health care policy at the Committee for a Responsible Federal Budget, a group that supports deficit reduction.

$3.9 trillion is ...

85%	All federal pandemic relief
1.8x	Wars in Iraq and Afghanistan (military spending)
2.4x	All federal student loan debt
3.5x	War in Iraq (military spending)
5x	All military spending in one year
6x	Walmart revenue FY23
14x	Veterans spending in one year
18x	Salaries of all public school teachers in one year
27x	Food stamps (SNAP) in one year
46x	Homeland security spending in one year

161x NASA spending in one year

Sources: New York Times analysis of data from the Congressional Budget Office, the White House Office of Management and Budget, and the departments of defense and education.

Those savings have affected Congress's appetite for other budgetary choices. Medicare itself might look very different if it had been consistently busting the budget. In 2011, near the beginning of the trend, congressional Republicans were talking seriously about changing the very structure of Medicare by converting it into a private voucher program to constrain its future cost. Mitt Romney's presidential platform in 2012 featured such a plan. Proposals of that sort have fallen out of favor in recent years.

The fact that spending has remained so much lower than expected "has allowed us to put these decisions off for a while," said Sherry Glied, the dean of the Wagner School of public service at N.Y.U., who has evaluated several proposed long-term options for managing Medicare's finances.

But Medicare's spending is unlikely to disappear as a concern for the budget and policymakers. An aging population means the number of Americans relying on the program is growing rapidly. And analysts continue to worry that the trend is an aberration, and that some new development — an effective Alzheimer's drug, a cultural turn away from cost cutting, the health burden of long Covid or some other chronic condition — will return Medicare spending to form. The Congressional Budget Office, which has lowered its forecasts repeatedly during the period in the face of lower spending, continues to expect growth to tick up again soon.

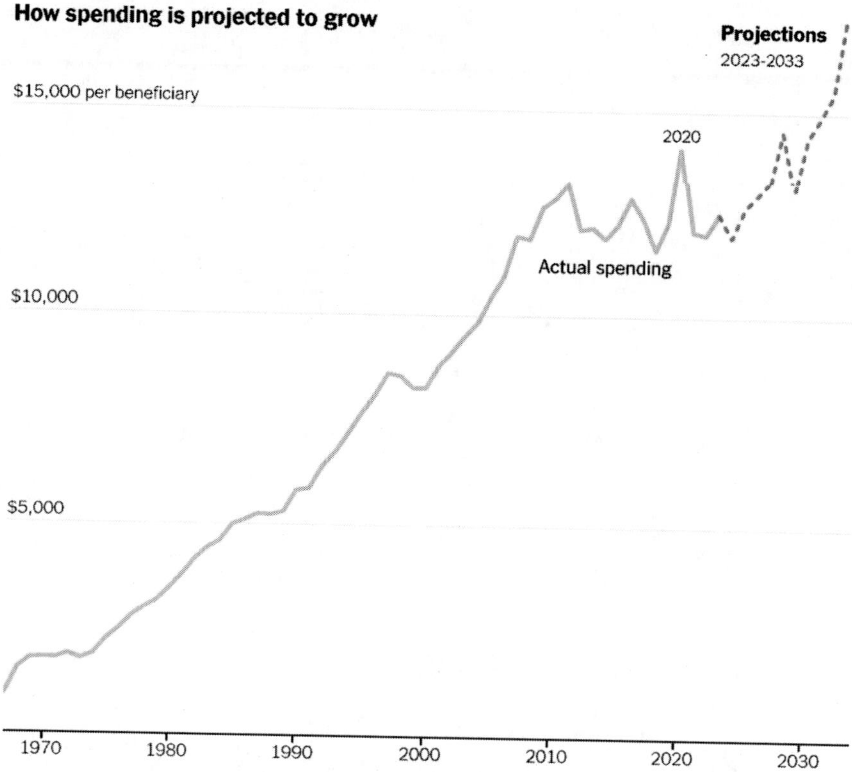

Sources: New York Times analysis of data from the Congressional Budget Office, the White House Office of Management and Budget, and the Medicare board of trustees. • Note: Mandatory Medicare outlays adjusted for inflation using the G.D.P. price index.

Medicare is growing more slowly than ever, but still more quickly than the rest of the federal budget. If the slowdown per beneficiary ends, it will strain the Medicare trust fund and drive up the federal debt — and may dominate the Washington policy conversation again. That means the uncertainty about the future has high stakes.

"I used to call this the trillion dollar question," Professor Buntin said. "But now it's more than a trillion dollars."

○

Index

A

acute stress, 83
aging population, 273, 274, 296, 299

B

baby boomers, 254, 275
bipartisan commitment, 220, 259
breast cancer, 16, 55, 116

C

capital gains, 175, 195, 222, 240, 255, 261, 262, 270, 274, 278, 288, 293, 315
chronic illness, 142, 240, 241
chronic obstructive pulmonary disease, 56
coronavirus, 77, 79, 81, 118, 120, 266
cost effectiveness, 91, 95
cost saving, 24, 28, 95, 109, 134, 162, 165, 171, 256

D

death rate, 13, 66
Department of Health and Human Services, 72, 73, 86, 92, 93, 96, 101, 107
diabetes, 10, 11, 55, 57, 240
dialysis, 90, 102, 105
disability, 89, 92, 100, 266
discrimination, 32, 89, 100, 149, 257
distress, 22, 71, 74, 83, 84

E

education, 33, 37, 43, 90, 91, 92, 96, 98, 101, 102, 103, 104, 125, 133, 150, 226, 272, 277
electrocardiogram, 19
equity, 10, 69, 70, 73, 80, 90, 92, 99, 101, 227, 230, 285
ethnicity, 41, 79, 80, 92, 99, 102, 103

H

health care costs, 10, 16, 33, 35, 152, 155, 176
heart attack, 11, 15, 55, 114, 115, 223, 264
heart disease, 240
high blood pressure, 10, 57
homelessness, 92, 100
human right, 2, 25, 32

I

income distribution, 46, 175, 245, 291
income inequality, 231, 235, 317
infant mortality, 42, 68, 102
insulin, 11, 33, 44

L

leukemia, 3
life expectancy, 2, 17, 41, 42, 57, 68, 121, 122, 225, 267
liver transplant, 157
longevity, 2, 12, 47, 58
long-term services and supports (LTSS), 24, 45, 47, 87, 165, 172, 173

lung disease, 11

M

Medicaid, 2, 16, 18, 19, 30, 36, 42, 44, 47, 52, 53, 54, 86, 88, 90, 93, 95, 102, 106, 118, 121, 127, 128, 129, 130, 131, 133, 134, 135, 138, 143, 144, 155, 161, 168, 169, 174, 219, 223, 249, 255, 272, 277, 295, 296, 313, 318
mental illness, 3, 33, 34, 235
money laundering, 294
mortality rate, 42
multiple sclerosis, 55

N

net investment, 233, 272, 316, 318
nursing care, 14, 69, 73, 74, 112

O

occupational health, 69, 72, 75
oligopolies, 122, 128

P

participants, 134, 159, 298, 304
patient care, 13, 14, 26, 64, 66, 68, 69, 71, 72, 74, 75, 77, 83, 97, 103, 104
payroll, 40, 46, 174, 195, 226, 231, 239, 245, 265, 268, 269, 270, 278, 279, 280, 290, 296, 299, 314, 316, 317, 319, 320, 321, 322
persons with disabilities, 224
pharmaceutical, 4, 5, 62, 91, 105, 108, 140, 162
pharmaceuticals, 62
physical health, 236
physicians, 19, 61, 63, 64, 65, 75, 91, 94, 96, 105, 112, 114, 124, 127, 128, 129, 137, 138, 140, 167, 168, 174, 303
population, 52, 65, 66, 94, 102, 106, 138, 159, 163, 169, 218, 229, 231, 235, 236, 269, 316
post-traumatic stress disorder, 74
poverty, vii, 18, 99, 102, 130, 232, 235, 267, 268, 277
pregnancy, 89, 100
premature death, 54, 223, 264
preparedness, 14, 69, 70, 75, 76, 79, 81, 85
prescription drugs, 3, 5, 28, 31, 49, 55, 62, 68, 87, 88, 93, 94, 108, 112, 162, 168, 170, 174, 220, 259, 297, 299, 300
prevention, 17, 22, 28, 33, 90, 91, 96, 101, 103, 122, 125, 241
professionals, 2, 13, 26, 48, 65, 67, 70, 92, 94, 98, 99, 103, 104, 128, 129, 313
prostate cancer, 223, 264
protection, 58, 65, 76, 148, 158
public health, 13, 14, 17, 26, 67, 74, 76, 79, 90, 97, 101, 102, 103, 106, 120, 122, 123, 125, 141, 210

Q

quality assurance, 87
quality of life, vii, 219, 257

R

race, 41, 79, 80, 89, 92, 99, 100, 102, 103, 290
racism, 79, 80
radiation treatment, 223, 264
reality, 71, 251, 291, 318
recall, 42, 246
regulations, 36, 86, 129, 147, 289
religion, 89, 100
respiratory therapist, 70, 85
restrictions, 46, 136, 137, 140, 173, 268
retirement, 23, 139, 218, 220, 221, 235, 245, 248, 257, 259, 261, 267, 275
retirement age, 221, 261
revenue, 30, 61, 63, 64, 71, 74, 75, 103, 104, 141, 144, 218, 219, 220, 222, 226, 230, 231, 233, 234, 237, 238, 239, 241, 242, 243, 245, 246, 248, 249, 250, 251, 256, 257, 258, 259, 261, 262, 265, 269, 273, 274, 275, 276, 279, 282, 285, 290,

291, 292, 295, 296, 297, 298, 304, 315, 316, 317, 318, 319

S

safety, 14, 18, 40, 41, 65, 66, 69, 70, 71, 72, 73, 74, 75, 76, 80, 82, 85, 94, 97, 99, 103, 107
sanctions, 293, 294
SARS-CoV, 78
savings, 11, 28, 47, 48, 49, 58, 60, 62, 63, 64, 93, 94, 106, 107, 108, 109, 110, 125, 141, 142, 160, 161, 162, 165, 175, 195, 221, 234, 241, 246, 256, 261, 266, 275, 292, 302, 303, 314
shortage, 38, 71, 72, 102, 104, 135, 136, 138
social security, 23, 37, 217, 218, 219, 220, 221, 222, 224, 226, 227, 229, 231, 235, 237, 238, 242, 248, 256, 257, 258, 259, 260, 261, 263, 265, 269, 272, 276, 280, 281, 295, 296, 298, 304, 305, 318, 319
society, 13, 27, 41, 67, 78, 79
socioeconomic status, 55, 92, 100, 102, 103
solution, 14, 17, 37, 43, 44, 70, 72, 77, 123, 127, 129, 132, 139, 152, 237, 241, 249, 268
stability, 230, 299, 304
structure, 97, 117, 230, 237, 249, 254, 287, 299, 300
substance abuse, 33, 34, 88
supply chain, 13, 37, 66, 176

T

tax base, 226, 227, 228, 231, 240, 246, 272, 273, 274, 276, 277, 278, 279, 280, 281, 283, 284, 285, 286, 287, 288, 289, 290, 292, 316
tax breaks, 31, 218, 257, 276, 277, 292
tax cuts, 95, 245, 248, 274, 275, 284, 285
tax evasion, 227, 231, 273, 274, 276, 281, 289, 291, 292, 293, 294
tax increase, 19, 145, 195, 197, 209, 221, 228, 234, 260, 317
tax rates, 218, 222, 251, 254, 257, 265, 273, 275, 276, 279, 288, 316, 318
tax system, 218, 220, 227, 228, 234, 237, 240, 251, 255, 257, 258, 271, 285
taxpayers, 133, 134, 147, 162, 196, 209, 210, 221, 225, 226, 233, 243, 244, 247, 261, 268, 269, 270, 273, 274, 276, 279, 284, 294, 297, 304, 305, 316, 317, 318
total costs, 229, 295
transactions, 27, 115, 274, 284, 294
transformation, 229, 282, 283
treatment, 8, 10, 13, 15, 16, 19, 33, 34, 35, 36, 38, 67, 77, 84, 88, 116, 144, 223, 236, 255, 264

U

uninsured, 2, 3, 10, 13, 16, 18, 23, 26, 33, 44, 49, 52, 53, 54, 58, 62, 63, 66, 77, 94, 104, 117, 127, 128, 129, 130, 131, 151, 161, 320
urban, 63, 97, 99, 101, 102, 104, 144
urban areas, 99, 101

V

vaccine, 35, 120
valuation, 320, 321, 322
violence, 73, 83, 84
vision, 5, 23, 34, 87, 112, 148, 155, 161, 171
vulnerability, 97, 103

W

wages, 16, 47, 50, 64, 76, 91, 102, 105, 109, 116, 122, 125, 135, 137, 175, 176, 226, 245, 269, 270, 278, 279, 314, 320
waiver, 152, 153, 154, 155, 156, 251
waste, 11, 22, 67, 133, 210, 273
wealth, 175, 196, 254, 277, 278, 287, 288, 293
welfare, 12, 58, 113

well-being, 14, 42, 67, 313
workforce, 22, 32, 69, 72, 73, 75, 76, 81, 92, 100, 101, 102, 120, 123, 137, 138, 142, 150, 282

Y

yield, 255, 256, 266
young people, 148, 150